The

Har

A Practical Guide for Clinicians

Fourth Edition

Gary S. Marshall, MD
Professor of Pediatrics
Chief, Division of Pediatric Infectious Diseases
University of Louisville School of Medicine

Foreword by Deborah L. Wexler, MD
Executive Director, Immunization Action Coalition

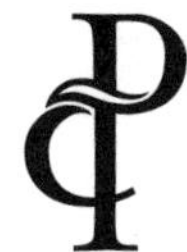

PROFESSIONAL
COMMUNICATIONS, INC.

Professional Communications, Inc.
A Medical Publishing & Communications Company

400 Center Bay Drive
West Islip, NY 11795
(t) 631/661-2852
(f) 631/661-2167

PO Box 10
Caddo, OK 74729-0010
(t) 580/367-9838
(f) 580/367-9989

For orders only, please call
1-800-337-9838
or visit our Web site at
www.pcibooks.com

ISBN: 978-1-932610-81-9

Printed in the United States of America

DISCLAIMER

The opinions expressed in this publication reflect those of the author. However, the author makes no warranty regarding the contents of the publication. The protocols described herein are general and may not apply to a specific patient. Any product mentioned in this publication should be taken in accordance with the prescribing information provided by the manufacturer.

This text is printed on recycled paper. 

TABLE OF CONTENTS

About the Immunization Action Coalition

Founded by Dr. Deborah Wexler in 1991, the Immunization Action Coalition (IAC) has grown to be the premier nongovernmental source of immunization education support materials for the nation's health care professionals, partnering with the Centers for Disease Control and Prevention (CDC) since the early 1990s.

Examples of IAC's highly respected, and much relied upon, free publications include its weekly email news service, *IAC Express*, sent to more than 45,000 opt-in subscribers; its Web sites, www.immunize.org and www.vaccineinformation.org, which host more than 20,000 visits per day; its periodicals, *Needle Tips* and *Vaccinate Adults*, which can be downloaded from the Internet; its official national repository for translations of the federally required patient handouts called Vaccine Information Statements; and its library of more than 250 separate educational pieces for health care professionals and their patients, furnishing approximately 2 million downloads per year.

CDC has recognized IAC for success in its mission to increase immunization rates by honoring IAC with the prestigious CDC *Partners in Public Health Award.*

Immunization Action Coalition
1573 Selby Avenue
Suite 234
Saint Paul, MN 55104
Phone: 651-647-9009
Email: admin@immunize.org

Web Site for Healthcare Professionals
www.immunize.org

Web Site for the Public
www.vaccineinformation.org

Web Site for Immunization Coalitions
www.izcoalitions.org

immunization
action coalition
IAC
immunize.org

Foreword

A few years ago, a colleague from the Centers for Disease Control and Prevention was giving a half-day training session to a large group of health care professionals. The program detailed many aspects of quality immunization delivery—administering vaccines properly, using only true contraindications, avoiding missed opportunities, addressing parents' concerns, and understanding all of the nuances of the child and adolescent immunization schedules. When the speaker began discussing the hepatitis B vaccine recommendations for low birth weight newborns, one seasoned physician stood up and said, "*That's it. This is just too much. This is just too much to know*!"

While we are all happy that vaccines can protect our patients and loved ones from so many diseases, most of us probably share some of this physician's sense of being overwhelmed. Vaccination is one of the most important actions we take to prevent illness in our patients and communities, but there is just *so* much to know to get it right!

I have dedicated most of my professional life to helping health care professionals "get it right," that is, give the right patient the right vaccine, at the right time, in the right amount, and in the right way. Having founded and fostered one of the most relied-upon immunization education organizations in the United States, I have fielded many immunization questions and have developed a deep appreciation for the complexity of managing all the actions that go into a quality immunization program. That is why I am so enthusiastic about Dr. Marshall's superb work, *The Vaccine Handbook: A Practical Guide for Clinicians*—more widely known as *The Purple Book*.

I invite you to explore and use this pocket-sized, "everything-you-ever-could-think-to-ask-about-vaccines" book in the following ways.

First, keep at least one copy in your office so your staff can find it when a question arises. Can't remember which age group is at risk for meningococcal disease and needs to be vaccinated? Need to know who gets a second dose of influenza vaccine? Or who has a special health condition and should not receive varicella vaccine? Or what to do if you accidently gave Tdap to a 15-month-old? *The Vaccine Handbook*'s Table of Contents tabs and the excellent indexing will help you find the answer.

In addition to using it as a quick reference, I urge you to look over the Table of Contents and explore the first section (*General Principles of Vaccinology and Vaccine Practice*) in depth. Sit down and start digging into it to see the wealth of information Dr. Marshall provides. Because, like you, I have to answer questions about vaccines, and I am thrilled to have this enormous amount of practical information compiled into one small, easy-to-read and easy-to-comprehend book. *The Purple Book* offers extensive coverage of vaccine immunology, federal vaccine financing and policy, and how the safety of US vaccines is assured. It even teaches us about coding and billing for vaccines. Chapter 4 details the gamut of activities involved in administering vaccinations in practice, with emphasis on storage and handling, vaccination technique, reminder and recall, how to use standing orders, and much more.

Several of these chapters are "must reading" for everyone involved in vaccinating patients in a medical practice. Certainly everyone in the office—including the receptionists—would benefit from reading Chapter 7 (*Addressing Concerns About Vaccines*). This key chapter provides answers to more than a dozen commonly asked questions that vaccine-hesitant parents and patients might ask, such as "Can too many vaccines overload the immune system?" and "Isn't natural immunity better than induced immunity?" and "Are alternative schedules a good idea?" During more than 20 years in the field of immunization education, I have not seen a book that is so brimming with state-of-the-science vaccine information. This book belongs in the hands of every medical student, physician-in-training, doctor, nursing student, and nurse who provides vaccines to patients, regardless of patient age or medical specialty.

EO Wilson, sociobiologist and two-time Pulitzer Prize winner, wrote, "*The world henceforth will be run by synthesizers, people able to put together the right information at the right time, think critically about it, and make important choices wisely.*" This is precisely what *The Vaccine Handbook* is designed to do—*synthesize*. As you learn and internalize this information, I believe you will be awed by your ability to prevent diseases that previously ravaged humankind.

Deborah L. Wexler, MD
Executive Director
Immunization Action Coalition

Preface

It has been 8 years since the first edition of *The Vaccine Handbook* was published. Much has changed since then. The number of vaccines packed into office refrigerators has increased—this is good news, because it means that several dreadful diseases, formerly having free rein, are now on their way out of the building. Along with this, however, has come great complexity and, in some cases, confusion. The world has seen a new pandemic, even as other diseases have faded into our collective memory. Still other diseases have temporarily resurged, if only to remind us that they are forgotten, not gone. New recommendations have come along and old recommendations have been modified. And we have never been healthier with respect to vaccine-preventable diseases.

Yet—to quote Al Stewart from the song *Nostradamus*—the more it changes, the more it stays the same. Providers still struggle to keep their footing on the shifting sands of products, guidances, rules, opinions, discoveries, regulations, marketing campaigns, reimbursement schemata, and media hype. Parents and patients are still bewildered, often in need of more information, sometimes downright defiant, but always interested in doing the right thing. And there is still much to be learned. Throughout all of this, the book you are reading has remained, well, purple.

And, one would hope, true to its original purpose—to synthesize authoritative information about vaccinology and vaccine practice into a concise, user-friendly, practical resource, suitable for the clinic or classroom, hospital ward, and even business office. If you are a pediatrician, family physician, internist, obstetrician, nurse, nurse practitioner, physician's assistant, student, resident, or even just an interested person, it may be just what the doctor ordered.

One goal we all share is to prevent disease and death without causing harm. Vaccines are a means to this end, and *The Purple Book* is intended to provide help along the way.

— **GSM**

Conventions Used in This Book

The nomenclature and abbreviations used in this book for disease agents and their respective vaccines are given in the *Appendix*. In general, standards set by the Advisory Committee on Immunization Practices (ACIP) are followed (http://www.cdc.gov/vaccines/recs/acip/downloads/vac-abbrev.pdf; accessed February 28, 2012), with some modifications. For example, the proteins used in protein-polysaccharide conjugate vaccines are added to the abbreviations as qualifiers, as in "Hib-T" for "*Haemophilus influenzae* type b vaccine, tetanus toxoid conjugate" and "Hib-OMP" for "*Haemophilus influenzae* type b vaccine, (meningococcal) outer membrane protein conjugate" (these are important to differentiate because the dosing schedules differ). To make things a little more complicated (but hopefully more accurate), there are times when vaccines are referred to in generic fashion, in which case the qualifier is dropped (eg, "Hib" for "*Haemophilus influenzae* type b conjugate vaccine," referring to both the "T" and "OMP" conjugates). Here's another example: "MCV4" refers to meningococcal conjugate vaccine, 4-valent, in general and including both available types, whereas "MCV4-D" refers specifically to the diphtheria toxoid conjugate (Menactra) and "MCV4-CRM" refers to the CRM_{197} conjugate (Menveo).

In general, the abbreviation for the agent (eg, "HAV" for "hepatitis A virus") is different from the vaccine (eg, "HepA," which means "hepatitis A vaccine"). In some cases, there is no abbreviation for the agent (eg, "human papillomavirus") so that an abbreviation can be used ("HPV") to refer to the vaccine (eg, "HPV" means "human papillomavirus vaccine"). The valency may get tacked on to the end, as in "HPV4," which means "human papillomavirus vaccine, 4-valent." For some vaccines (eg, rabies vaccine), the abbreviation was just made up (eg, "RAB"). Specific identifying characteristics, such as the cell type in which the vaccine was produced, may be indicated, as in "RAB-HDC," which means "rabies vaccine, human diploid cell."

Premixed combination vaccines are denoted by dashes between the components (eg, "DTaP-HepB-IPV" for Pediarix, which contains DTaP, HepB, and IPV). Combination vaccines that require reconstitution are denoted by a slash mark (eg, "DTaP-IPV/Hib-T," where the liquid DTaP-IPV is used to reconstitute the lyophilized Hib-T, creating the combination vaccine Pentacel). In general, vaccine trade names use initial capitals only, except where upper and lower case letters are interspersed in the name, as in "RotaTeq." Trademark symbols are not used. Uncommon abbreviations used in the book are defined in the text upon first use; commonly used abbreviations may be used in the text without definition but are listed in the *Appendix*.

In general, “age” means that the individual has passed one mark in time but has not yet reached the next relevant mark. For example, “2 months of age” means “at or beyond the 2-month birthday but not yet at the 3-month birthday.” Age intervals may be indicated by a dash or the word “to”; thus, “4-6 years of age” and “4 to 6 years of age” mean “4 years of age through 6 years of age,” or “from the 4th birthday until the day before the 7th birthday.” As far as time is concerned, “weeks” are 7 days and, up to 4 months, “months” are 28 days; at 4 months and beyond, “months” are “calendar months,” meaning an interval to the same date in the appropriate month. For example, for an infant vaccinated on January 6, an interval of 6 months would be on July 6. These definitions are particularly relevant when referring to age indications for vaccines and minimum intervals (eg, **Table 5.1**).

Many organizations provide guidance regarding immunizations. The most generally applicable, authoritative recommendations come from the ACIP, the American Academy of Pediatrics (AAP), and the American Academy of Family Physicians (AAFP). The recommendations from these organizations are usually very similar, and as such, ACIP recommendations (as of the February 2012 meeting) are referenced in this book. Any differences with the recommendations of other agencies, or the respective package inserts, are highlighted.

Disclaimers

Care has been taken to confirm the accuracy of the information presented herein and to describe generally accepted practices. However, the author, editor, and publisher are not responsible for errors or omissions or for any consequences from application of the information in this book and make no warranty, expressed or implied, with respect to the currency, completeness, or accuracy of the contents of the publication. Application of this information in a particular situation remains the professional responsibility of the practitioner.

The author, editor, and publisher have exerted every effort to ensure that drug selection and dosage set forth in this text are in accordance with current recommendations and practice at the time of publication. However, in view of ongoing research, changes in government regulations, and the constant flow of information relating to drug therapy and drug reactions, the reader is urged to check the package insert and published or posted recommendations for each drug or vaccine discussed, being aware that there may be changes in indications, dosage, or schedule, and that added warnings and precautions may have been issued. This is particularly important when the recommended agent is a new or infrequently employed drug. Some drugs and medical devices presented in this publication may have Food and Drug Administration (FDA) clearance for limited use in restricted research settings. It is the responsibility of health care providers to ascertain the FDA status of each drug or device planned for use in their clinical practice.

Some of the material from the first edition (*The Vaccine Handbook: A Practical Guide for Clinicians*; 2004, Lippincott Williams & Wilkins; Philadelphia, PA), contributed by Drs. Penelope Dennehy, David Greenberg, Paul Offit, and Tina Tan, is retained here with the respective authors' express permission. In addition, some of the material in this book was previously published in *The Vaccine Quarterly* (©2007-2010, Wolters Kluwer Health) and is reprinted here with permission.

About the Author

Dr. Marshall received his undergraduate degree from the University of Pennsylvania and his medical degree from Vanderbilt University. After completing a pediatric residency at Vanderbilt in 1986, he entered a fellowship in infectious diseases at the Children's Hospital of Philadelphia. In 1989, he joined the Department of Pediatrics at the University of Louisville School of Medicine, where he is now Professor of Pediatrics, Chief of the Division of Pediatric Infectious Diseases, and Director of the Pediatric Clinical Trials Unit. Dr. Marshall also serves as an attending physician at Kosair Children's Hospital and participates in an outpatient infectious diseases practice. He is the recipient of the Outstanding Clinical Professor Award, Educator of the Year Award, and the Peer Clinician-Teacher Excellence Award from the Department of Pediatrics, as well as the Distinguished Educator Award from the School of Medicine and the Educational Achievement Award from the Kentucky Medical Association. Dr. Marshall is a member of the Society for Pediatric Research and the Pediatric Infectious Diseases Society and has authored over 130 scientific papers, many in the areas of vaccine development, advocacy, and education.

Acknowledgements

The author is deeply indebted to Drs. David Greenberg (now at Sanofi Pasteur), Penny Dennehy (Brown University), Tina Tan (Northwestern University), and Paul Offit (Children's Hospital of Philadelphia) for their contributions to the first edition, and to Drs. Sharon Humiston (University of Rochester) and Jim Conway (University of Wisconsin) for their helpful suggestions on the book's intervening editions. Appreciation is also extended to the many other people who contributed cumulatively to this work, through conversation and comment, including Dr. Litjen Tan (American Medical Association); Dr. Bruce Gellin (National Vaccine Program Office); Dr. Michelle Goveia (Merck Vaccines); Dr. Geoffrey Evans (Health Resources and Services Administration); and Drs. Yabo Beysolow, Andrew Kroger, and Bill Atkinson (Centers for Disease Control and Prevention). Finally, the author would like to thank Dr. Deborah Wexler from the Immunization Action Coalition for writing the *Foreword* and for her organization's determination to spread the word about preventing disease through vaccination.

Dedication

For Cherie, Emily, and Cullen.
And for Grandpop, who recently asked
what do you think about this shingles vaccine?

1 Introduction to Vaccinology

Immunization

Immunization is the process of protecting individuals from disease by making them immune. This is most often accomplished *actively* through *vaccination*, the delivery of *antigens* (substances on the microbe that are foreign to the host, contained in *vaccines*) for purposes of stimulating an immune response. It can also be accomplished *passively* by the administration of antibodies. While not technically correct in all instances, the terms *vaccination* and *immunization* are often used interchangeably.

Table 1.1 shows one approach to classifying vaccines that are used in humans. Broadly speaking, vaccines are either *live* or *inactivated*; **Table 1.2** lists general characteristics of live and inactivated vaccines. These have very real consequences in practice, affecting storage conditions, scheduling, expected efficacy, contraindications, and the potential for adverse reactions.

■ Live Vaccines

Live vaccines replicate in the host and generate immune responses that mimic those induced by natural infection. They are generally *attenuated*, or weakened, in some fashion such that they cause subclinical infection with very little risk of disease. Several approaches to attenuation are represented in our current repertoire of vaccines.

- *Serial passage*—This is the classical method of attenuating viruses, dating back to the 1930s when Thieler passaged YF virus in eggs 200 times in order to weaken it. For viruses, serial passage is now most often accomplished in animal or human cell cultures. The mechanisms of attenuation are not clear but probably involve the accumulation of deletions and mutations that, while adapting the virus to growth in vitro, render the virus less fit (but still capable of replicating) in vivo. Sabin developed the modern prototype live-attenuated virus vaccine by passaging the poliovirus serially in monkey cells and demonstrating that oral administration of the attenuated virus protected against polio. Serial passage also was used to attenuate measles, mumps, and rubella viruses for use in vaccines. The virus used to make VAR was originally isolated from a child in Japan in the early 1970s. It was serially passaged in human embryonic lung, embryonic guinea pig, and WI-38 (human diploid) cells in order to achieve attenuation, and it is currently produced in MRC-5 (human diploid) cells. The most recent example of the use of serial

TABLE 1.1 — Classification of Vaccines Currently Available in the United States

Live			Inactivated				
	Attenuated			Component			
Nonattenuated	Classical	Engineered	Whole Agent	Toxoid	Purified	Engineered	Recombinant
Adenovirus[a]	MMR[b]	LAIV[c]	HepA	Diphtheria	Anthrax[d]	Hib[e]	HepB[f]
	RV1[g]	RV5[g]	IPV	Tetanus	IIV[h]	MCV[e]	HPV[i]
	Smallpox	Ty21a[j]	JEV		MPSV[k]	PCV[e]	
	VAR		RAB		Pertussis (acellular)[l]		
	YFV				PPSV[k]		
	ZOS				TViPSV[k]		

Listed vaccines are administered parenterally unless otherwise noted. The following vaccines never were or are no longer available in the United States: BCG (tuberculosis)—live-attenuated, classical bacterial; cholera—inactivated, whole cell; cholera (CVD 103-HgR)—live-attenuated, engineered, orally administered; cholera (WC/rBS)—inactivated, whole agent plus recombinant-derived subunit, orally administered; OPV (polio)—live-attenuated, classical viral; influenza (whole virus)—inactivated, whole agent; hepatitis B (plasma-derived)—inactivated, whole agent; Lyme disease (rOspA)—inactivated, recombinant-derived subunit; Hib polysaccharide—inactivated, purified subunit; pertussis (whole cell)—inactivated, whole agent; plague—inactivated whole agent; typhoid—inactivated whole agent.

[a] The vaccine strains are not intrinsically attenuated but they do not produce disease because they are administered by the enteric route.
[b] Contains a mixture of classically-attenuated measles, mumps, and rubella viruses.
[c] Influenza virus engineered to attenuation, then reassorted to include hemagglutinin and neuraminidase of circulating influenza strains.
[d] Produced from cell-free filtrate.

[e] Protein-polysaccharide conjugate. Valency varies. For example, Hib contains only one polysaccharide derived from the capsule of *H influenzae* type b, whereas MCV contains polysaccharides derived from the capsules of 4 different *N meningitidis* serogroups. Carrier proteins also vary. For example, Hib uses either tetanus toxoid or an outer membrane protein from *N meningitidis*; MCV uses either diphtheria toxoid or CRM_{197}, a mutant diphtheria toxin.

[f] HBsAg expressed in yeast.

[g] RV1 contains a classically-attenuated human rotavirus strain and is monovalent. RV5 contains bovine-human reassortants and is 5-valent. Both are orally administered.

[h] Contains physically-purified hemagglutinin and neuraminidase from influenza virus.

[i] Human papillomavirus L1 protein expressed in yeast (HPV4) or baculovirus (HPV2); these vaccines are 4-valent and 2-valent, respectively.

[j] Mutagenized *S typhi*, selected for attenuation, orally administered.

[k] Contains physically-purified polysaccharides. Valency varies. For example, MPSV contains polysaccharides derived from the capsules of 4 different *N meningitidis* serogroups, whereas PPSV contains polysaccharides from 23 different *S pneumoniae* serotypes.

[l] All pertussis vaccines contain physically-purified, inactivated pertussis toxin (arguably, this could be classified as a toxoid) and filamentous hemagglutinin; some also contain pertactin and fimbriae.

TABLE 1.2 — Generalizations About Live and Inactivated Vaccines

Characteristic	Live Vaccines	Inactivated Vaccines
Immune response	Humoral and cell-mediated	Mostly humoral[a]
Primary immunization	1 dose usually sufficient[b]	Multiple-dose series usually necessary[c]
Booster dose	Usually not necessary[d]	Usually necessary
Adjuvant	Not neceessary	May be necessary[e]
Route of administration	IN, PO, or SC	IM or SC
Duration of immunity	Potentially lifelong	Booster doses may be necessary[f]
Person-to-person transmission	Possible[g]	Not possible
Inactivation by passively acquired antibodies	Likely[h]	Possible[i]
Use in immunocompromised hosts	May cause disease	May not be immunogenic
Use in pregnancy	Fetal damage theoretically possible[j]	Fetal damage theoretically unlikely
Rationale for storage requirements	Maintain viability	Maintain stability
Administration on the same day	Acceptable[k]	Acceptable[l]
Interval between doses of the *same* vaccine given in sequence	Minimum intervals apply[m]	Minimum intervals apply[n]
Interval between doses of *different* vaccines given in sequence	Minimum intervals apply[m]	No minimum intervals[o]

[a] Inactivated vaccines may stimulate limited humoral responses. For example, polysaccharide vaccines (eg, MPSV and PPSV) induce short-lived IgM responses and do not result in immunologic memory. Engineering can overcome these limitations, as in the conjugation of polysaccharides to protein carriers. Protein vaccines can induce memory responses that are T-helper cell dependent.

[b] Live oral vaccines such as RV1, RV5, and typhoid Ty21a are given in multiple-dose series.

[c] Some inactivated vaccines, such as PPSV in older adults, are given as a single dose. In this case, individuals have probably been previously primed by natural exposure to *S pneumoniae*.

[d] Although 1 dose of MMR or VAR may be sufficient to induce long-lasting immunity, second doses are given before school entry to ensure that children who did not seroconvert to the first dose have another chance to do so. Since immunity to varicella zoster virus can wane after immunization in some individuals, the second dose of VAR may also serve as a booster.

[e] Hib-T, IIV, MCV4-D, MCV4-CRM, MPSV4, PPSV23, IPV, and RAB do not contain adjuvants.

[f] Long-term protection has been demonstrated for some inactivated vaccines, such as HepA and HepB, in the absence of booster doses.

[g] This phenomenon is relevant for OPV, where horizontal transmission probably contributes to immunity at the population level but also on rare occasion causes disease in contacts. Transmission of vaccinia from smallpox vaccinees represents a real risk to susceptible close contacts. Transmission of VAR, LAIV, and RV has been documented but is extremely rare. Transmission of MMR, Ty21a, and YFV has not been documented.

[h] Passively acquired maternal antibodies may interfere with the “take” (replication) of MMR and VAR, which is why these vaccines are not given in the first year of life. Passively acquired antibodies do not affect the take of vaccines administered at mucosal surfaces (LAIV, RV, Ty21a).

[i] Passively acquired maternal antibodies may interfere with the “take” (immunogenicity) of HepA, which is why this vaccine is not given in the first year of life. To avoid antigen-antibody interactions, antibody-containing products are not administered at the same site as inactivated vaccines.

[j] The possibility of fetal infection leads to the general recommendation that live vaccines not be given during pregnancy, although there are some exceptions (see *Chapter 6: Vaccination in Special Circumstances—Pregnancy*).

Continued

TABLE 1.2 — *Continued*

[k] Separate sites are always used for simultaneous administration. The only example of two live vaccines that cannot be given at the same time are varicella and smallpox (the concern is increased complications of smallpox vaccination).

[l] Separate sites are always used for simultaneous administration. The only example of two inactivated vaccines that cannot be given at the same time are MCV4-D and PCV13 in anatomically or functionally asplenic children (the concern is reduced response to pneumococcal antigens).

[m] Replication of the first live vaccine can interfere with replication of a second live vaccine that is given within 4 weeks.

[n] Proper spacing between the doses is necessary to maximize the immune response.

[o] The AAP suggests a minimum interval of 1 month between Tdap and MCV4-D if the vaccines are not given on the same day (the concern here is that both vaccines contain diphtheria toxoid [it is used as the carrier protein in MCV4-D]—too many doses of diphtheria toxoid in sequence can cause increased reactogenicity). However, the ACIP does not recommend a minimum interval.

passage is the human rotavirus vaccine RV1, which was derived from a strain of rotavirus that circulated in Cincinnati in the late 1980s. That virus was initially passaged 26 times in Vero (African green monkey kidney) cells in order to achieve attenuation.

Attenuation of bacteria dates back to the mid 1800s, when Pasteur protected animals from anthrax using a form of the bacterium that had been weakened using chemicals. In vitro passage also has been used to attenuate bacteria. For example, Bacille Calmette-Guérin (BCG), a vaccine that protects against disseminated tuberculosis, was a strain of *Mycobacterium bovis* (which is related to *M tuberculosis*) originally isolated from a cow in 1908 and passaged over 200 times in culture (BCG is used throughout the world but is no longer available in the United States).

- *Heterologous host*—This method dates back to the late 1700s, when Jenner used cowpox to protect humans from smallpox. The modern smallpox vaccine, consisting of a virus called vaccinia, is not the cowpox virus per se but rather a hybrid of cowpox and variola virus (the scientific name for smallpox) that does not exist in nature. Nevertheless, Jenner established the principle that animal viruses can induce immunity to human diseases. Cowpox is not necessarily attenuated for humans—it does cause lesions, as does vaccinia (in fact, if smallpox vaccination does not result in a lesion, it is not considered to have been effective). However, other animal viruses are naturally attenuated for humans. For example, RV5 was derived from a bovine strain of rotavirus (WC3) that can replicate in humans but does not cause disease. It also does not induce sufficient protective antibody to human strains, so it had to be altered to express immunogenic surface proteins of human rotaviruses. This was accomplished through *reassortment*, whereby the parental strain was cocultured with natural human strains. Bovine viruses that "accidentally" packaged genes for the human G or P proteins (the dominant protective antigens) were selected and propagated. The vaccine strains, then, consist of viruses that in every way are identical to the naturally attenuated bovine virus, except for the fact that each one expresses an immunogenic human protein instead of the corresponding bovine protein.
- *Engineered attenuation*—Today, the attenuated phenotype can be engineered into vaccines. A good example of this is the oral typhoid (Ty21a) vaccine, which was derived from *Salmonella typhi* strain Ty2 after treatment with a mutagenic agent and selection for attenuation. Another example is LAIV. Here, influenza virus was serially passaged in chick embryo cells at successively lower temperatures, selecting for mutants that grow well in the cold (77°F [25°C)]). As it happens, these

strains grow poorly at core body temperature. After intranasal inoculation, they replicate well in the relatively cooler nasal passages, thereby generating broad-based systemic and mucosal immune responses. Their attenuation comes in the fact that they cannot replicate in the lower airways and therefore cannot cause pneumonia or more serious influenza syndromes. Each year, a new set of live-attenuated viruses must be constructed, incorporating genes for the hemagglutinin and neuraminidase (the dominant protective antigens) for the strains anticipated in the next season. This can be accomplished through reassortment, as described earlier, or through direct transfer of the genetic material.

- *Altered site of infection*—The attenuated phenotype can be achieved by something as simple as using an unnatural route of inoculation. The best example of this is the adenovirus vaccine used in the military, which consists of enteric-coated tablets, one containing live (intrinsically nonattenuated) adenovirus type 4, and the other, type 7. These viruses are pathogenic in the respiratory tract but when given in the gastrointestinal tract, they replicate, stimulating an immune response without causing disease.

■ Inactivated Vaccines

Inactivated vaccines may consist of whole, inactivated microbial agents or specific microbial components that are derived through physical, chemical, or molecular means.

- *Whole agent*—Inactivated *whole agent* vaccines date back to the late 1800s, when Pasteur used killed rabies virus (derived from dried rabbit spinal cords) to protect animals and, eventually, humans against rabies. Salk developed the modern prototype inactivated whole-virus vaccine by growing the poliovirus in cell culture, purifying it, inactivating it with formaldehyde, and demonstrating that intramuscular injection of the inactivated virus protected against polio. HepA, JEV, and RAB are made in much the same way. The modern prototype whole bacterial vaccine is whole-cell pertussis, which was made from suspensions of cultured *Bordetella pertussis* organisms that were killed and detoxified. Because it contained every antigen from the live organism, this vaccine was both effective and reactogenic.
- *Component*—These vaccines use only a part of the pathogen instead of the whole organism. *Toxoids*, for example, are protein toxins elaborated by bacteria that are immunogenic but have been chemically modified to reduce pathogenicity. The only current toxoid vaccines are those for diphtheria and tetanus (inactivated pertussis toxin is generally not referred to as a toxoid). Other component vaccines are made from *purified subunits* of the organism. The original HepB, for

example, consisted of HBsAg that was purified from the blood of persistently infected individuals (these individuals overproduce HBsAg, which is released from the liver into the plasma). Of course, steps were taken to inactivate any live virus that might have also been present. In order to reduce reactogenicity of the whole cell pertussis vaccine, specific immunogenic proteins—filamentous hemagglutinin, pertactin, and fimbriae (in addition to inactivated pertussis toxin)—were purified from whole organisms and formulated into acellular vaccines. For *S pneumoniae*, *H influenzae*, *N meningitidis*, and *S typhi*, it was known that the capsular polysaccharide was the immunogenic part of the bacterium. Subunit vaccines were therefore developed using capsular polysaccharide that was stripped from the cell and purified.

Pure polysaccharide vaccines, however, induce only short-term immunity, do not produce immunologic memory, and are not immunogenic in young infants. *Engineered subunits*, in the form of protein-polysaccharide conjugates, are necessary to overcome these problems *(see below)*. Subunits can also be produced through *recombinant DNA* technology. The prototype here is the recombinant-derived HepB, in which the gene for HBsAg was inserted into yeast cells, which produce large quantities of the protein for purification. A similar method was used to produce HPV. In this case, the gene for the L1 protein was expressed in either yeast cells (HPV4) or insect cells using a baculovirus vector (HPV2). The nice thing about L1 is that it spontaneously aggregates into virus-like particles, which in every way look like viruses on the outside and are immunogenic but which carry no genetic material and are, therefore, incapable of replicating.

In classical vaccinology, the immunogenic subunits of a pathogen are identified, physically purified, and injected into animals to measure the immune response. Vaccines of the future may be developed using *reverse vaccinology*.[1] Here, rather than starting with the phenotype (the antigens), one starts with the genotype (the genes), looking for ones that code for molecules that are likely to be important in immunity (eg, cell surface expression and critical roles in infectivity or pathogenicity). The genes are then excised, expressed in some fashion to produce the antigens, and screened for immunogenicity in animals. This approach has been used, for example, to identify proteins that could be used in vaccines against *N meningitidis* serogroup B.[2]

■ Passive Immunization

Passive immunization is the process by which short-term protection from disease is conferred through the administration of antibodies. This process occurs naturally during the last 2 months of pregnancy, when large quantities of IgG are transferred across the placenta to the fetus, and it explains the relative protection that newborns enjoy against invasive *S pneumoniae* and *H influenzae* type b infections, among others. Passive immunization is necessary for patients with humoral immune defects who cannot synthesize their own antibody; in these cases, *polyclonal immune globulin* is used. Polyclonal immune globulin is also used to prevent certain specific infections, such as measles and hepatitis A, because the level of antibody to these agents is sufficiently high in the general population from whom the immune globulin is derived.

Passive immunization also is useful for persons at risk for particular infections; in such cases, *hyperimmune globulins*, derived from donors with high antibody levels to the pathogen, are used. One example is varicella zoster immune globulin (VariZIG), which is used for prevention of chickenpox in exposed immunocompromised individuals. Another example is hepatitis B immune globulin (HBIG), which is used in neonates born to mothers who are chronic hepatitis B carriers and also in other susceptible individuals who are exposed to the virus. Hyperimmune globulins contain antibodies to pathogens besides the one they target; this is true because the individuals from whom they are derived, while selected for their high antibody levels to specific pathogens, also have antibodies to other agents. Antibodies also can be *engineered* for prevention of specific diseases, as in the case of RSVmAB (Synagis), a monoclonal antibody that has the effector (constant) region of human IgG but the combining (antigen recognition) region of a mouse monoclonal antibody specific for the RSV F protein (which mediates fusion of the viral envelope to the host cell membrane—blocking this prevents infection). *Antitoxins*, also known as *heterologous hyperimmune sera*, are also used for passive immunization. These are produced in animals like horses and target toxins such as diphtheria, botulinum, and tetanus.

Passively acquired antibodies can inactivate parenterally administered live-attenuated viral vaccines. Thus, MMR and VAR are not given in the first year of life in order to avoid inactivation by maternal antibodies, and administration is deferred if a person receives blood products (which contain antibodies; see **Table 5.2**). Passively acquired antibodies do not appear to interfere with vaccines administered at mucosal surfaces, which is why RV can be given as early as 6 weeks of age. ZOS, by definition, is designed to boost immunity in persons who already have had varicella and therefore likely still have antibodies to varicella zoster virus (VZV); the vaccine contains enough virus to overcome interference by pre-existing antibody. Interestingly, maternal antibodies may interfere with the take of HepA, which is an inactivated vaccine; for this reason, vaccination is recommended in the second year of life. Maternal antibodies may interfere with the take of other inactivated vaccines but this is of little practical significance.[3]

1

RSVmAB, which is specific for RSV alone, does not inactivate live vaccines. YFV (which is also live-attenuated) does not appear to be inactivated by commercially available polyclonal immune globulin products in the United States, since the amount of YF virus antibody in the donors from whom these products are derived is low.

Basic Vaccine Immunology

Vaccines are designed to generate pathogen-specific antibodies and T-cells by stimulating the *adaptive immune system*, which recognizes and remembers specific pathogens and learns to respond to them more strongly after each exposure. What follows is a simplified version of the immune mechanisms that underpin vaccination—in essence, what you need to know to understand how vaccines work.[4] These concepts shed light on the differences between various types of vaccines, the duration of protection, dosing schedules, and other aspects of vaccine practice that are delineated elsewhere in this book.

■ Antibodies

Antibodies are proteins that bind to 3-dimensional patterns, or *epitopes*, that are present on antigens. They constitute the humoral, or soluble, arm of the adaptive immune system, and are produced as several different immunoglobulin *isotypes* (IgG, IgA, IgM, IgE, IgD) that differ in function. A given antibody with a given antigenic specificity can be produced as one of several different isotypes. Antibody binding is *specific* in that each antibody molecule binds best to one particular epitope; any given antigen may express many different epitopes, and any given microbe may have hundreds of different antigens. Binding of antibodies to a virus or toxin can lead to *neutralization*, ie, the blocking of ligands or receptors that are critical for infectivity or toxicity. Binding of antibodies to a bacterium can lead to *opsonization* (coating of the organism) so that it can be pulled out of circulation by cells of the reticuloendothelial system or so that it can be killed by *complement-mediated lysis* (fixing of complement proteins on the surface, forming a *membrane attack complex* that kills the organism). Binding of antibodies to a virus-infected cell can lead to *antibody-dependent cell-mediated cytotoxicity*, whereby the infected cell is flagged for destruction by natural killer cells, monocytes, and eosinophils.

Antibodies are the only element of the adaptive immune system that can *prevent* viral infection because they can neutralize the virus before it has a chance to replicate in cells. They are also the mainstay of protection against bacterial invasion since they facilitate destruction of the inoculating organism before it has a chance to reproduce. The battle between antibodies and pathogens takes place at different sites. At mucosal surfaces, where most pathogens try to gain entry, secretory IgA and serum IgG antibodies that leak across from the vascular compartment are important. Live vaccines that replicate at mucosal surfaces (eg, LAIV) have the advantage of inducing strong local IgA responses that can neutralize pathogens before invasion. Vaccines given parenterally are not as good at generating secretory IgA at mucosal surfaces, although this does happen. A vaccine that induces high levels of serum IgG not only can protect against bloodstream invasion or infection in extravascular spaces, but also can block infection at mucosal sites before the organism gains a foothold.

Antibodies are produced by plasma cells, which are derived from B lymphocytes or B-cells. B-cells have immunoglobulins on their surface (mostly IgM, also referred to as the *B-cell receptor*) that express one and only one antibody specificity. During ontogeny, genetic rearrangements lead to a diversity of B-cell clones, each with its own unique antibody specificity (those B-cells that emerge from this process with receptors that recognize self antigens are deleted). People are, therefore, walking around with millions of B-cells, each pre-committed to recognizing one and only one epitope. Theoretically, humans even have B-cells capable of responding to the *Andromeda* strain,[5] should it ever happen to (again) fall to earth. The point is that the B-cell repertoire presumably covers every possible antigen that is not self. When a given B-cell finds its antigenic match, it becomes activated and proliferates; this is known as *clonal expansion.* The daughter cells eventually differentiate into plasma cells, the factories that secrete large amounts of antibody.

There are two basic pathways through which antibody production occurs, and the differences between them are important to understanding how vaccines work.

■ The Extrafollicular Reaction

The extrafollicular reaction is best exemplified by the immune response to polysaccharides (**Figure 1.1**). A precommitted B-cell encounters its polysaccharide match (at the site of inoculation with a vaccine or perhaps in a lymph node to which the vaccine antigen was transported), leading to activation, proliferation, and rapid differentiation into plasma cells, which migrate to the red pulp of the spleen and intramedullary areas of lymph nodes. There the plasma cells begin producing antibodies. It is important to understand that these are *germline* antibodies, ie, antibodies transcribed from genes that were present in the B-cell to begin with. Germline antibodies have low affinity for their corresponding antigens because the genes from which they are transcribed, their sequence of amino acids, the shape of their combining site,

FIGURE 1.1 — Polysaccharide Antigens and the Extrafollicular Reaction

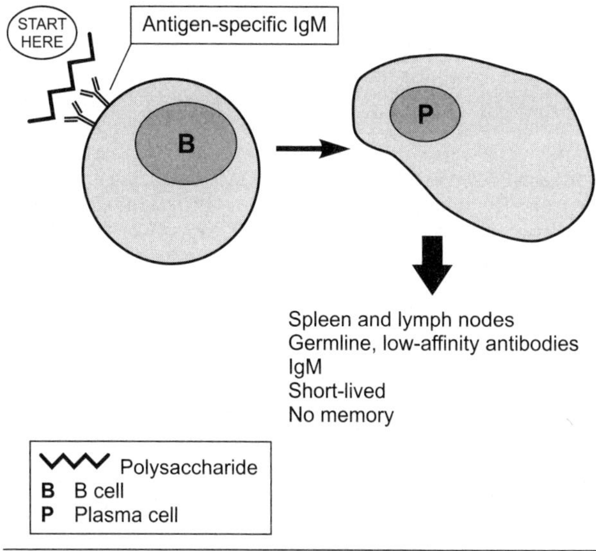

See text for explanation.

and thus their ability to bind to the antigen was determined by a random process way back when the person was a fetus. These B-cells (and their genes) were selected during ontogeny because they recognized nonself antigens, not because they would someday bind especially tightly to those particular antigens. Furthermore, most of the antibodies produced in the extrafollicular reaction are of the same isotype that was present on the B-cell surface, namely IgM, which does not offer the functional benefits of other isotypes such as IgG. Finally, the plasma cells produced through the extrafollicular reaction ultimately die out—no more antibodies produced, no more protection, no ability to remember the encounter and respond more quickly or decisively the next time.

This is called the *extrafollicular reaction* because it takes place outside of the germinal centers of lymph nodes. Antigens that elicit this response are called *T-cell independent* because the responding B-cells differentiate without much T-cell interaction. The characteristics of T-cell independent responses—rapid production (days to weeks) of short-lived, low-affinity, predominantly IgM antibodies without induction of memory—are hallmark features of the response to pure polysaccharide antigens, such as those in the original *H influenzae* vaccine, PPSV, and

MPSV. To compound the problem with polysaccharides, children <2 years of age do not mount robust T-cell independent responses, making these vaccines poor immunogens in that age group.

There is one other problem with polysaccharides—*hyporesponsiveness*.[6] This refers to the observation that individuals who initially receive pure polysaccharide vaccines seem to respond less well to polysaccharide challenge, as if they have permanently "used up" some of the pre-existing polysaccharide-specific B-cell pool—this phenomenon has been referred to as *original polysaccharide sin*. Interestingly, hyporesponsiveness might even be naturally induced—infants receiving PCV7 have decreased responses to the *S pneumoniae* serotypes they are colonized with at the time they are immunized, suggesting that colonization—a natural form of exposure to capsular polysaccharide—also induces hyporesponsiveness.[7]

It is important to point out that there is some crossover between immunologic pathways. For example, some degree of T-cell help *(see below)* may be available to extrafollicular B-cells, such that some isotype switching occurs and some memory may be generated.

■ The Germinal Center Reaction

Underpinning the adaptive immune system is the much more primitive *innate immune system*, capable of initiating the battle against invading microorganisms in a nonspecific fashion. Cells of the innate immune system—most notably dendritic cells and monocytes—carry receptors that recognize conserved patterns among pathogens (*pathogen-specific molecular patterns*) that are not found in self tissues. Among these are *Toll-like receptors* (TLRs), each of which recognizes a different pattern. TLR3, for example, recognizes double-stranded viral RNA; TLR7 binds single-stranded RNA, TLR9 binds double-stranded DNA, and TLR5 binds bacterial flagellins.[8] Engagement of pattern-recognition receptors activates the cell, which then secretes *cytokines* (intercellular communication molecules) that activate and recruit other cells, setting up an inflammatory reaction. The end result might be destruction of the invader through processes such as phagocytosis. Importantly, this is a one-time occurrence—once the pathogen is destroyed, there is no memory of the encounter that might facilitate a response the next time around.

Why do vaccinologists care about innate immunity if it provides no memory? The answer lies in the fact that activation of the innate immune system can trigger an adaptive immune response. The key link is provided by *antigen-presenting cells* (APCs), the most important of which are dendritic cells (**Figure 1.2**). Immature APCs circulate through the body or reside in tissues (immature dendritic cells in the dermis are called *Langerhans cells*). When a pathogen-specific molecular pattern is encountered—in the form, for example, of an injected vaccine—the

FIGURE 1.2 — Antigen-Presenting Cells and the Germinal Center Reaction

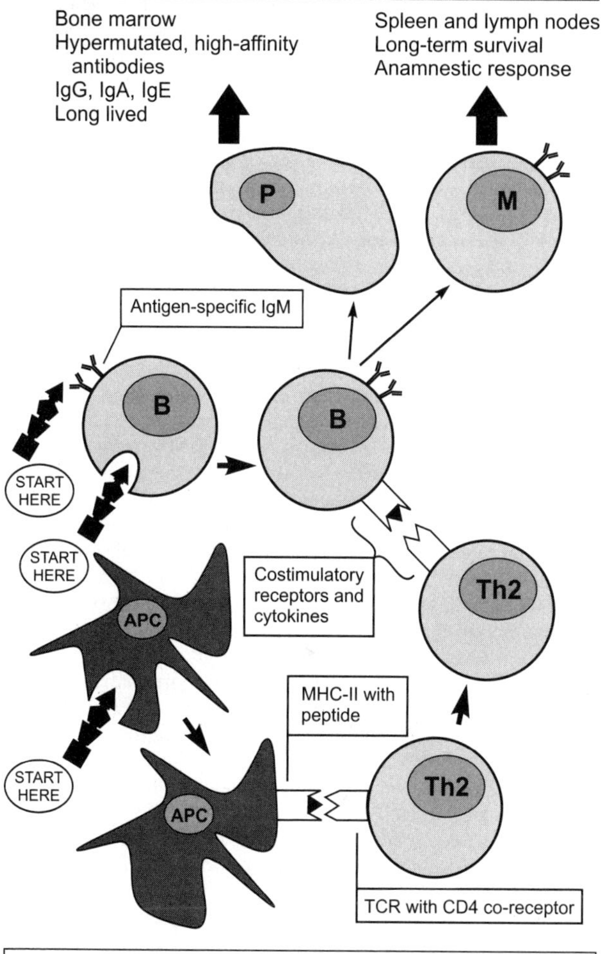

Protein	
APC	Antigen-presenting cell
B	B cell
M	Memory B cell
MHC-II	Class II major histocompatibility complex molecule
P	Plasma cell
TCR	T-cell receptor
Th2	Helper T cell type 2

See text for explanation.

APCs begin to mature, express new receptors on their surface, and migrate through lymphatic vessels to regional lymph nodes. Some of them also engulf the vaccine antigens, degrade the proteins into small peptides, load the peptides into the groove of *major histocompatibility complex* (MHC) *class II molecules* (MHC-II), and express those molecules on their surface (MHC molecules are also referred to as *human leukocyte antigens* or HLAs).

The mature APCs are now activated (secreting proinflammatory cytokines and expressing costimulatory molecules on the surface), flagged (by the surface expression of antigen-derived peptides in the context of MHC-II), and have migrated to the follicular region of the lymph node. At this stage, the APCs are ready to engage immature *helper T lymphocytes* (Th-cells) by interacting with the *T-cell receptor* (TCR) and the *CD4 coreceptor* (both are on the Th-cell). Each Th-cell is predetermined to recognize a particular peptide/MHC-II flag by virtue of its TCR and CD4 molecule (like the surface receptor of B-cells, the TCR has a unique antigenic specificity; the diversity of TCRs is generated during fetal development by a random process, much like the generation of germline antibodies, and those T-cells that emerge from this process with receptors that recognize self antigens are deleted or inactivated). Through soluble cytokines and costimulatory receptor-ligand interactions, contact with the right APC results in activation and maturation of the Th-cell into one of two antigen-specific subtypes: Th1- or Th2-cells. Th2-cells have some direct antimicrobial functions, particularly against parasites. More importantly, though, Th2-cells seek out their unique B-cell matches in order to help them make antibody (to the antigen from which the peptide in the MHC groove was originally derived). B-cells are primed to be helped by engulfing some of the bound antigen, digesting the proteins, and presenting the peptides on their surface in the context of MHC-II, much like dendritic cells do.

Th1-cells also have direct antimicrobial functions. More importantly, though, Th1-cells seek out *cytotoxic T-cells* (Tc-cells) and macrophages, coaxing them into performing cytotoxic functions *(see below)*. Several factors determine whether a Th-cell differentiates into a Th1 or Th2-cell during immunization; among these are the dose of antigen, route of administration, and the effect of *adjuvants (see below)*. These factors, therefore, also determine whether humoral or cellular responses predominate.

The interaction between B-cells and Th-cells takes place in the germinal centers of lymph nodes, hence the name of the reaction. The signals provided by Th2-cells, as well as the persistence of antigen shuttled there by APCs, drive B-cells to undergo massive clonal proliferation—producing millions of daughter cells capable of making the same antibodies. As they proliferate under these conditions, the B-cells undergo a process of somatic hypermutation, whereby the genes encoding the immunoglobulin combining region mutate at exceptional rates, randomly producing a spectrum of antibodies with varying affinities for the antigen. Those B-cells expressing high-affinity antibodies are selected for and clonally expanded. The end result is a set of dominant B-cell clones that produce high-affinity antibodies, ones that bind the antigen better than the germline antibodies produced in the extrafollicular reaction. The only problem is that this process takes a week or two to get rolling.

Two other things happen in the germinal center. First, signals from Th2-cells drive *isotype switching* (from IgM to other isotypes) as B-cells transform into plasma cells. The end result is large numbers of plasma cells that migrate to the bone marrow and produce high-affinity IgG, as well as other isotypes. Second, Th2-cells drive the parallel evolution of *memory B-cells*, which migrate to the spleen and lymph nodes and wait there—sometimes for decades—until they again encounter the antigen, at which time they rapidly proliferate and differentiate into plasma cells that produce antibody. This is called the *anamnestic response*. Memory Th-cells are also generated, but their numbers wane with time.

The germinal center reaction has many implications for vaccination.

- *Stimulating innate immunity*—The more innate immunity is stimulated, the more robust the adaptive immune response will be. For example, intradermal vaccination may stimulate more robust responses than intramuscular injection because there are more immature dendritic cells lying in wait in the dermis.[9] As another example, we know that live viral vaccines are more immunogenic than inactivated ones. One reason is that live viruses can disseminate and encounter dendritic cells at multiple sites, ultimately establishing multiple foci of germinal center reactions. Live vaccines also carry more recognizable pathogen-specific molecular patterns that are capable of activating innate immune cells.
- *Adjuvants*—Adjuvants are substances that potentiate the immune response to vaccine antigens.[10] Whereas they are necessary for some inactivated vaccines to engender robust immune responses, there is no predicting which antigens will need adjuvants and which ones will not (adjuvants are not necessary for live vaccines because live vaccines are capable of stimulating innate immune responses on their own). In fact, similar vaccines may differ with regard to adjuvants—take, for example, the *H influenzae* type b conjugate vaccines: Hib-OMP (PedvaxHIB) contains an adjuvant, whereas Hib-T (ActHIB, Hiberix) does not. For many decades, the only adjuvant used in human vaccines was alum, an amorphous mixture of aluminum salts that presumably works by inducing inflammation at the injection site,[11] and/or retaining antigen

at the site and promoting uptake by dendritic cells,[12] and/or activating an intracellular immune response system called the Nalp3 inflammasome.[13] In 2009, the door to newer adjuvants was opened with the licensure of HPV2 (Cervarix), which contains AS04, an adjuvant composed of 3-*O*-desacyl-4'-monophosphoryl lipid A (MPL, a derivative of bacterial lipopolysaccharide) adsorbed to an aluminum hydroxide salt.[14] MPL activates TLR4 on APCs, promoting cytokine expression, antigen presentation, and migration of APCs to lymph nodes. Adjuvants may allow for *antigen sparing*. For example, an adjuvanted version of IIV was just as immunogenic as a nonadjuvanted version, even though it contained one fourth the amount of antigen (as might be expected, though, the adjuvanted vaccine produced more local and systemic symptoms, but these were transient and mild to moderate in intensity).[15] Taking this observation one step further, a study involving nearly 5000 children demonstrated that an IIV adjuvanted with MF59, an oil-in-water emulsion, was 75% more efficacious than an unadjuvanted IIV.[16] Finally, adjuvants may cause *epitope spreading*, a broadening of the antibody repertoire such that more epitopes on a given antigen are recognized.[17]

- *Priming and boosting*—Ultimately, the magnitude and duration of the antibody response to inactivated vaccines depends on the immunologic set point following primary immunization. In other words, the more germinal centers that are formed, the more long-lived plasma cells and memory B-cells there will be. In addition to optimizing antigen dose and using adjuvants, *primary immunization* is enhanced by multiple doses of the vaccine given in succession, classically separated by 1 or 2 months (as in the 2-, 4-, and 6-month schedule for primary DTaP immunization). These doses are given too soon to exploit memory responses, but they do drive the process of affinity maturation in the germinal centers. Following priming, vaccine schedules take advantage of anamnestic responses, which boost the level of high-quality antibody (**Figure 1.3**).[18] The need to wait until the germinal center reaction is complete explains the longer interval between the primary series of a vaccine and the booster doses (as in the 15- to 18-month dose of DTaP). The response to booster doses of vaccine mimics what happens when the natural pathogen is encountered.
- *Specificity*—Hypermutated, high-affinity antibodies specifically target single epitopes. For this reason, most inactivated vaccines are very specific in the protection they afford. For example, IPV contains formalin-inactivated, disrupted viral particles from three different serotypes of poliovirus because the antigens from any given serotype do not induce antibodies that will neutralize the other serotypes. Germinal center

FIGURE 1.3 — Time Course of Antibody Responses

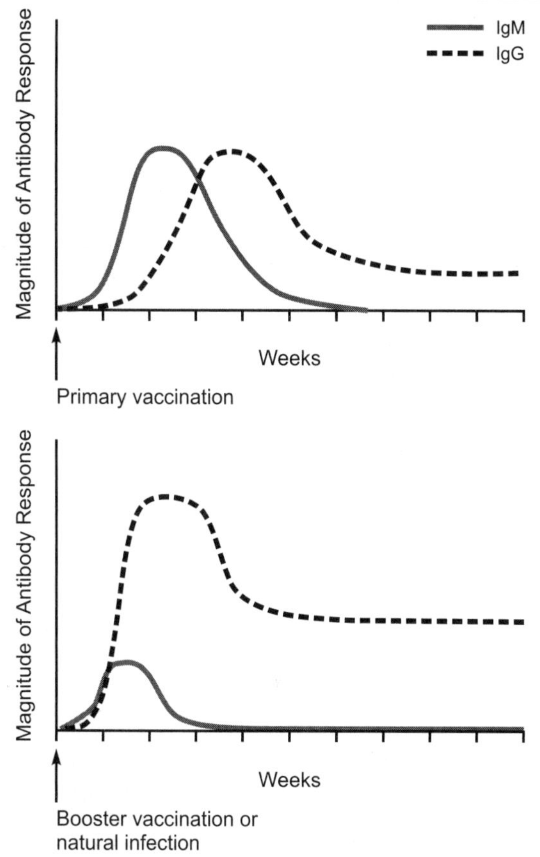

See text for explanation.

reactions by and large generate *homotypic* responses, ones directed against the antigen used as the vaccine. *Heterotypic*, or *cross-protective*, responses occur only if there is sufficient similarity between the antigens of different strains, or if there is a common antigen between them. Tc-cells offer much more potential for cross-strain protection *(see below)*.

- *Persistence of antibody*—The germinal center reaction peaks in several weeks, after which it is terminated. The mechanisms by which serum antibodies persist for long periods of time—something so critical to maintaining protection—are not yet worked out.[19] Some models suggest that there is more or less constitutive differentiation of memory B-cells into plasma cells, stimulated by persistent antigen, reinfection, or exposure to cross-reactive antigens. Other models propose there is nonspecific, or so-called "bystander," activation of memory B-cells. These models have important implications for vaccine programs. For example, early studies of VAR showed persistent if not *rising* titers of antibody over time. But these studies were done at a time when the wild-type virus was still circulating; therefore, immunized individuals might have experienced repeated subclinical reinfections with natural virus, coaxing memory B-cells to differentiate into plasma cells and boosting antibody production. As transmission of natural varicella decreased, some studies began to show waning immunity over time (this observation made it less likely that antibody persisted because of boosting from periodic reactivation of latent vaccine virus). Although initially intended to immunize those who failed to seroconvert after the first dose (so-called *primary vaccine failures*), the second dose of VAR also serves to boost immunity in those individuals whose antibody levels have fallen low enough to allow *take*, or replication of the vaccine virus.

Other models suggest that plasma cells derived from the germinal center reaction can live for a very long time. Either way, for some vaccines, it is necessary to periodically conjure up the anamnestic response through booster vaccination. One thing is clear—to prevent infections with a short incubation period (*N meningitidis* is a good example), one must have a sufficient amount of circulating antibody at the time of encounter with the pathogen. Anamnestic responses, while brisk, are not fast enough to be of much help when dealing with rapidly replicating bacteria. They may be sufficient, however, for pathogens with longer incubation periods. Thus, for example, although antibodies to HBV, and along with them protection from *infection*, may wane with time, protection against *disease* does not wane—there is plenty of time for memory responses to kick in before the virus can do damage.

- *Making better immunogens*—As mentioned above, polysaccharides are poor immunogens. Vaccinologists have learned, however, to harness the power of the germinal center reaction to enhance their immunogenicity (**Figure 1.4**). The polysaccharides are chemically attached to protein carriers—among the variety of carriers used are an outer-membrane protein from *N meningitidis* (Hib-OMP [PedvaxHIB]), a mutant diphtheria toxin called CRM_{197} (PCV13-CRM [Prevnar], MCV4-CRM [Menveo]), tetanus toxoid (Hib-T [ActHIB, Hiberix]), and diphtheria toxoid (MCV4-D [Menactra]). B-cells that are pre-committed to producing anti-*polysaccharide* antibody are stimulated by their encounter with the antigen. They also

FIGURE 1.4 — Response to Protein-Polysaccharide Conjugate Vaccines

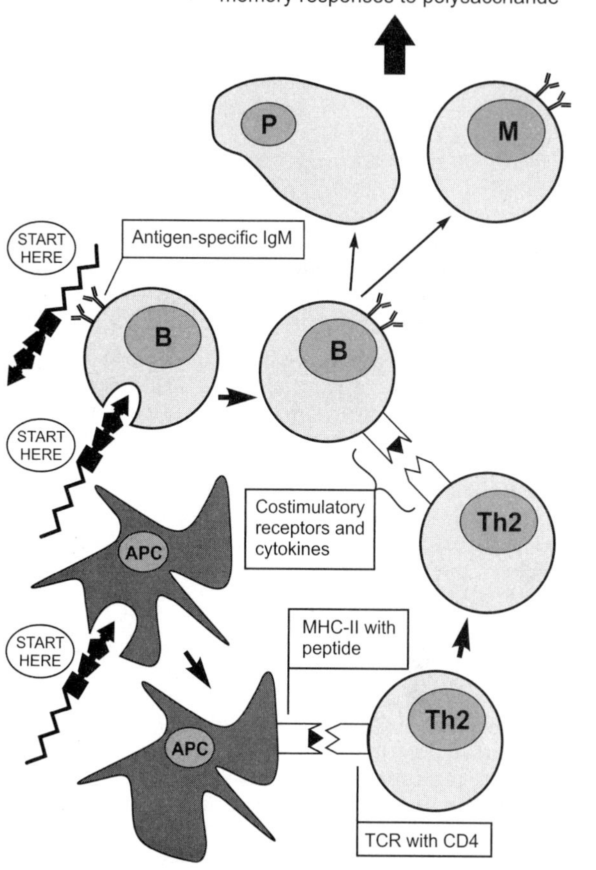

	Protein-polysaccharide conjugate		
APC	Antigen-presenting cell	**MHC-II**	Class II major histocompatibility complex molecule
B	B cell	**P**	Plasma cell
M	Memory B cell	**TCR**	T-cell receptor
		Th2	Helper T cell type 2

See text for explanation.

engulf the bound antigen, digest it, and present peptides from the *protein* portion of the vaccine on their surface in the context of MHC-II (polysaccharides cannot be presented in this context). So what you have is a B-cell committed to making anti-*polysaccharide* antibodies that is displaying a *peptide/MHC-II* flag on its surface. All it takes now is for APCs to display the same peptides in the context of MHC-II, stimulating Th2-cells, which then find their B-cell matches and help them make antibody through the germinal center reaction. In essence, the Th2-cells "think" they are helping B-cells make antibodies to the protein antigen from which the peptides were derived but, in fact, the flagged B-cells make *polysaccharide* antibody. By converting a *T-cell independent* response to a *T-cell dependent* one, the shortcomings of polysaccharides as antigens are overcome. **Table 1.3** summarizes the advantages of protein-polysaccharide conjugate vaccines.

■ Cytotoxic T Cells

Tc-cells are the main effectors of the adaptive cellular immune response. Like Th-cells, they express the TCR on their surface, which has a unique antigenic specificity encoded in the germline. Unlike Th-cells, which express CD4, Tc-cells express the CD8 coreceptor, which directs engagement with *MHC class I molecules* (MHC-I). Like MHC-II, MHC-I loads pathogen-derived peptides into its groove and presents those peptides on the cell surface. However, instead of coming from the digestion of exogenous proteins that were engulfed by the cell, the peptides loaded into MHC-I are actually made inside the cell—by infecting viruses or other intracellular pathogens.

MHC-I is expressed on APCs as well as on all nucleated host cells. Naïve Tc-cells, predetermined to recognize a particular peptide/MHC-I flag, engage infected APCs that express those particular peptides in the context of MHC-I (**Figure 1.5**). While this leads to activation of the Tc-cell, the Tc-cell does not become a killer until it receives additional signals—those coming in the form of cytokines from Th1-cells, which in turn have been activated by engagement of APCs expressing pathogen-derived peptides in the context of MHC-II (Th1-cells have other functions as well, such as activation of macrophages). The respective, critical role of the two different types of Th-cells is obvious—Th2-cells help B-cells produce high-quality antibodies and memory cells, and Th1-cells help Tc-cells become killers (and memory cells as well).

What does a Tc-cell kill? Remember that Tc-cells recognize peptides in the context of MHC-I, and all cells express MHC-I. Therefore, Tc-cells find and destroy infected cells that express pathogen-derived peptides on their surface in the context of MHC-I. How does a Tc-cell kill? One mechanism is through the release of *cytotoxins* that create holes in the cell membrane. In

TABLE 1.3 — Advantages of Protein-Polysaccharide Conjugate Vaccines

	Type of Vaccine	
Property	**Polysaccharide**	**Protein-Polysaccharide Conjugate**
B-cell response	T-cell independent	T-cell dependent
Pathway	Extrafollicular	Germinal center
Antibody generation in young infants	No	Yes
Induction of immune memory	No	Yes
Anamnestic or booster responses	No	Yes
Long-term protection	No	Yes
Reduced carriage of the organism at mucosal surfaces	No	Yes[a]
Herd immunity	No	Yes[b]

[a] Robust serum IgG levels allow for leakage onto mucosal surfaces, where colonizing bacteria are killed.
[b] Fewer colonized people means less transmission of the pathogen from person to person, indirectly protecting people who are not immune.

FIGURE 1.5 — Cytotoxic T-Cell Response

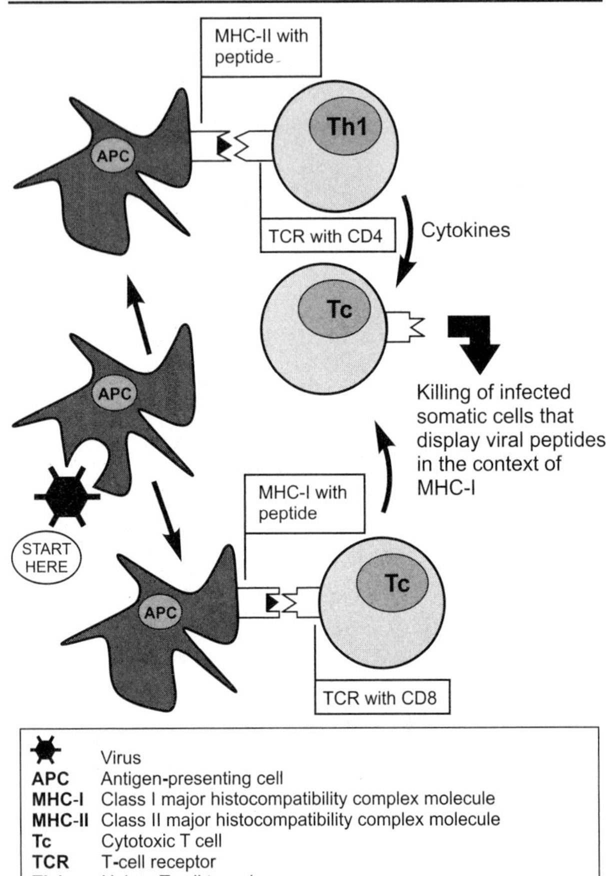

(virus symbol)	Virus
APC	Antigen-presenting cell
MHC-I	Class I major histocompatibility complex molecule
MHC-II	Class II major histocompatibility complex molecule
Tc	Cytotoxic T cell
TCR	T-cell receptor
Th1	Helper T cell type 1

See text for explanation.

addition, Tc-cells can induce *apoptosis*, or programmed cell death, through the release of certain enzymes and through cell-surface receptor-ligand interactions.

It is important to point out that there is some crossover between the immune mechanisms delineated above. For example, some exogenous peptides can be presented to a limited extent in the context of MHC-I; therefore, some inactivated vaccines can induce Tc responses.

The unique characteristics of Tc-cells and their generation have several implications for vaccination:

- *Viruses vs bacteria*—Tc-cells are much more important in controlling viral rather than bacterial infections. The reason is simple—most bacteria are capable of replicating outside of cells, and therefore do not generate APCs or somatic cells flagged with peptide/MHC-I ("somatic cells" refers to all cells in the body except gametes, or sex cells). Viruses, on the other hand, can only replicate by usurping the host cell machinery for protein synthesis. Therefore, infected APCs and somatic cells are routinely flagged with peptide/MHC-I—unless the virus has evolved a mechanism to cloak the infected cell in anonymity by preventing the surface expression of peptide/MHC-I (cytomegalovirus and adenovirus, for example, evade the immune response in this fashion).

  Vaccines against bacterial pathogens are designed to maximize high-quality antibody production (some part of this involves the generation of large pools of Th2-cells). The ideal vaccine for a viral infection would maximize high-quality antibody production, as well as lead to the generation of Tc-cells.
- *Preventing vs limiting infection*—Tc-cells operate *after* infection has taken place; they limit but do not prevent infection. Unlike antibody, a Tc-cell cannot kill a free virion that lands on a mucosal surface or enters the bloodstream. It must first wait until a cell is infected and expressing viral peptides. If a vaccinated person is exposed to a virus, the first line of defense is the antibody that resides at the site of inoculation or in the immediate local environment. That antibody could neutralize the virus, thus preventing *infection*. If it does not, and the virus gains entry into cells and begins to replicate, memory Tc-cells are called into action to destroy those cells, thus preventing *disease*. Antibody may also play a role in the destruction of infected cells through antibody-dependent cell-mediated cytotoxicity.

  Differences between VAR and ZOS, both of which contain the same live-attenuated strain of VZV, are instructive. First, the main goal of ZOS is to expand the pool of memory Tc-cells. By definition, people who get herpes zoster (shingles) are already infected with VZV (herpes zoster is the reactivation of endogenous, natural VZV that has been latent in the person since he or she had chickenpox). Early in the process of reactivation, infected cells begin to express viral peptides on their surface, and the idea is to have Tc-cells ready to pounce on those cells before the disease can manifest. Second, in order for the vaccine itself to stimulate Tc-cells, it must first infect host cells so that its peptides can be expressed in the context of MHC-I. The reason ZOS has so much more virus in it (14 times the amount in VAR) is precisely the fact that it must avoid neutralization by any naturally occurring antibody in order to gain entry into host cells.

- *Live vs inactivated vaccines*—Because they replicate within cells, live viral vaccines are much better at inducing Tc-cells than are inactivated vaccines. This is in addition to other factors that have already been mentioned, such as their enhanced ability to stimulate innate immune responses and their ability to amplify and disseminate antigens.
- *Cross-protection*—B-cells recognize epitopes that are conformational in nature, in essence 3-dimensional structures that are presented on antigens on the pathogen surface. A good example of such an antigen is the hemagglutinin (H) molecule of influenza virus, a glycoprotein that protrudes from the viral envelope and mediates attachment to cells. IIV is very good at eliciting antibodies to H that can block infectivity—but those antibodies are specific to the strain of influenza virus that was used to make the vaccine. If antigenic drift occurs during a given season—that is, if the H of the prevailing virus has a slightly different sequence and conformation—the vaccine will not be as effective.

  Tc-cells, on the other hand, recognize peptides that are derived from any protein made by the pathogen, some of which are more conserved between strains than are surface molecules. Just like IIV, LAIV elicits strain-specific antibodies directed at H. However, it can also induce Tc-cells that recognize peptides derived from the nucleocapsid of the virus. The advantage here is that nucleocapsid proteins are well conserved from one strain to another. Thus LAIV can induce Tc-cell responses capable of limiting infection due to strains whose H has drifted from the vaccine strain.

Additional Concepts

■ Correlates of Protection

Ideally, vaccines are shown to be effective in randomized, blinded, placebo-controlled trials, where one group of subjects gets vaccine, another gets placebo, and the measured outcome is *efficacy*, or ability to prevent disease (or infection). This works if the disease is prevalent, such that the number of subjects needed in a clinical trial is within reach. For diseases that are relatively rare, demonstrating efficacy may not be feasible.[20] In these situations, *immunogenicity*, or the ability to generate an immune response, is relied upon as a predictor of efficacy. Such predictors may be *correlates* of immunity, that is responses that are closely related to protection, or *surrogates* of immunity, qualifiable immune responses that, while not in themselves protective, nevertheless can substitute for the true correlate.[21] As will be seen, however, the connection between immunogenicity and efficacy is not that straightforward.

1

Correlates of protection against a disease are useful for other reasons as well. For example, it may not be possible to study vaccine efficacy in every population that will ultimately be targeted for immunization. How can we be sure that a vaccine demonstrated to be effective in one age group will be effective in another, or, for that matter, in persons of different ethnic groups, those with underlying medical conditions, or those living in different geographic areas? If we knew which immunologic tests predicted protection, we could be reassured that if the immunologic criteria were met, protection would likely ensue. Immune correlates or surrogates also drive preclinical development, in the sense that scientists choose antigens, delivery systems, and dosing schedules that maximize immune responses thought to be important in protecting people from disease. Correlates also are critical to quality assurance—each new production lot of vaccine cannot be studied for efficacy, but it *can* be studied for immunogenicity and, in particular, for its ability to generate responses that are relevant in some way to protection. Likewise, there are many vaccination scenarios that must be studied in practice. For example, a new vaccine might be effective in clinical trials, but in real life, it needs to be given concomitantly with other vaccines. It would be very difficult to study efficacy under every permutation of concomitant use; instead, investigators rely on correlates to determine if concomitant use is likely or unlikely to compromise protection. For new combination vaccines, noninferiority (with respect to a relevant immune response) to concomitant administration of the separate vaccines must be demonstrated (see *Chapter 2: Vaccine Infrastructure in the United States—Vaccine Development and Licensure*).

Table 1.4 shows some generally accepted quantitative correlates of protection after vaccination. For some diseases, there are generally accepted, albeit imperfect, correlates of protection. For example, studies in the prevaccine era showed that children who had naturally occurring antibody to the *H influenzae* capsular polysaccharide (polyribosylribitol phosphate [PRP]) in amounts ≥0.15 mcg/mL were protected from invasive *H influenzae* disease; those with levels <0.15 mcg/mL were not. Studies utilizing the pure (unconjugated) PRP vaccine showed that antibody levels ≥1.0 mcg/mL immediately following vaccination correlated with protection against disease. So, which is the correlate of protection, 0.15 mcg/mL or 1.0 mcg/mL? Some have referred to 0.15 mcg/mL as the "short-term" correlate of protection, meaning that this is the level of circulating anti-PRP antibody you need at any given time to kill *H influenzae* that happens to gain entry into the bloodstream; 1.0 mcg/mL is referred to as the "long-term" correlate of protection, meaning that this is the amount of antibody

TABLE 1.4 — Generally Accepted Correlates of Protection After Vaccination

Disease	Test	Correlate of Protection
Diphtheria	Toxin neutralization	0.01-0.1 IU/mL
Hepatitis A	Enzyme-linked immunosorbent assay	10 mIU/mL
Hepatitis B	Enzyme-linked immunosorbent assay	10 mIU/mL
H influenzae (polysaccharide vaccine)	Enzyme-linked immunosorbent assay	1 mcg/mL
H influenzae (conjugate vaccine)	Enzyme-linked immunosorbent assay	0.15 mcg/mL
Influenza	Hemagglutination inhibition	1:40 dilution
Japanese encephalitis	Plaque reduction neutralization	1:10 dilution
Lyme	Enzyme-linked immunosorbent assay	1100 EIA U/mL
Measles	Microneutralization	120 mIU/mL
N meningitidis (serogroup C)	Serum bactericidal assay using human complement	1:4 dilution
Polio	Serum neutralization	1:4-1:8 dilution
Rabies	Serum neutralization	0.5 IU/mL
Rubella	Immunoprecipitation	10-15 mIU/mL
S pneumoniae	Enzyme-linked immunosorbent assay	0.20-0.35 mcg/mL (for children)
	Opsonophagocytosis	1:8 dilution
Tetanus	Toxin neutralization	0.1 IU/mL
Varicella	Serum neutralization	1:64 dilution
	Glycoprotein enzyme-linked immunosorbent assay	5 IU/mL

Adapted from Plotkin SA. *Pediatr Infect Dis J*. 2001;20:63-75.

you need after vaccination with a pure polysaccharide vaccine to be protected for a long time. The question is, what antibody levels are necessary immediately after vaccination with a *conjugate* Hib vaccine to achieve long-term protection? One cannot directly infer this from studies of polysaccharide vaccine, because conjugate vaccines induce higher quality antibodies.

The situation becomes even more complex. Protection may be mediated before the organism enters the bloodstream, at the site of mucosal colonization. Little is known, however, about mucosal correlates of protection. How much secretory IgA or extravascular IgG is enough to prevent colonization? What role does prevention of colonization play in prevention of disease? How about the role of inoculum size (assuming there is a correlate of protection necessarily assumes there is an average inoculum)?

Another example of the problem with interpreting correlates of protection comes from observations made with HepB. Studies suggest that circulating levels of HBsAb ≥10 mIU/mL at the time of exposure to HBV perfectly predict protection from infection. In this sense, then, HBsAb ≥10 mIU/mL is a correlate of protection. However, studies also show that antibody wanes with time—often to levels <10 mIU/mL—even though protection does not. Therefore, there must be another (unmeasured) correlate of long-term protection.

One also needs to ask how antibodies are being measured. Clearly, quantitation of high-avidity antibodies that kill or opsonize *H influenzae* would correlate more closely with protection than measurement of antibodies that bind to PRP in an enzyme-linked immunosorbent assay. Similarly, we are much more interested in the levels of serum bactericidal antibodies to *N meningitidis*, a functional immune response endpoint, than we are in quantitating antibody binding to the capsular polysaccharide; bactericidal assays, however, are difficult to standardize. Quantitation of antibodies that neutralize viruses in vitro might be more relevant than measurement of antibodies that bind to viral proteins—unless one knows exactly which proteins are involved in generating neutralizing antibody. Even then, there is no guarantee that a protein-binding assay will measure antibodies that bind to the neutralizing epitopes, and that binding to those epitopes actually correlates with neutralization in a functional assay. For some infections (eg, tetanus), antibodies to the *organism itself* are not relevant, but antibodies to *toxins produced by the organism* are. The situation becomes even more complex when one considers that for some diseases, protection may be mediated as much by Th- and Tc-cells as by antibody. In as much as Th-cells help B-cells make antibodies, antibody levels may be an indirect measure of cellular immunity.

Fortunately, vaccine development does not depend on establishing immunologic correlates of protection. For example, there is no consensus on correlates of protection against rotavirus (candidates include mucosal IgA and T-cells), even though highly effective vaccines have been developed. Likewise, debate continues about the correlates of protection against pertussis. Most agree that antibody to pertussis toxin is necessary; some say it is sufficient, but some say immunity is incrementally enhanced by antibodies to filamentous hemagglutinin, pertactin, and fimbriae. No one really agrees on the actual levels of antibody that are necessary. Yet pertussis vaccines in various iterations have been in use since the 1940s—licensed based on demonstrated efficacy against disease in clinical trials.

Interestingly, the newest pertussis vaccine, Tdap, was licensed without proof of efficacy—and despite the fact that there are no agreed-upon correlates of protection. For both available products (Boostrix and Adacel), the basis for licensure was the demonstration of levels of antibodies to pertussis antigens that were similar to the levels found in infants who had received DTaP, a vaccine already proved to be effective against disease. Similarly, MCV4-D was licensed because the levels of antibody following vaccination were equivalent to those achieved after immunization with MPSV4, which was known to be protective. MCV4-CRM, in turn, was licensed after demonstration of noninferiority with MCV4-D.

■ Herd Immunity

Vaccines protect people in two ways. First, they stimulate adaptive immunity in vaccinated individuals. The level of protection depends on the quality, magnitude, and duration of the individual's response. Since no vaccine is 100% effective, even vaccinated individuals can become infected—*if* they are exposed. Exposure, in turn, depends on transmission of the pathogen from person-to-person (an exception is tetanus, which is acquired from the environment, not other people). What if transmission were interrupted because there were enough immune individuals in the population? Then everyone—susceptible vaccinated and unvaccinated individuals alike—would be indirectly protected.

The term *herd immunity* was coined in 1923 by Topley and Wilson in drawing a distinction between (but acknowledging the relatedness of) the immunity of individuals and protection of the community in which the individuals live. It refers to the fact that susceptible members of "the herd" are protected by the presence and proximity of immune members who prevent propagation of the infection (**Figure 1.6**).[22] For every disease that is transmitted from person to person, there is a *herd immunity threshold*—a critical proportion of the population that must be immune in order to prevent sustained disease transmission (**Figure 1.7**). Although simple in concept, the herd immunity threshold depends on a complex interplay of many factors, including contagiousness

FIGURE 1.6 — Herd Immunity

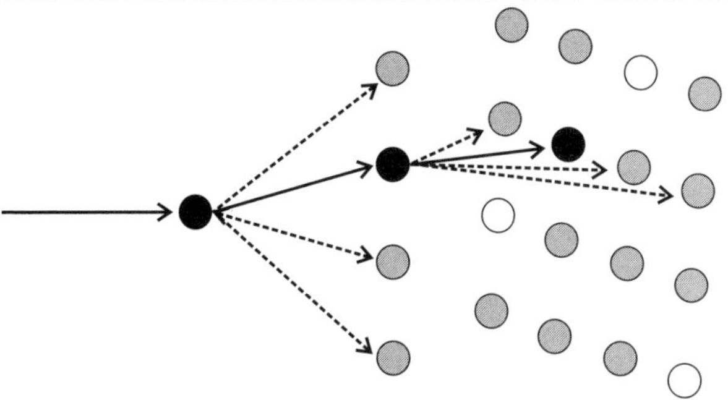

The figure illustrates introduction of a hypothetical infection (solid arrows) into a population with 75% immunity. The infection has a basic reproduction number (R_0) of 4, meaning that the first case (the first black circle) would result in 4 secondary cases if all members of the population were susceptible. Here, however, there is only one secondary case (second black circle) because 3 out of 4 individuals are immune (gray circles) and transmission to them is unsuccessful (dashed arrows). Similarly, the secondary case gives rise to only one tertiary case. The 3 open circles represent susceptible individuals who do not get infected because of herd immunity.

Adapted from Fine P, et al. *Clin Infect Dis*. 2011;52:911-916.

FIGURE 1.7 — Herd Immunity Threshold

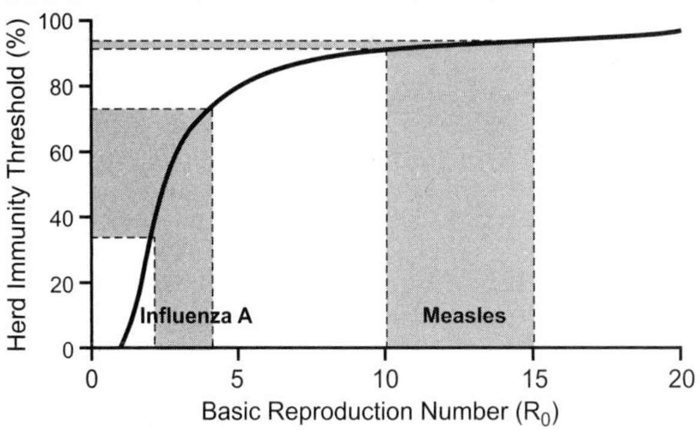

The figure illustrates the relationship between the basic reproduction number (R_0) and the herd immunity threshold for measles and influenza A. Because measles is more contagious (has a higher R_0), the herd immunity threshold is higher (a larger proportion of the population must be immune in order to prevent sustained transmission). This model assumes a randomly mixing homogenous population.

Adapted from Zepp F. *Vaccine*. 2010;28S:C14-C24.

of the pathogen, often expressed as the basic reproduction rate (R_0)—the number of secondary cases that arise from an index case when all members of the population are susceptible. Other factors include the mode of transmission (eg, fecal-oral vs respiratory droplet), how people interact with each other, and whether the disease is endemic or comes in epidemic waves. Ideally, one would want to know what proportion of a population needs to be vaccinated in order to protect the entire population. This will depend on the above factors, as well as on the efficacy of the vaccine and the reality that neither vaccination nor exposure is evenly distributed within a population. For example, there may be pockets of susceptible individuals (eg, undervaccinated inner-city residents) or foci of close contact (eg, college dormitories).

In addition, the microbial ecology of the pathogen must be taken into account. For measles virus, there is no carrier state and there is no reservoir per se. Thus a vaccine that prevents individual infection will prevent transmission and amplify the protective effect on individuals through herd immunity. For *H influenzae*, in contrast, there *is* a reservoir—the nasopharynx of young children. A vaccine that prevents invasive infection but not nasopharyngeal colonization arguably would not result in herd immunity, since transmission could still occur from vaccinated children who remain colonized. Fortunately, protein-polysaccharide conjugate vaccines are very effective at reducing colonization. In the case of Hib, herd immunity effects are dramatic. A Danish study, for example, estimated that by 3.5 years of age, the protection afforded unvaccinated children through herd immunity was about the same as the direct protection afforded through vaccination, approximately 94%.[23]

Figures 1.8 and **1.9** give modern-day examples of herd immunity in action. In the early 1990s, the incidence of hepatitis A in Butte County was six times higher than in California as a whole. Beginning in 1995, children 2 through 17 years of age were routinely immunized with HepA. Within 5 years, the incidence of hepatitis A had fallen dramatically among children, as one might have expected (**Figure 1.8**). However, the incidence also had fallen in all other age groups—groups that were not targeted for immunization. Preventing hepatitis A in children was enough to prevent transmission to, and infection among, adults. Economic models suggest that herd immunity effects more than double the cost savings from universal HepA immunization of young children.[24]

Similarly, **Figure 1.9** illustrates the impact that routine childhood PCV7 immunization had on *S pneumoniae* meningitis in unimmunized older individuals. In this case, herd immunity was mediated by decreases in nasopharyngeal colonization among vaccinated children.[25] However, there is a cautionary tale to tell here. Vaccination only affects colonization with vaccine sero-

FIGURE 1.8 — Average Annual Age-Specific Incidence of Hepatitis A in Butte County, California

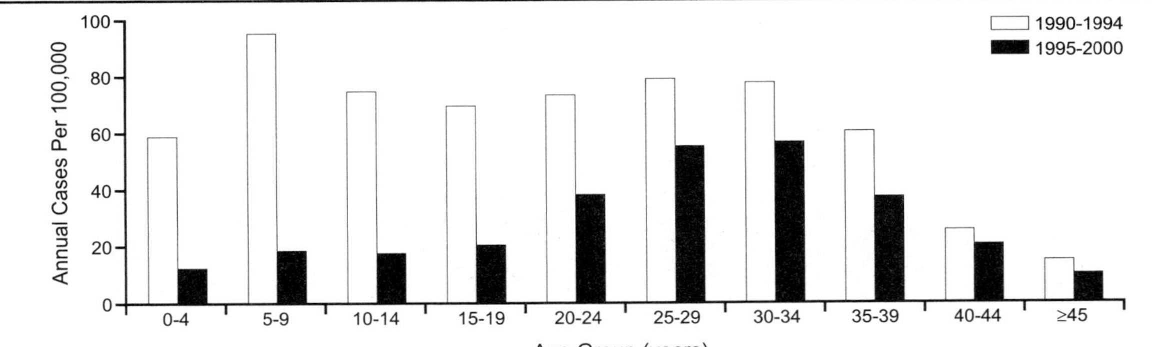

White columns show the years 1990-1994, prior to implementation of an immunization program. Black columns show the years 1995-2000, when a universal immunization program for children was implemented. The decrease in incidence among older individuals who were not being vaccinated is the result of herd immunity.

Adapted from Averhoff F, et al. *JAMA*. 2001;286:2968-2973.

FIGURE 1.9 — Mean Annual Incidence of Pneumococcal Meningitis Due to PCV7 Serotypes (4, 6B, 9V, 14, 18C, 19F, and 23F) at United States Surveillance Sites

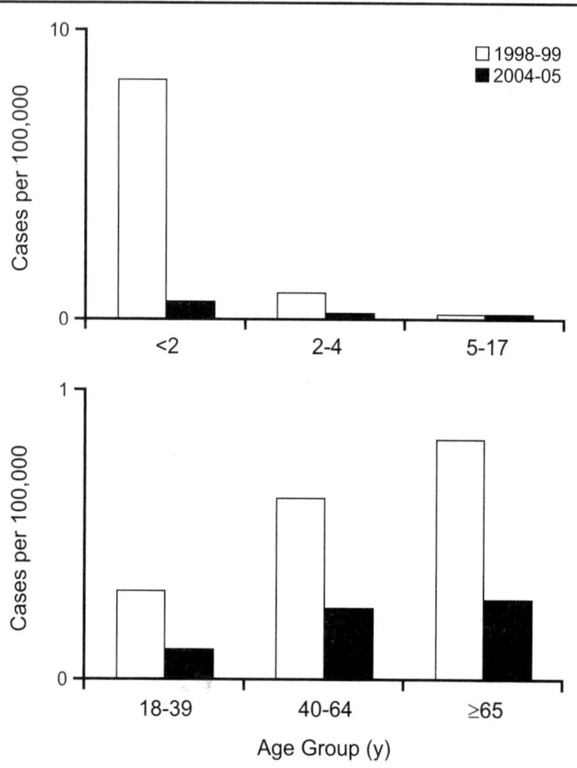

Routine use of PCV7 at 2, 4, 6, and 12-15 months of age was introduced in 2000. The dramatic reduction in incidence among children *(top panel)* was due to both direct and herd effects. The reduction seen in adults was due to herd effects alone, since adults were not being immunized with PCV7 (note the difference in scale between the two panels).

Adapted from Hsu HE, et al. *N Engl J Med.* 2009;360:244-256.

types. When these serotypes disappear from the nasopharynx, other serotypes take over, something called *serotype replacement*.[26] Some of those serotypes—19A, for example, in the case of *S pneumoniae*—are themselves capable of causing invasive disease. In fact, invasive disease due to nonvaccine serotypes *increased* in the PCV7 era, although the overall rate of invasive disease (all serotypes included) declined.[27] The challenge is to stay one step ahead of the organism by developing vaccines that include the emerging serotypes, which, in the case of PCV7, has been accomplished with the licensure of PCV13. Interestingly, widespread *H influenzae* serotype replacement has not occurred in the Hib vaccine era, despite similar effects of Hib on nasopharyngeal colonization with that organism.[28,29] However, the possibility for serotype replacement still exists, as demonstrated by the emergence of *H influenzae* type f disease in Ontario between 1989 and 2007.[30]

Dramatic herd effects have also been seen in the United Kingdom[31] and Canada[32] with the introduction of serogroup C meningococcal conjugate vaccines.

■ Genetics of Vaccine Responses and Adverse Events

Immune responses depend on the interplay of various cells that engage each other through MHC molecules loaded with peptides derived from the pathogen (or vaccine). The genes encoding MHC molecules demonstrate a large degree of diversity, such that one person's MHC molecules might be better able to present a given peptide than another person's. Thus, for example, individuals with a particular HLA allele called DQB1*0303 appear to be less competent at producing mumps antibody after 2 doses of vaccine than those who possess other alleles.[33] Other HLA alleles, however, such as DRB1*0301, DRB1*0801, DRB1*1201, and DRB1*1302, are associated with lower lymphoproliferative responses. Polymorphisms in cytokine and cytokine receptor genes may also predict immune responses. In addition, polymorphisms may also predict breakthrough disease; for example, children who develop invasive *H influenzae* disease despite immunization may have polymorphisms in the *TIRAP* gene, which encodes a protein involved in intracellular signal transduction from TLR2 and TLR4, or polymorphisms in the promoter region of the *IL-10* gene.[34] Importantly, these polymorphisms are not something you would necessarily know about ahead of time, since they (probably) do not result in a particular disease phenotype.

Genetic analyses might someday be used to predict which individuals are at risk for adverse reactions to vaccines. One study, for example, showed that specific haplotypes in the IL-1 gene complex on chromosome 2 and the *IL18* gene on chromosome 11 were associated with fever after smallpox vaccination.[35] The application of genetic analyses to the prediction of immune responses and adverse events has been termed *vaccinomics*.[36] It has been said that we are at the cusp of a new "golden age" of vaccinology, where vaccinomics, combined with advances in immunology and bioinformatics, will propel us beyond the empiricism of yesterday to a future of directed vaccine development and use.[37]

Goals of Immunization Programs

Some historians believe that smallpox killed more people since civilization began than all other infectious diseases combined. Although global eradication through vaccination was conceived by Jenner as early as 1801, it did not become a real possibility until 1967, when the following factors converged: 1) the World Health Assembly resolved to eradicate the disease and increased funding was secured; 2) large amounts of stable, lyophilized vaccine became available and reference testing centers were established; 3) a highly effective bifurcated needle was adopted for administration; and 4) the strategy of ring vaccination was developed, wherein active cases were hunted down and their contacts vaccinated. As a result, the last natural case of smallpox on the planet occurred in 1977 (the last case in the United States was in 1949), and on December 9, 1979, the WHO certified that smallpox had been eradicated (the only other disease to ever be eradicated from the face of the earth is rinderpest, a viral infection of cattle[38]). It was remarked that smallpox eradication was one of the few things that needed to be done only once in the history of the world.

Vaccination programs progress from *control* of disease to *elimination* of disease and infection to *eradication*, defined as a permanent reduction to zero of the worldwide incidence of infection as the result of deliberate efforts.[39] Because there is no reservoir of variola virus in nature and there is no human carrier state, the elimination of smallpox was felt to be definitive. In the United States, routine vaccination of civilians ceased in 1972, health care personnel (HCP) in 1976, and military personnel in 1990. Until 2001, the only persons in the United States who continued to be vaccinated were laboratory and animal care workers with potential exposures to orthopox viruses and HCP conducting clinical trials with recombinant vaccinia virus vaccines. Between 1984 and 2001, no country routinely immunized civilians.

The terrorist attacks of September 11, 2001, raised the concern that the end game for smallpox should not have been eradication but rather *extinction*, where the specific agent no longer exists in nature or the laboratory. After eradication, worldwide stocks of variola virus were consolidated at the CDC and the Institute of Virus Preparations in Moscow (now the Russian State Centre for Research on Virology and Biotechnology, Koltsovo, Novosibirsk Region, Russian Federation). It is now known that the Soviet Union had an active program to weaponize variola virus, and with the political unrest and economic hardship that ensued in Russia during the 1990s, it remained possible that the virus and the technology to deliver it may have fallen into the hands of terrorists or rogue nations. Even a single case of smallpox anywhere in the world would strongly imply an intentional release and would be considered an international medical and strategic emergency. The destruction of remaining lots of variola virus was debated in the 1990s, but on December 20, 2001, the WHO gave the virus a stay of execution in order to facilitate research into molecular diagnosis, genetic analysis, serologic assays, animal models, antiviral drugs, and vaccines.

The idea of destroying the last remaining stocks of variola virus, once crucial research is completed, was reaffirmed at the 64th World Health Assembly held in May 2011.[40] The issue will again be discussed at the 67th Assembly in 2014, and perhaps then an execution date will be set. Until then the debate will continue.[41,42]

Many diseases have been *controlled* through vaccination. Beyond smallpox, three diseases—polio, measles, and rubella—have been *eliminated* from the United States, meaning that indigenous cases no longer occur. Because infection can still be imported from outside the country, elimination should be viewed as a step along the way to the ultimate goal of global eradication. Worldwide efforts to eliminate and ultimately eradicate hepatitis B, measles, rubella, and polio are under way. One could argue, though, that in the post-9/11 era, the ultimate goal should be *extinction*. Even that, however, may not be enough—the genome of polio virus is known, and live virus could theoretically be reconstructed from the raw genetic materials.

What does it take to eliminate or eradicate a vaccine-preventable disease? First, it takes favorable disease characteristics, including a readily recognizable clinical syndrome, easy diagnosis, few subclinical infections, a short period of contagion, absence of persistence and nonhuman reservoirs, little strain variability, and lifelong immunity after natural infection. Then it takes a safe, effective, stable, easily stored and transported, cheap vaccine. Then it takes political will and the collaboration of governments, organizations, and many individuals. Finally, eradication takes money—while it requires intensive effort and expense over a short period of time, eradication can be viewed as very cost-effective when you consider that once achieved, vaccination may no longer be necessary.

■ Public Health Impact of Vaccines

It is difficult to summarize the tremendous impact that vaccines have had on our general well-being. Vaccination ranks among the top ten great achievements in public health during the 20th century and is partially responsible for the dramatic increase in life expectancy that was seen during that period of time.[43] Great public health benefits continued to be realized on a global scale in the first decade of the 21st century.[44] **Table 1.5** shows the impact on specific diseases by comparing the peak number of

TABLE 1.5 — Annual Morbidity and Mortality From Vaccine-Preventable Diseases

Disease	Historical Peak		2004-2006[a]	
	Cases	Deaths	Cases	Deaths
Vaccine Programs Initiated Before 1980				
Diphtheria	30,508	3065	0	0
Measles	763,094	552	55	0
Mumps	212,932	50	6584	0
Pertussis	265,269	7518	15,632	27
Poliomyelitis (acute)	42,033	2720	0	0
Poliomyelitis (paralytic)	21,269	3145	0	0
Rubella	488,796	24	11	0
Congenital rubella syndrome	20,000	2160	1	0
Smallpox	110,672	2510	0	0
Tetanus	601	511	41	4
Vaccine Programs Initiated After 1980				
Hepatitis A	254,518	298	15,298	18
Hepatitis B	74,361	267	13,169	47
Invasive:				
H influenzae type b	>20,000	>1000	<50	<5
S pneumoniae	64,400	7300	41,550	4850
Varicella	5,358,595	138	612,768	19

[a] For programs initiated before 1980, reported cases in 2006 and deaths in 2004 are given; for programs initiated after 1980, estimates for cases and deaths in 2006 are given.

Adapted from Roush SW, Murphy TV; Vaccine-Preventable Disease Table Working Group. *JAMA*. 2007;298:2155-2163.

cases and deaths in the prevaccine era to data from 2004 to 2006. The decline in cases for almost all of these diseases has been nothing short of spectacular, although a few things are worth pointing out. Pertussis, for example, declined to historic lows in the 1970s but resurged after 1980, reaching a peak around 2004. Some part of this was more awareness, active surveillance, and better diagnostic tools, such that more cases were being detected. Part of it was also the fact that immunity induced by childhood vaccination wanes, and that until recently there were no vaccines available to boost immunity in adolescents and adults. **Table 1.5** also reflects the abrupt resurgence of mumps that occurred in the Midwest in 2006, which was probably due to a virus imported from Europe. That outbreak, which disproportionately affected young adults, was driven by waning vaccine-induced immunity and the close-contact living situation of college students.

New strategies have been adopted for diseases that have stubbornly persisted. For example, HepA targeted at high-risk individuals and communities could only bring us so far; the adoption of a universal childhood immunization program in 2006 has brought the number of cases down much further. Similarly, the one-dose VAR program initiated in 1995 was very successful, but, because of breakthrough disease in vaccinees (primary vaccine failure), could only bring us so far; the adoption of a routine 2-dose childhood schedule and catch-up immunization for everyone else should close the deal. In the case of invasive *S pneumoniae* disease, the licensure of PCV13 should take care of many of the serotypes that emerged after 2000, when PCV7 was licensed; however, it is likely that more serotypes will need to be added in the future.

The number of vaccines in our armamentarium has grown exponentially (**Figure 1.10**), and studies have shown that the *clinically preventable burden*—the proportion of disease aborted by a preventive service in usual practice—is higher for the routine childhood immunization schedule than for virtually every other routine public health intervention.[45] Vaccines also make economic sense—a study of the 2001 US birth cohort showed that for every $1 spent on routine childhood immunizations (which at the time did not include RV, HepA, PCV, influenza vaccine, MCV, or HPV), $5 was saved in direct costs and an additional $11 was saved in societal costs.[46]

FIGURE 1.10 — Vaccine-Preventable Diseases Timeline

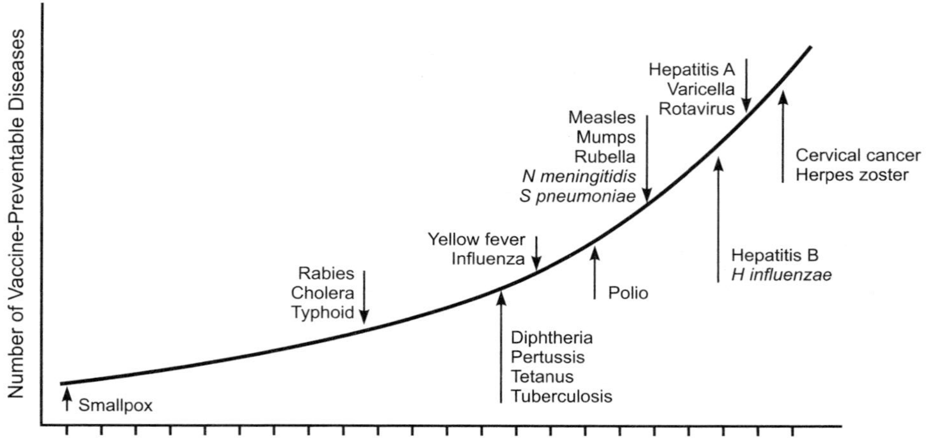

The figure shows the era when the first vaccine for each disease or pathogen was developed.

Adapted from Fine P, et al. *Clin Infect Dis*. 2011;52:911-916.

REFERENCES

1. Rappuoli R. *Vaccine*. 2001;19:2688-2691.
2. Pizza M, et al. *Science*. 2000;287:1816-1820.
3. Sarvas H, et al. *J Infect Dis*. 1992;165:977-979.
4. Moser M, et al. *Vaccine*. 2010;28S:C2-C13.
5. Crichton M. *The Andromeda Strain*. New York, NY: Knopf Publishing; 1969.
6. O'Brien KL, et al. *Lancet Infect Dis*. 2007;7:597-606.
7. Dagan R, et al. *J Pediatr*. 2010;10:1570-1579.
8. Iwasaki A, et al. *Science*. 2010;327:291-295.
9. Arnou R, et al. *Vaccine*. 2009;27:7304-7312.
10. Garcon N, et al. *Sci Amer*. 2009;301:72-79.
11. Noe SM, et al. *Vaccine*. 2010;28:3588-3594.
12. de Veer M, et al. *Vaccine*. 2010;28:6597-6602.
13. Eisenbarth SC, et al. *Nature*. 2008;453:1122-1127.
14. Garcon N, et al. *Expert Opin Biol Ther*. 2011;11:667-677.
15. Roman F, et al. *Vaccine*. 2010;28:1740-1745.
16. Vesikari T, et al. *N Engl J Med*. 2011;365:1406-1416.
17. Khurana S, et al. *Sci Transl Med*. 2010;2:1-7.
18. Pichichero ME. *Pediatrics*. 2009;124:1633-1641.
19. Amanna IJ, et al. *N Engl J Med*. 2007;357:1903-1915.
20. Qin L, et al. *J Infect Dis*. 2007;196:1304-1312.
21. Plotkin SA. *Pediatr Infect Dis J*. 2001;20:63-75.
22. Fine P, et al. *Clin Infect Dis*. 2011;52:911-916.
23. Hviid A, et al. *Vaccine*. 2004;22:378-382.
24. Armstrong GL, et al. *Pediatrics*. 2007;119:e22-e29.
25. Millar EV, et al. *Clin Infect Dis*. 2008;47:989-996.
26. van Gils EJM, et al. *JAMA*. 2010;304:1099-1106.
27. Miller E, et al. *Lancet Infect Dis*. 2011;11:760-768.
28. Ladhani S, et al. *Lancet Infect Dis*. 2008;8;275-276.
29. MacNeil JR, et al. *Clin Infect Dis*. 2011;53:1230-1236.
30. Adam HJ, et al. *Vaccine*. 2010;28:4073-4078.
31. Ramsay ME, et al. *BMJ*. 2003;326:365-366.
32. Kinlin LM, et al. *Vaccine*. 2009;27:1735-1740.
33. Ovsyannikova IG, et al. *Pediatrics*. 2008;121:e1091-e1099.
34. Ladhani SN, et al. *Clin Infect Dis*. 2010;51:761-767.
35. Stanley SL, et al. *J Infect Dis*. 2007;196:212-219.
36. Poland GA. *Clin Pharmacol Ther*. 2007;82:623-626.
37. Poland GA, et al. *Vaccine*. 2010;28:3509-3510.
38. Normile D. *Science*. 2010;330:435.
39. Hinman A. *Annu Rev Pub Health*. 1999;20:211-229.

40. Sixty-fourth World Health Assembly closes after passing multiple resolutions. World Health Organization Web site. http://www.who.int/mediacentre/news/releases/2011/world_health_assembly_20110524/en/index.html. Accessed November 8, 2011.
41. Lane JM, et al. *Vaccine*. 2011;29:2823-2824.
42. Weinstein RS. *Emerg Infect Dis*. 2011;17:681-683.
43. CDC. *MMWR*. 1999;48:243-248.
44. CDC. *MMWR*. 2011;60:814-818.
45. Coffield AB, et al. A*m J Prev Med*. 2001;21:1-9.
46. Zhou F, et al. *Arch Pediatr Adolesc Med*. 2005;159:1136-1144.

2

Vaccine Infrastructure in the United States

Vaccine Development and Licensure

A great deal of effort is involved in vaccine development. The biology of the infectious agent and pathogenesis of the disease must be elucidated. Correlates of immunity, and the laboratory tools to measure them, must be developed. Animal models of vaccine efficacy need to be investigated. Issues such as immunopotentiation, formulation, and delivery need to be worked out, and consistent test lots must be produced. As illustrated in **Figure 2.1**, these steps take place in academia, industry, governmental research institutions, and/or collaborations between these groups.

Once candidate vaccines are ready for testing in humans, the process is rigorously overseen by the Food and Drug Administration (FDA).[1] In general, the financial risk of clinical development is borne by industry. The risk is substantial—for example, the estimated, inflation-adjusted, capitalized, total research and development costs for RotaTeq (RV5) were as high as $644 million[2]—and there was no guarantee that the investment would pay off. It is important to understand that no vaccines reach the public without industry, since pharmaceutical companies—not academic medical centers or government agencies—manufacture and distribute the final products.

The FDA group that sets the standards for vaccine development is the Center for Biologics Evaluation and Research (CBER). The World Health Organization (WHO) provides guidance for products that are used internationally. Laboratory testing for vaccine purity and consistency is required before and after licensure. An intensive search is performed for adventitious agents (with improved technology there have been some unexpected findings; see *Chapter 7: Addressing Concerns About Vaccines—Do Vaccines Contain Adventitious Agents?*). Potency tests are applied and biochemical identity is assured. Manufacturers are required to conform to Good Manufacturing Practices (GMPs), a vast collection of rules and guidances that cover everything from raw-materials quality assurance to record keeping, cleanliness standards, personnel qualifications, in-house testing, process controls, warehousing, and distribution. They must also adhere to Good Laboratory Practices (GLPs), an analogous set of guidances for the laboratory that involves everything from assay reproducibility to interpretation. Several large lots of vaccine (each containing tens of thousands of doses) with identical potencies

FIGURE 2.1 — Schematic of the Process of Vaccine Development and Licensure in the United States

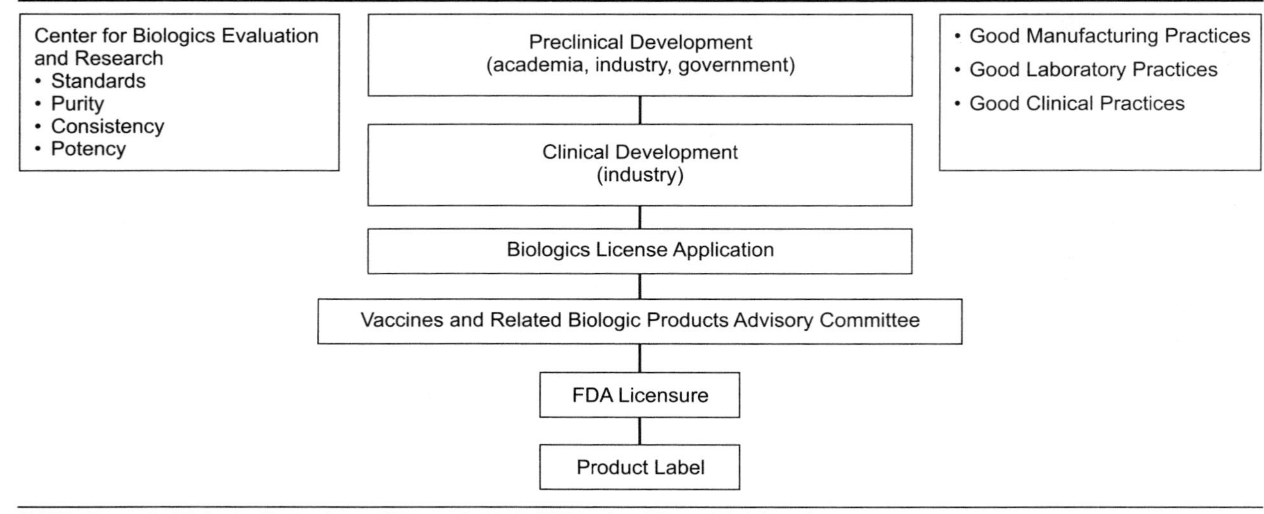

CBER, Center for Biologics Evaluation and Research; FDA, US Food and Drug Administration.

and demonstrated safety must be produced in a manner that is consistent and reliable. In addition, manufacturers are required to provide information regarding appropriate storage and handling. Fulfilling the requirements of CBER may take 5 and 10 years.

2

After a candidate vaccine is approved as an investigational new drug for use in clinical trials, studies for safety, immunogenicity, and (if possible) efficacy are performed. Good Clinical Practices (GCPs) set the standard for the conduct of clinical trials (GCPs, GMPs, and other guidance on vaccine and drug development can be found on the web site of the International Conference on Harmonisation of Technical Requirements for Registration of Pharmaceuticals for Human Use[3]). Some trials are conducted by the National Institutes of Health (NIH) through Vaccine and Treatment Evaluation Units; as of October 2012, there were eight such funded units, most of them at academic medical centers. Other studies, generally involving more mature candidate vaccines, are conducted at academic medical centers or private offices by pharmaceutical companies (or clinical research organizations contracted by these companies) using local principal investigators who are overseen by institutional review boards. Strict federal guidelines apply regarding the protection of human subjects and the management of potential conflicts of interest.

Prelicensure trials proceed in three phases, followed by a postmarketing phase (**Figure 2.2**):

FIGURE 2.2 — Sequential Stages in the Testing of Vaccines in Humans

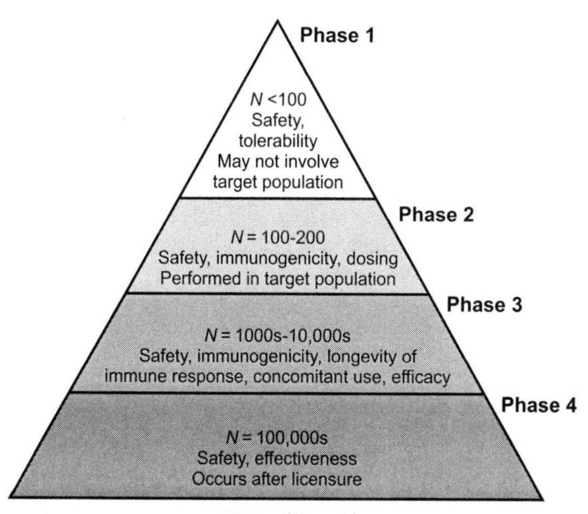

- *Phase 1*—These trials usually involve <100 volunteers and are intended to provide basic information on safety and tolerability. Because of their small size, they can detect only common adverse events. Subjects are often not drawn from the intended vaccine target population. For example, pediatric vaccine candidates might undergo initial testing in adults until basic safety is assured.
- *Phase 2*—These trials enroll hundreds of subjects and provide information about the vaccine's immunogenicity, dosing, and common side effects. Studies are performed in the proposed target group and may also provide some information on immunogenicity.
- *Phase 3*—These studies enroll thousands to tens of thousands of subjects, using sample sizes large enough to ensure that questions about safety and efficacy (or surrogates of efficacy) will be answered—these are often referred to as *pivotal studies*. Subjects are carefully followed for adverse events in the immediate postvaccination period, sometimes as long as 42 days out. Longer periods of observation allow for assessment of persistence of immune responses, protection from disease, and insidious side effects. Large trials also evaluate the consistency of responses and look at concomitant use with other vaccines. This phase of development includes the transfer of manufacturing to full-scale facilities, which must operate under GMPs and are subject to rigorous inspections (the plant itself must be licensed).

  Phase 3 trials of vaccines for diseases that previously were not vaccine-preventable include placebo recipients; therefore, efficacy against disease can be determined. Phase 3 trials of new versions of existing vaccines generally pit the new vaccine against the existing one. Here, prevention of disease may not be a feasible end point, since the disease itself may be unusual. The end point, therefore, may be immunogenicity, the inference being that if the new vaccine is as immunogenic as the existing one (which is known to be protective), it should provide equal protection; these are often called *immunogenicity bridging* studies. *Noninferiority* is statistically defined for each study and is usually agreed upon before the trial is conducted.

  Pressure to make sure that vaccines are as safe as possible before licensure has driven the size of phase 3 trials upward—the studies that went into the licensure of RV5 and RV1, for example, each involved about 70,000 children, more than any other prelicensure studies since the Salk vaccine trials of the early 1950s. As illustrated in **Table 2.1**, huge numbers of subjects are needed to detect adverse events that have a low background rate in the general population and a rare association with vaccination. For example, assuming that a

TABLE 2.1 — Number of Subjects Needed to Test for Increased Relative Risk of an Adverse Event Relative to Background Rates

	Rate in vaccinated population		
Background rate in general population	**2-fold higher**	**10-fold higher**	**100-fold higher**
1 in 10,000	141,000	5,500	500
1 in 100,000	1,238,000	53,500	2,500
1 in 1,000,000	12,951,500	532,500	23,500

Adapted from Evans D, et al. *J Infect Dis*. 2009;200:321-328. Assumes a 5% risk of committing a Type I error and 90% power to detect a difference.

given event occurs in 1 out of 100,000 people in the general population, a clinical trial would need to enroll 1,238,000 subjects in order to detect a 2-fold higher rate of the event in vaccinees. Such trials are obviously not feasible, necessitating postmarketing safety surveillance mechanisms *(see below)*.

- *Phase 4*—Prelicensure trials cannot detect very rare side effects, adverse events with delayed onset, or potential reactions in culturally or ethnically diverse populations. Formal postmarketing studies are designed to detect such rare events. Guidance for postmarketing activities is provided by Good Pharmacovigilence Practices (GPPs), which are analogous to GCPs. These studies are supplemented by the surveillance systems described below. Postmarketing studies also may look at *effectiveness*, that is to what extent a vaccine reduces disease in real life (not to be confused with *efficacy*, which is how the vaccine performs in the context of a controlled clinical trial). Effectiveness assesses the net balance between the benefits and risks of a vaccination program, not just the potency of the vaccine itself. It is affected by many things, including coverage rates, storage conditions, herd immunity, etc, and is determined by ecological, case-control, indirect cohort, or case-cohort studies.[4]

After Phase 1 through 3 studies are completed, the manufacturer submits a Biologics License Application (BLA) to the FDA. The BLA contains all of the data necessary to determine if a license should be granted, which, technically, is permission to introduce a product into interstate commerce. The BLA file is not submitted blindly—rather, its content is determined in a dynamic process of evaluation and negotiation between CBER and the manufacturer. Around the time of the BLA submission, the manufacturing facilities are inspected and all aspects of vaccine production are evaluated. Once the BLA is accepted, the formal evaluation process begins—a process that generally takes a year or two, depending on whether supplemental information or additional studies are requested. In 1992, the Prescription Drug User Fee Act (PDUFA) went into effect, authorizing the FDA to collect fees from manufacturers submitting a file. The continued reauthorization of PDUFA has allowed FDA to expand its staff and shorten the time to approval—the current goal is to act on 90% of standard new BLAs within 10 months. If, after review, a product is deemed not ready for approval, the FDA issues a Complete Response Letter, which describes specific deficiencies and outlines recommended actions that could lead to licensure.

Sometimes the manufacturer is invited to present the entire case for licensure to the Vaccines and Related Biological Products Advisory Committee (VRBPAC), especially if the vaccine is the first in a class or if there are questions about safety or efficacy.

VRBPAC consists of 12 core voting members appointed by the FDA Commissioner. Although most members have recognized expertise in fields related to vaccinology, one member who is identified with consumer interests may be appointed. In addition, a nonvoting representative of the pharmaceutical industry also may be invited, ensuring that all interested parties have input into vaccine licensure decisions. VRBPAC makes recommendations to the FDA Commissioner regarding whether to license the product, what the indications should be, and whether any additional data are needed.

Along with licensure of the vaccine, the FDA also approves a *package insert* (PI), synonymously referred to as the *product information* or *label*. The PI contains official indications, statements about efficacy, contraindications, warnings, precautions, and adverse events. When people refer to *labeled indications*, they are referring to the specifics contained in the PI. The labeled indications are based on the data in the BLA. So, for example, if the studies on file only include persons in a certain age group, the label specifies approved use only in that age group. That will not change, even if new studies are published, unless the manufacturer submits a supplemental BLA that is subsequently approved. The PI also determines how a vaccine can be advertised and marketed. Company field representatives must restrict their claims about the product to the information contained in the PI. Likewise, promotional programs must remain within the label, and it must be specified during continuing medical education programs when off-label uses of a product are mentioned.

In 2006, the FDA issued new rules on the content and format of PIs, intending to make them more informative and user friendly.[5] Among the changes were a Highlights section, providing immediate access to the most important information and listing the original date of approval, recent major changes, and contact information in the event of adverse reactions. A Table of Contents was added and the PI was reordered so as to place the most frequently consulted material (eg, Indications and Usage, Dosage and Administration, Dosage Forms and Strengths) up front. Even with these improvements, it is important to understand that the PI is a regulatory document and its content is largely prescribed. For example, adverse events that have been reported postlicensure are listed, *whether or not there is evidence of a causal relationship with vaccination*; this can lead to unnecessary concern on the part of parents, patients, and providers.

It is also important to understand the difference between the *labeled indications* and the *official recommendations*, which sometimes differ from each other (**Table 2.2**). The labeled indications are derived strictly from the PI and are based on the information in the BLA; the recommendations, on the other hand, derive from authoritative professional bodies *(see below)*. One question

TABLE 2.2 — Notable Differences Between Product Labels and Official Recommendations

Vaccine(s)	Product Label(s)	ACIP Recommendation(s)
Many products	Limited information on concomitant administration of other vaccines	Virtually all vaccines can be given concomitantly (see *Chapter 5: General Recommendations—Rules by Which to Vaccinate*)
HepB-Hib-OMP (Comvax) and DTaP-HepB-IPV (Pediarix)	Indicated for infants of HBsAg-negative mothers	May be used to complete HepB series in infants of HBsAg-positive mothers
Hib-T (Hiberix)	Booster immunization, 15 months to 4 years of age	Booster immunization, 12 months to 4 years of age
JE-VC (Ixiaro)	Indicated for persons ≥17 years of age	May be used in children and adolescents
MCV4-D (Menactra)	Contraindicated in persons with a history of Guillain-Barré syndrome	May be used in persons with a history of Guillain-Barré syndrome
MCV4-D (Menactra) and MCV4-CRM (Menveo)	One dose for persons 2 to 55 years of age[a]	Routine booster dose for adolescents 2-dose primary series for persons with reduced immune response Revaccination every 5 years for high-risk persons
MMR (M-M-R_{II})	Indicated for persons ≥12 months of age	Use in infants 6 to 12 months of age before international travel (does not count as part of routine series)
MMR (M-M-R_{II}) and VAR (Varivax)	Contraindicated in primary or acquired immunodeficiency states	May be used in certain primary and acquired immunodeficiency states
PCV13 (Prevnar 13)	Indicated for persons 6 weeks to 71 months and ≥50 years of age	One dose for high-risk persons 6 to 18 years of age

RAB (Imovax Rabies and Rabavert)	5-dose series for postexposure prophylaxis	4-dose series for postexposure prophylaxis
RV1 (Rotarix)	First dose beginning at 6 weeks of age, last dose ≤24 weeks of age	First dose 6 weeks to 14 weeks 6 days of age, last dose <8 months 0 days of age
RV5 (RotaTeq)	First dose at 6 to 12 weeks of age, last dose ≤32 weeks of age	First dose 6 weeks to 14 weeks 6 days of age, last dose <8 months 0 days of age
Tdap (Adacel)	Booster immunization, 11 to 64 years of age	Use in children 7 to 10 years of age who are not complete on pertussis immunization; may be given to adults ≥65 years of age
Tdap (Boostrix)	Booster immunization, ≥10 years of age	Use in children 7 to 9 years of age who are not complete on pertussis immunization
Tdap (Adacel and Boostrix)	5-year interval since last DTaP or Td	No minimum interval since last DTaP or Td
ZOS (Zostavax)	Consider separating from PPSV23 by 4 weeks due to reduced immune response	ZOS and PPSV23 may be administered at the same time

[a] The label for MCV4-CRM does allow for a second dose in children 2 to 5 years of age who are at continued high risk for meningococcal disease.

2

is which of the two—the label or the recommendations—sets the reference standard in malpractice litigation? Most people would agree that the recommendations supersede the label in this respect because they are based on a more comprehensive dataset and they represent the opinion of medical peers.

Policy and Recommendations

Figure 2.3 gives an overview of the various agencies and committees involved in making and executing vaccine policy in the United States. The Centers for Disease Control and Prevention (CDC) includes the National Center for Immunization and Respiratory Diseases (NCRID), an interdisciplinary program that merges vaccine-preventable disease science and research with immunization program activities. NCIRD provides leadership in the planning, coordination, and conduct of immunization activities throughout the country. It assists health departments in implementing immunization programs, supports establishment of vaccine supply contracts for state and local programs through the Vaccines For Children (VFC) Program, assists in the development of information-management systems, administers research and operational programs, provides clinician educational programs, and supports surveillance for vaccine-preventable diseases.

The ACIP is the principal body that makes recommendations for vaccine use.[6] It provides advice and guidance to the Secretary of Health and Human Services, the Assistant Secretary, and the Director of the CDC regarding the most appropriate application of vaccines and related agents to control communicable diseases in the civilian population. ACIP recommendations also provide an evidence base for providers and programs regarding how vaccines should be used. There are 15 voting members who are appointed by the Secretary; persons who are knowledgeable about consumer perspectives and/or social and community aspects of immunization programs are included, as are infectious diseases specialists. In addition, there are eight *ex officio* members representing a variety of other governmental agencies involved in vaccine policy, distribution, and financing, as well as 26 nonvoting liaison members from professional organizations. Rigorous safeguards are in place to minimize actual or perceived conflicts of interest.

The committee meets three times each year. In making its recommendations, the ACIP considers a product's labeled indications and dosing schedule, disease burden, safety data, feasibility, programmatic issues, equity of access, stewardship of public funds, and input from other stakeholder groups. In 2008, a standardized approach to the presentation of health economics studies was adopted.[7] Oftentimes, data that are not included in the BLA are considered, which explains why the recommendations may differ from the label. The process usually involves the formation

FIGURE 2.3 — Governmental Agencies and Advisory Committees Involved in Vaccine Development, Policy, and Implementation

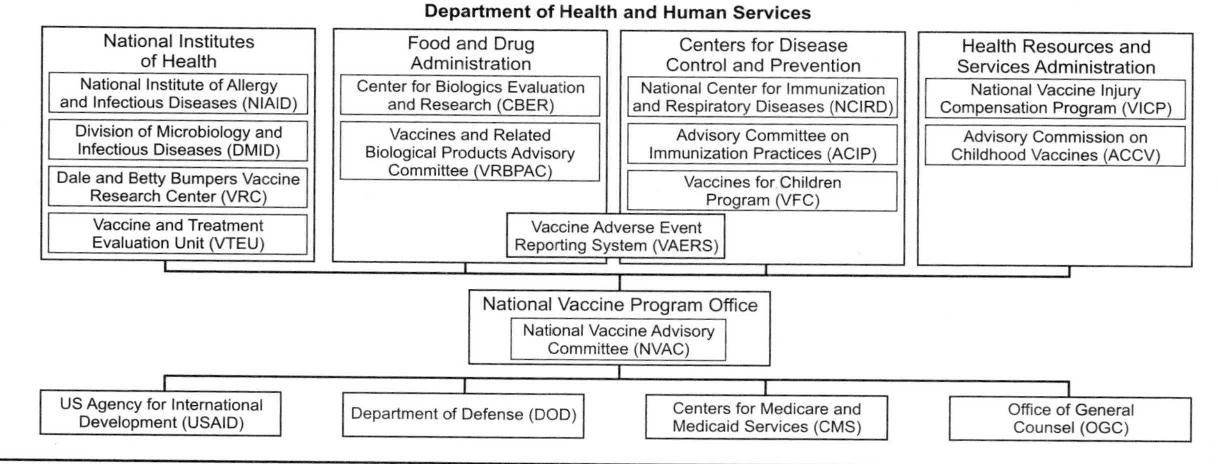

of working groups on specific topics; these groups are chaired by ACIP members but often include outside experts. For some issues, such as vaccination during pregnancy and breastfeeding, specific guiding principles have been adopted.[8]

There are four permanent working groups:

- *Harmonized Schedule for Children and Adolescents*—This group recommends changes to the routine childhood and adolescent schedules, which are published every January. Since 1995, the ACIP schedule has been harmonized in its characteristic graphic layout with the recommendations of the American Academy of Pediatrics (AAP) and the American Academy of Family Physicians (AAFP).
- *Adult Immunization Schedule*—This group recommends changes to the routine adult schedule, which are also updated every year. The adult schedule is endorsed by the AAFP, the American College of Physicians, and the American Congress of Obstetricians and Gynecologists.
- *Influenza Vaccines*—This group makes recommendations regarding influenza immunization for the upcoming influenza season, which are usually published in late spring or summer.
- *General Recommendations on Immunization*—Every 3 to 5 years, the ACIP publishes a document entitled *General Recommendations on Immunization*, commonly referred to as the "General Recs," which provides background and technical guidance regarding vaccination.[9] Specific topics include timing and spacing of doses, contraindications and precautions, administration technique, storage and handling, special situations, record keeping, and adverse-event reporting, among others. These topics are elaborated upon in *Chapter 5: General Recommendations*.

Provisional recommendations are posted within a few weeks of ACIP meetings on the CDC Web site.[10] Final recommendations and informational items ("Notice to Readers") are published periodically in the *Morbidity and Mortality Weekly Report (MMWR)* and on the CDC Web site. Importantly, the final published recommendations may differ slightly from the provisional recommendations because the latter must undergo review and approval by the CDC Director. A comprehensive summary of ACIP recommendations is released every few years in a book entitled *Epidemiology and Prevention of Vaccine-Preventable Diseases*, commonly known as the "Pink Book."[11]

There are several varieties of ACIP recommendations. First, there are recommendations *for routine immunization*, whereby every person in the specified age group should be vaccinated (eg, all children should receive PCV13 at 2, 4, 6, and 12 to 15 months of age). Second, there are recommendations for *catch-up immunization*, which apply to defined cohorts and time periods (eg, a second dose of VAR should be given to all persons who previously received one dose). Third, there are *risk-based immunization* recommendations, which apply to persons with specific risk factors for the disease or complications (eg, MCV4 should be given to persons with functional or anatomic asplenia). Occasionally, there are *recommendations against routine immunization*, which specify that a vaccine should not be routinely administered in certain situations (eg, MCV4 should not be *routinely* given to healthy children 2 through 10 years of age, even though it is licensed in that age group). Finally, there are *permissive statements*, which allow for use of a vaccine but do not make a recommendation (eg, the 2010 statement that HPV4 *may be used* in boys for prevention of genital warts; in October 2011, use of HPV4 in male adolescents became a *routine recommendation*).

In October 2010, the ACIP adopted an evidence-based system based on the GRADE approach, which stands for **G**rading of **R**ecommendations, **A**ssessment, **D**evelopment and **E**valuation.[12] Recommendations will be classified as either Category A—applying to all persons in age- or risk-based groups (using language such as *recommend, recommend against, should, should not*), Category B—a call for individual clinical decision making (using language such as *may* and *suggest*), or a third category—no recommendation or unresolved issue. In addition, the evidence behind recommendations will be ranked, from 1—randomized controlled trials or overwhelming evidence from observational studies, to 4—clinical experience and observations or controlled or observational studies with major limitations. It may not be widely known, but ACIP meetings are convened by the ringing of a bell that bears the inscription "May the ACIP Recommendations Always Ring Clear," presented to the committee by Dr. Sam Katz in 1993, when he stepped down as Chairman. The new framework should foster that goal.

The AAP Committee on Infectious Diseases also develops policy recommendations on the use of vaccines, subject to approval by the AAP Board of Directors. While these are developed independently, every attempt is made to achieve congruity with the ACIP recommendations. From time to time, however, there are subtle but important differences. For example, early in the Tdap program, the AAP recommended immunization of pregnant teenagers in the second or third trimester, while ACIP did not. AAP recommendations are included in the *Report of the Committee on Infectious Diseases*, a comprehensive summary of infectious diseases that is published every 3 years and is commonly called the "Red Book."[13] The AAP also partners with the CDC in the Childhood Immunization Support Program, with goals to promote quality improvement and best immunization practices, improve delivery, and enable effective communication.

The ACIP has one other important function: it determines which vaccines should be added to the VFC program *(see below)*. In order for a vaccine to be covered under the VFC program, a specific resolution must be passed. Resolutions may be passed even when the ACIP position on a given vaccine is permissive.

The National Vaccine Program Office (NVPO) was created in 1986 to coordinate the activities of all federal agencies in developing and implementing the National Vaccine Plan. In so doing, the NVPO strives to improve collaboration with the commercial vaccine industry, global organizations, consumer groups, and academic institutions. The Plan, created in 1994 and updated in 2010,[14] has five main goals:

- Develop new and improved vaccines
- Enhance the vaccine safety system
- Support communications to enhance informed vaccine decision-making
- Ensure a stable supply of, access to, and better use of recommended vaccines in the United States
- Increase global prevention of death and disease through safe and effective vaccination.

The National Vaccine Advisory Committee (NVAC) makes recommendations to the NVPO regarding the supply of safe and effective vaccines, research priorities, areas of cooperation, and ways to achieve optimal prevention of infectious diseases through vaccine development while minimizing adverse reactions. The 17 members include physicians, researchers, and people involved in manufacturing and public health, and representatives from parent organizations.

Monitoring Delivery

Once vaccines are licensed and recommended for use, delivery to the appropriate people needs to be monitored. *Coverage* refers to the proportion of eligible persons who receive a recommended vaccine. *Timeliness* assesses whether vaccinated persons received the recommended doses of a vaccine within the recommended age range, measured as the proportion of individuals who receive the vaccine on time or as the cumulative number of days a given vaccine or vaccine series is delayed. Both coverage and timeliness are important measures of the quality of immunization care. Through effective monitoring, racial and ethnic disparities can be discovered, underserved groups can be identified, the effectiveness of intervention programs can be assessed, uptake of new vaccines and the effect of shortages can be tracked, and correlates of quality can be determined.[15]

■ National Immunization Survey (NIS)

Conducted annually since 1994, the NIS is a random digit dialing telephone survey of households in the United States. Historically focused on vaccine coverage among children 19 to 35 months of age, it was expanded in 2006 to include adolescents 13 to 17 years of age (NIS-Teen) and again in 2007 to include adults (NIS-Adult). Respondents provide information about vaccinations as well as sociodemographic information. For those who give permission, validating data are obtained from the providers. The survey includes all 50 states and selected urban and county areas. **Figure 2.4** shows the NIS coverage rates for children 19 to 35 months of age over the past decade.

The 2010 report included data from 17,004 provider-reported vaccination records.[16] Coverage rates for most routinely recommended vaccine series were ≥90%, with the following exceptions: ≥4 DTaP, 84.4%; ≥4 PCV, 83.3%; ≥2 HepA, 49.7%; RV series, 59.2%; birth dose of HepB, 64.1%; and the full Hib series 66.8% (this reflects a shortage of vaccine from 2007-2009). Coverage for the 4:3:1:3:3:1:4 series (≥4 DTaP, ≥3 IPV, ≥1 MMR, ≥3 Hib,

FIGURE 2.4 — Immunization Coverage Rates Among Children 19 to 35 Months of Age

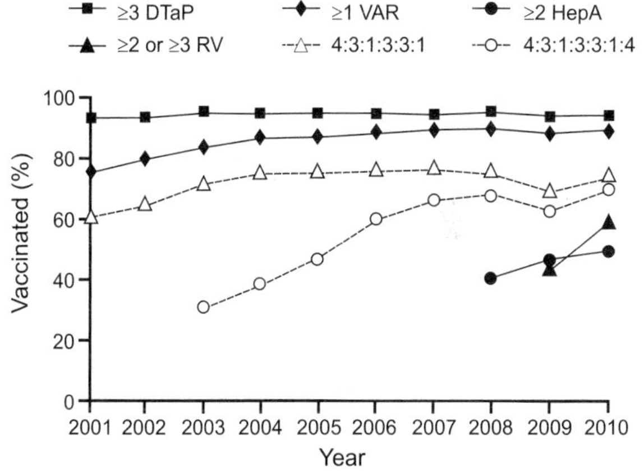

The graph shows the percentage of children who received the indicated vaccines. Solid lines and markers represent selected individual vaccines. Dashed lines and open markers represent combined vaccine series. Coverage rates for RV depend on the product (≥2 doses for RV1 and ≥3 doses for RV5). 4:3:1:3:3:1, ≥4 DTaP + ≥3 IPV + ≥1 MMR + ≥3 Hib + ≥3 HepB + ≥1 VAR; 4:3:1:3:3:1:4, 4:3:1:3:3:1 + ≥4 PCV.

Data from CDC. *MMWR* 2006;55:988-993; CDC. *MMWR*. 2010;60:1157-1163.

≥3 HepB, ≥1 VAR, ≥4 PCV) was 70.2%. Coverage for the full series excluding Hib ranged from 82.7% in Wisconsin to 61.3% in Nevada. Importantly, <1% of children were completely unimmunized, which is reassuring given the pervasiveness of vaccine hesitancy (see *Chapter 7: Addressing Concerns About Vaccines*). For most vaccines, disparities based on race or ethnicity were not seen, although disparities based on poverty persisted (**Figure 2.5**).

Figure 2.6 shows the NIS-Teen coverage rates over the past few years. Data from 19,488 provider-reported vaccination records were included in the 2010 report.[17] Coverage rates for the three routine adolescent vaccines increased compared with 2009: Tdap, from 55.6% to 68.7%; MCV4, 53.6% to 62,7%; and ≥1 HPV, 44.3% to 48.7%. Coverage for ≥3 HPV was only 32.0% and was unfortunately low in some of the states with high rates of cervical cancer.[18] Also disappointing was coverage for ≥2 VAR among adolescents without a history of chickenpox, which was only 58.9%.

NIS data have been instrumental in uncovering poor timeliness as an issue in vaccine delivery, one that is masked by good coverage rates. A study using 2003 NIS data and involving 14,810

FIGURE 2.5 — 4:3:1:3:3:1 Coverage Rates Among Children 19 to 35 Months of Age by Race and Poverty Level

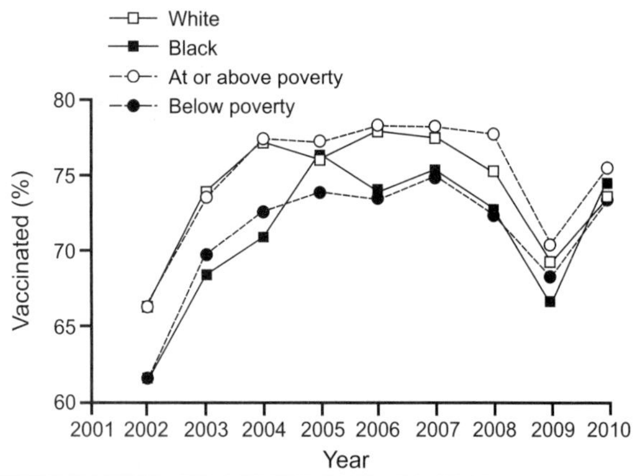

The graph shows the percentage of children who received the 4:3:1:3:3:1 vaccine series. Solid lines and squares show coverage rates stratified by white or black race. Dashed lines and circles show coverage rates stratified by poverty level. 4:3:1:3:3:1, ≥4 DTaP + ≥3 IPV + ≥1 MMR + ≥3 Hib + ≥3 HepB + ≥1 VAR.

Data from US Vaccination Coverage Reported via NIS. CDC Statistics and Surveillance Web site. http://www.cdc.gov/vaccines/stats-surv/nis/#nis. Accessed September 4, 2011.

FIGURE 2.6 — Immunization Coverage Rates Among Adolescents 13 to 17 Years of Age

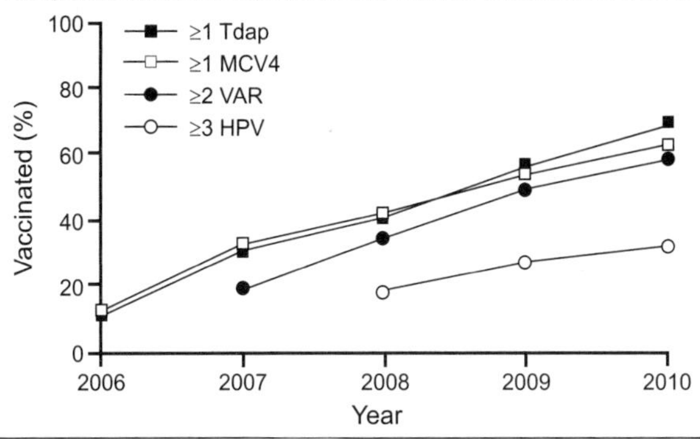

The graph shows the percentage of adolescents who received the indicated vaccines. Tdap rates include adolescents down to 10 years of age. VAR rates are for persons without a history of varicella disease.

Data from CDC. *MMWR* 2007;56:885-888; CDC. *MMWR* 2009;58:997-1001; CDC. *MMWR*. 2011;60:1117-1123.

children showed that during the first 2 years of life, children spent a median of 172 days underimmunized; 37% of underimmunized children had cumulative delays of >6 months.[19] Eighteen percent of children who were considered fully covered by 24 months of age were actually undervaccinated for >6 months. In some states, <5% of children had received the 4:3:1:3:3 (≥4 DTaP, ≥3 IPV, ≥1 MMR, ≥3 Hib, ≥3 HepB) series exactly as recommended. Poor timeliness could leave children vulnerable to disease.

NIS data rely on provider-reported vaccination histories, which may be incomplete. In addition, coverage estimates for state and local areas may be imprecise because of small sample size.

■ Behavioral Risk Factor Surveillance System (BRFSS)

This state-level, random digit dialing telephone survey of noninstitutionalized civilians 18 years of age and older has been conducted by the CDC since 1984. More than 350,000 adults are surveyed every year, making the BRFSS the largest ongoing health survey in the world. The data obtained are very useful for issues such as influenza and pneumococcal vaccine coverage. The BRFSS showed that influenza vaccine coverage during the 2010-2011 season for persons ≥65 years of age was only 67.4%; coverage for pneumococcal vaccination was 68.6%. These rates represent no gains over previous years. Moreover, influenza vaccine coverage for persons 50 to 64 years of age was only 44.5%, and for high-risk persons 18 to 49 years of age only 39%.[20]

School Surveys

Retrospective school entry surveys are the most common form of state and local level surveillance. Coverage data are collected from the health records of randomly selected schools, and an assessment is made of vaccine coverage. Audits are performed to validate school entry data. The data necessarily lag several years behind current performance because children are 5 or 6 when they enter school. In addition, no information on the timing of immunizations is obtained. A recent study looked at coverage rates for kindergarten students during the 2009-2010 school year.[21] Coverage for most vaccines was >90%, although some states fell below the *Healthy People 2020* goal of ≥95%. In particular, in half of the states coverage for 2 doses of MMR was <95%. In the majority of states, nonmedical exemption rates were <3%.

Other Methods

Many other methods are used to estimate immunization coverage, including:

- *National Health Interview Survey (NHIS)*—This survey covering a broad range of health issues has been conducted by the CDC's National Center for Health Statistics since 1957. The current sample size target is 35,000 households containing about 87,500 persons. The NHIS is an important source of information about adult vaccine coverage.
- *Special area and population surveys*—These studies involve small geographic units such as counties or census tracts or specific populations in a local area, such as Medicaid participants. Largely supported by federal grants, special surveys can target needy groups and ensure accountability within the public and private health care sectors. The National Nursing Home Survey, which is conducted on an episodic basis, is an example of a targeted survey.
- *Healthcare Effectiveness Data and Information Set*—The National Committee for Quality Assurance, an independent nonprofit organization, monitors the performance of managed health care plans through HEDIS, a set of standardized measures. Immunization rates on preschoolers, children, adolescents, and adults are captured through administrative claims, encounter data, and chart review.

Monitoring Effectiveness

Vaccine-preventable disease activity is monitored in order to assess the effectiveness of immunization programs. Efforts are coordinated by the CDC's Epidemiology Program Office and the NCIRD, in collaboration with groups such as the Council of State and Territorial Epidemiologists. Over 60 diseases are now reportable through the National Notifiable Disease Surveillance

System (NNDSS).[22] Disease reporting by the states is voluntary, and reporting of diseases within states is mandated through legislation or regulation; for these reasons, the list of notifiable diseases varies from state to state. Reporting to the CDC occurs weekly through the National Electronic Telecommunications System for Surveillance; the CDC analyzes the data and launches investigations when appropriate. Active surveillance systems are in place for certain diseases such as measles, mumps, rubella, congenital rubella syndrome, diphtheria, tetanus, pertussis, poliomyelitis, and varicella. Laboratory-based surveillance programs, such as that for influenza, supplement these programs. Additional surveillance for invasive bacterial infections, such as those due to *S pneumoniae*, *H influenzae*, and *N meningitidis*, is accomplished through the Active Bacterial Core surveillance (ABCs) system, which is part of the CDC's Emerging Infections Program Network.[23] This system stores demographic information on cases and collects bacterial isolates for further laboratory testing.

The New Vaccine Surveillance Network (NVSN) was established in 1999 to evaluate the impact of new vaccines and new recommendations.[24] The network initially consisted of three academic medical centers but has since expanded to seven (referred to as the NVSN-Extended System). These sites conduct inpatient and outpatient surveillance for vaccine-preventable diseases, including seasonal surveillance for acute respiratory illness and acute gastroenteritis. Special targeted studies look at vaccine effectiveness.

Other systems contribute to our understanding of changes after immunization programs are implemented. For example, the impact of rotavirus vaccine has been monitored using the National Respiratory and Enteric Surveillance System (NREVSS), a passive laboratory system that provides data on rotavirus testing. A similar program, the National Rotavirus Strain Surveillance System (NRSSS), looks at the geographic occurrence of rotavirus genotypes over time.

The Vaccine Safety Net

No medical intervention is 100% safe. For therapeutic interventions—antibiotics, for example—there is an inherent tolerance for risk, because without therapy, the infection will intensify. Preventive interventions such as vaccines, in contrast, are usually given to people who are perfectly healthy; as a consequence, the tolerance for adverse events is much lower. Moreover, everyone gets vaccines but only selected people get medicines. Therefore, the consequences of even rare adverse events are significant at the population level. It has been said that when a medicine is given, *disease is treated*, but when vaccines are given, *nothing happens*. The truth is, of course, that disease prevention through vaccination is something happening, just as is treating pneumonia with antibiotics. The difference is that with antibiotics, it is about what you see happen (*the pneumonia improves*), whereas with vaccines, it is about what you do not see happen (*disease does not occur*).

Monitoring for safety begins as soon as a candidate vaccine is proposed for testing and continues throughout its life cycle.[25,26] Prelicensure evaluation is described earlier in this chapter. Aspects of postlicensure safety monitoring are described below. Many examples of the safety net in action are described in *Chapter 7: Addressing Concerns About Vaccines—Specific Concerns*.

■ Vaccine Adverse Event Reporting System (VAERS)

VAERS is a postmarketing surveillance system created by the National Childhood Vaccine Injury Act of 1986 and coadministered by the FDA and the CDC. Anyone can submit a report about any event that they feel is related to vaccination, and reporting of certain events is mandated by law (see *Chapter 3: Standards, Principles, and Regulations—National Childhood Vaccine Injury Act*). Information from VAERS reports is entered into a database, and selected serious events and deaths are compiled and analyzed. Between 1991 and 2001, a total of 128,717 reports were received, representing approximately 11.4 reports per 100,000 net doses distributed.[27] The most common adverse events reported were fever (25.8%), injection site hypersensitivity (15.8%), rash (11.0%), injection site edema (10.8%), and vasodilatation (10.8%). Approximately 14% of reports described serious adverse events. Most reports were from vaccine manufacturers (36.2%), health departments (27.6%), and providers (20.0%). The proportion reported by providers increased from 11.4% in 1991 to 35.3% in 2001. Overall, only 4.2% of reports were filed by parents or patients.

A significant limitation of VAERS is that it only receives information regarding vaccinated persons in whom an adverse event occurs. Because it does not receive information about the number of vaccine doses administered or the occurrence of adverse events in unvaccinated persons, causal relationships between vaccines and particular adverse events cannot be established.[28] In addition, underreporting, poor data quality, incomplete reports, differences between public and private sector reporting rates, lack of consistent diagnostic criteria for disease, and simultaneous administration of multiple vaccines limit the information that can be derived from VAERS. Moreover, significant reporting biases exist. For example, increased reporting is seen immediately after licensure and when particular vaccines are "in the news." As another example, many of the reports of autism following administration of thimerosal-containing vaccines have been filed by attorneys. For all of the above reasons, VAERS is vital for hypothesis *generation*, but not useful for hypothesis *testing*.

Despite these limitations, VAERS is the only surveillance system that covers the entire US population, and it includes the largest number of case reports temporally associated with vaccination. It serves to generate the signal that triggers further investigation, and can provide early warning of potential problems, including new, rare, or unusual adverse events. A good example of the utility of VAERS data was in prompting investigation of the relationship between the rhesus rotavirus vaccine and intussusception (see *Chapter 7: Addressing Concerns About Vaccination—Do Rotavirus Vaccines Cause Intussusception?*). Unfortunately, VAERS data have also been misunderstood by the media and misused by antivaccine activists, who have made the erroneous supposition that temporal association means causation.

■ Vaccine Safety Datalink (VSD)

The VSD is an active surveillance system created by the CDC in 1990 and operated by the CDC's Immunization Safety Office.[29] Information regarding vaccination, medical outcomes, birth history, and census is collected through large, linked, computerized databases from eight managed care organizations across the country. Approximately 8.8 million people of all ages are studied through this process, amounting to 3% of the entire US population. Given these numbers, relatively rare adverse events can be detected. Since the VSD includes control data (including information about unvaccinated persons, as well as data on individuals in the weeks preceding vaccination), it is an excellent place to test hypotheses and determine if relationships between vaccines and adverse events are causal or coincidental.[30] The database is replete with information, including demographics, hospitalizations, outpatient and emergency room visits, and mortality; pharmacy, laboratory, and radiology data also can be collected to validate outcomes and vaccination history. Electronic improvements have led to the ability to conduct near-real time analyses.

■ Clinical Immunization Safety Assessment (CISA) Network

Before the creation of the first CISA centers in 2001, there was no coordinated effort to evaluate and treat vaccine adverse events in individual patients. The CISA network is a partnership between six academic medical centers and the CDC that systematically evaluates patients who experience adverse events after immunization. Major goals include developing research protocols for the evaluation and management of adverse events, studying the pathophysiologic basis of such events and determining risk factors, developing evidence-based guidelines for vaccination of high-risk persons, and serving as a resource for clinical vaccine safety questions.[31] CISA centers have been involved in evaluating adverse reactions after Dose 5 of DTaP, examining the role of genetics in the immune response to VAR, and elucidating risk factors for apnea after immunization of infants in the neonatal intensive care unit, among other things.

Brighton Collaboration

The Brighton Collaboration, launched in 2000, is an international organization that aims to facilitate the development, evaluation, and dissemination of high-quality information about the safety of vaccines.[32] Participants are volunteers from patient care, public health, pharmaceutical, regulatory, scientific, and professional organizations. The primary objective is to develop standardized definitions of adverse events following immunization, which enhance comparability of data. In addition, Brighton aims to establish guidelines for collection, analysis, and presentation of safety data. As of October 2011, Brighton had developed 25 case definitions for adverse events following immunization, including, for example, definitions of common events like fatigue and fever as well as less common events like hypotonic hyporesponsive episode and acute disseminated encephalomyelitis.[33] In addition, protocols for collection, analysis and presentation of data in pre- and postlicensure clinical studies[34] and surveillance systems[35] had been published.

Defense Medical Surveillance System (DMSS)

The DMSS is a central repository of medical surveillance data for the US military operated by the Department of Defense (DOD). The health records of approximately 1 million men and women in uniform are available to study adverse events following immunization.[36] The Veterans Administration has also been involved in surveys among veterans and Veterans Administration employees.

Special Surveillance Efforts

The 2009 H1N1 influenza immunization campaign, during which tens of millions of individuals were vaccinated in a short period of time, called for unprecedented safety surveillance efforts, especially in light of the association between the 1976 swine flu vaccine and Guillain-Barré syndrome (GBS) (see *Chapter 7: Addressing Concerns About Vaccines—Do Vaccines Cause Guillain-Barré Syndrome?*). Existing systems were enhanced and new systems were deployed in this effort, including: VAERS reporting, facilitated by vaccination report cards and collaboration with the American Academy of Neurology; near-real time rapid-cycle analysis by the VSD; surveillance through the Vaccine Analytic Unit, a collaboration between the CDC, FDA, and DOD; GBS case finding through the Emerging Infections Program, a collaboration between the CDC and state health departments; the Real Time Immunization Monitoring System, a Web-based active surveillance system developed by Johns Hopkins University and sponsored by the CDC; surveillance through the Indian Health Service; near real time active surveillance of Medicare recipients; and the Post-Licensure Rapid Immunization Safety Monitoring Network, which linked health plan and Immunization Information Systems data to survey for unexpected risks.[37] Through these efforts, tens of millions of vaccinees were monitored for potential safety issues.

■ Ad-Hoc Committees and Task Forces

From time to time, ad-hoc committees and task forces are constituted to address particular issues. The National Childhood Vaccine Injury Act of 1986, for example, mandated the establishment of the Task Force on Safer Childhood Vaccines, comprising representatives of several PHS agencies. The charge was to make recommendations promoting the development of safer vaccines and assuring improvement in licensing, manufacturing, processing, testing, labeling, warning, use instructions, distribution, storage, administration, field surveillance, adverse reaction reporting, recall of reactogenic lots, and research. The task force report, released in 1998, emphasized the need to assess and address public concerns about the risks and benefits of vaccines, conduct research on the biological basis for vaccine reactions, foster partnership between stakeholders, enhance the ability to detect adverse events, and improve coordination of effort between agencies.[38]

Another good example of an ad-hoc committee is the Immunization Safety Review Committee (ISRC), convened in 2001 by the Institute of Medicine (IOM), a private, nonprofit, nongovernmental organization of distinguished scholars. The ISRC reviewed nine different vaccine safety hypotheses, assessing each for scientific plausibility based on epidemiologic and clinical evidence of causality and experimental evidence for biologic mechanisms, considering as well the significance of the issue in a broader societal context. In no case was a causal relationship between a vaccine and one of the hypothesized adverse events accepted, except for the 1976 swine influenza vaccine and GBS.[39] Many of the safety concerns addressed by the ISRC are covered in *Chapter 7—Addressing Concerns About Vaccines*.

In August 2011, the IOM released a new Consensus Report that looked at eight specific vaccines and over 150 vaccine-adverse event pairs.[40] For the vast majority, the evidence was inadequate to accept or reject a causal relationship. Conclusions regarding the remaining vaccines and events are listed in **Table 2.3**.

Financing

Table 2.4 shows how the total cost for all routinely recommended vaccines during childhood has skyrocketed, the direct result of more vaccines, more doses, and increased cost per dose. Layered on top of the purchase price for vaccines are the costs associated with administration, from personnel time, storage, and equipment to wastage and insurance.

TABLE 2.3 — 2011 Institute of Medicine Consensus Report[a]

Finding	Vaccine(s)	Adverse Event
Evidence convincingly supports a causal relationship	Any injectable vaccine	Deltoid bursitis
		Syncope
	VAR	Disseminated varicella
		Disseminated varicella with pneumonia, meningitis, or hepatitis in immunodeficient persons
		Vaccine strain reactivation
		Vaccine strain reactivation with meningitis or encephalitis
	MMR	Measles inclusion body encephalitis in immunodeficient persons
		Febrile seizures
	Influenza, HepB, meningococcal, MMR, TT, VAR	Anaphylaxis[b]
Evidence favors acceptance of a causal relationship	HPV	Anaphylaxis
	MMR	Transient arthralgia in children and adult females[c]
	Certain Canadian IIV preparations	Oculorespiratory syndrome
Evidence favors rejection of a causal relationship	MMR	Autism and type 1 diabetes
	DTaP, DT, TT	Type 1 diabetes
	IIV	Bell's palsy and exacerbation of asthma

[a] For 135 vaccine-adverse event pairs, the evidence was inadequate to accept or reject a causal relationship.
[b] For HepB, anaphylaxis is attributed to yeast allergy.
[c] For adult females, arthralgia is attributed to the rubella component of the vaccine.

Adapted from Adverse effects of vaccines: evidence and causality. Institute of Medicine Web site. http://www.iom.edu/Reports/2011/Adverse-Effects-of-Vaccines-Evidence-and-Causality.aspx. Accessed October 6, 2011.

TABLE 2.4 — Cost of Vaccines (US$) in the Routine Childhood Schedule

Sector	1987	2003	2009	2011
Public	34	437	1403	1670
Private	116	705	1918	2189

The table shows the total cost of all recommended childhood and adolescent vaccines for a person born in the given years. The cost of the HPV series and yearly influenza vaccine is included beginning in 2009. Public and private sector costs are from Hinman AR, et al. *Clin Infect Dis.* 2004;38:1440-1446, and CDC Vaccine Price List. Centers for Disease Control and Prevention Web site. http://www.cdc.gov/vaccines/programs/vfc/cdc-vac-price-list.htm. Accessed October 5, 2011. The least expensive vaccination strategies and products were used in the calculations, although preference was given to combination vaccines where applicable.

The system for financing immunizations in the United States rests on a unique partnership between the public and private sectors. More than half of the purchase cost is borne by public entities, whereas most of the vaccinating is done in private settings. As seen in **Figure 2.7**, only 47% of the purchase cost of routine childhood vaccines is borne by the private sector; most of this is reimbursed through private insurance, but some comes directly out-of-pocket. Historically, many states had laws requiring insurers to cover childhood immunizations, at least to some degree. Some mandated coverage in accord with the recommended childhood immunization schedule, while others made reference to appropriate pediatric vaccines. Some states prohibited deductibles and coinsurance, and while self-insured employers may have been exempt from such regulation, federal statutes prohibited employers providing vaccine coverage as of May 1, 1993 from reducing that coverage. Before 2010, insurance plans differed in terms of which vaccines they covered for both children and adults and to what extent they reimbursed for vaccine administration.

The health care reform law enacted in March 2010 (officially called the Patient Protection and Affordable Care Act [PL 111-148]) contains many provisions aimed at improving immunization delivery. For one, the law requires new employer and individual health plans to cover all ACIP recommended immunizations, without deductible, copay, or coinsurance, when delivered by in-network providers. This includes vaccines recommended for adults. In addition, states are given authority to purchase adult vaccines with state funds through federally negotiated contracts.[41]

■ Children

Public sector funds for vaccination include the following sources:

- *The Vaccines for Children (VFC) Program*—Created in 1993, VFC is a federal program that guarantees immuniza-

FIGURE 2.7 — Childhood Vaccine Doses According to Funding Source, 2007

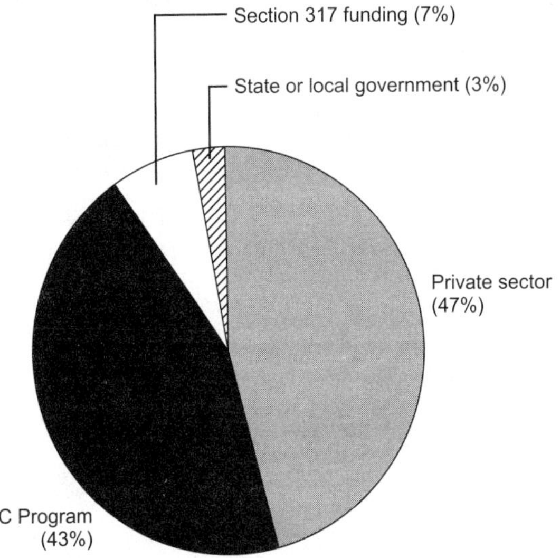

Includes vaccines for children 0 to 6 years of age, excluding influenza vaccine.

Data from Shen AK, et al. *Pediatrics*. 2009;124:S540-S547.

tion services for children 18 years of age and younger who are 1) Medicaid-eligible; 2) uninsured; 3) underinsured and receiving immunizations at federally-qualified health centers (FQHCs) or rural health clinics (RHCs); or 4) American Indian or Alaska Native. Through this program, vaccines are purchased by the CDC at reduced rates and provided to participating private practices and public clinics free of charge. Providers are prohibited from charging the patient for the vaccine itself. Whereas they *can* charge patients administration fees, within limits established by the Centers for Medicare and Medicaid Services, they cannot *deny* vaccination if the patients cannot pay the fee (claims for these fees can still be submitted to Medicaid for those children who are enrolled). There are no regulations regarding charges for the visit itself or other services.

Any private provider who sees eligible children can participate in the program; this has resulted in a shift toward private sector delivery of vaccines, establishing an anchor point for the medical home for many children. Covered vaccines are determined by ACIP resolutions; such resolutions may pertain to routinely recommended or permissively recommended vaccines, with some differences on the resulting actions (**Table 2.5**). Even when a VFC resolution is passed, significant delays in securing a federal contract may occur. During such delays, state Medicaid programs must cover ACIP-recommended vaccines. Common questions about the VFC program are addressed in **Table 2.6**.

VFC is an *entitlement program*, which means that Congress is obliged to appropriate the funds necessary to purchase the covered vaccines, no matter how much they cost. However, there are an increasing number of children who are falling out of the system, namely those who qualify for VFC because their private insurance does not cover all routinely recommended vaccines (the *underinsured*) but who must receive their VFC vaccines at FQHCs or RHCs (with health care reform, the number of immunization-underinsured persons should decrease). The simple fact is that many of these children do not get to these sites, and the fall-back position—namely, to receive the uncovered vaccines at the local health department—is less of an option as the other public funding sources become more inadequate. Importantly, there is no VFC-equivalent program for adults.

- *Section 317 Funds*—States, territories, protectorates, and several designated cities may purchase vaccines through block grants under Section 317 of the Public Health Service Act. The majority of these funds are used for childhood immunization, but adolescent and adult programs may be supported as well. Section 317 funds also may be used to support infrastructure and programmatic activities such as quality assurance, immunization information systems (IISs), disease surveillance, and school- or community-based delivery services. The main intent of the 317 program is to provide vaccines to people who fall outside of the VFC program. The problem is that this program—in contrast to VFC—represents *discretionary federal spending*. The amount allocated by Congress, therefore, varies from year to year, and as the costs of vaccination have increased, so has the financing gap.[42]
- *State and Local Funds*—States may appropriate funds to support both childhood and adult immunizations, but in general the contribution of this source to the whole funding picture is small (**Figure 2.7**). The State Children's Health Insurance Program (SCHIP), enacted in 1997, is a federal block grant program targeted to low-income children who are not eligible for Medicaid and are otherwise uninsured. States can use SCHIP funds to expand Medicaid or to create separate, freestanding children's insurance programs.

TABLE 2.5 — Actions Required Under VFC Resolutions

Action	ACIP Recommendation	
	Affirmative	**Permissive**
Provider *expected to* offer the vaccine proactively to VFC-eligible children	Yes	No
Provider *may* offer the vaccine proactively to VFC-eligible children	Yes	Yes
Provider *expected to* vaccinate VFC-eligible children on request	Yes	Yes, if the provider stocks the vaccine; if not, the child should be referred
Immunization programs *expected to* promote the recommendation	Yes	No
Uptake is taken as a measure of provider or program performance	Yes	No

Adapted from Rodewald LE. ACIP Summary Report, October 21-22, 2009. CDC Web site. http://www.cdc.gov/vaccines/recs/acip/downloads/min-oct09.pdf. Accessed October 5, 2011.

TABLE 2.6 — Common Questions About the VFC Program

Question	Answer
Are providers required to post a sign stating that eligible children will not be denied vaccine?	No.
Can a provider refuse to administer VFC vaccine to an eligible child?	Private VFC providers, unless otherwise required by state law, do not have to vaccinate walk-ins who are not established patients. For established patients, vaccination cannot be denied because of inability to pay the administration fee.
How does a medical or health savings account affect eligibility?	Patients with such accounts must also be insured. If their insurance does not cover vaccines, they can receive VFC vaccine at FQHCs or RHCs.
Is an uninsured child eligible if his parents plan to insure him in the near future?	Yes. Eligibility is determined on the day of vaccination. Eligibility screening must take place at every vaccination visit.
Are all children from birth through 18 years of age who are enrolled in Medicaid automatically eligible?	Yes.
What about children who have Medicaid as a secondary insurance?	Yes, they are also eligible.
If a child starts a vaccine series at 18 years of age, can the series be completed with VFC vaccine if he turns 19?	No.
Are American Indian/Alaska Native children still eligible for VFC vaccine even if they have insurance?	Yes.

If a child's insurance covers a percentage of the cost of vaccination, can he receive VFC vaccine?	No.
Can all children at a school-based clinic receive VFC vaccine?	No. They must still be screened for eligibility (this can be incorporated into the consent process).
If a child has exceeded his insurance coverage for provider visits in a given year, is he considered underinsured for VFC purposes?	Yes.

Adapted from VCF: frequently asked questions. Centers for Disease Control and Prevention Web site. http://www.cdc.gov/Vaccines/programs/vfc/projects/faqs-doc.htm. Accessed October 5, 2011.

As of 2006, 18 states and territories had some type of universal purchase policy. Under these plans, federal, state, and local monies are used to purchase recommended childhood vaccines at the CDC-negotiated price. The vaccines are then distributed to providers free of charge for administration to children, regardless of insurance status. Supporters argue that universal purchase removes financial barriers to immunization, improves coverage rates, reinforces the concept of the medical home, increases immunization rates, improves efficiency, reduces overhead at the provider level, and facilitates participation in IISs. Detractors argue that public funds should not be used to pay for vaccines that insurers would otherwise cover. In addition, concerns have been raised about potential restrictions on product choice and provider autonomy, as well as loss of financial incentives for manufacturers to bring new vaccines to market.

■ Adults

Most private insurance plans cover vaccination of adults.[43] Medicare, an entirely federal insurance program for adults 65 years of age and older, covers influenza vaccine, PPSV23, and HepB (for persons of any age with end-stage renal disease or other high-risk conditions) under Part B (medical insurance). Other vaccines (eg, ZOS) may be covered under Part D (prescription drug coverage), depending on the plan, but there may be requirements for prior authorization to determine medical necessity. Moreover, Part D involves pharmacies, not physicians. So providers may opt to write a prescription and have a pharmacist administer the vaccine, or purchase and administer the vaccine and bill the patient directly so that Medicare can then be petitioned for reimbursement. In general, Medicare reimbursement includes the cost of administration.

The vast majority of Section 317 funds are used to purchase vaccines for children, not adults. Medicaid is a source of vaccine funding for adults, but coverage and reimbursement rates vary widely from state to state. States also may use their own funds to purchase vaccines for adults, but only a minority of states do so. Finally, some vaccine manufacturers have assistance programs for qualifying patients.

■ The Future of Vaccine Financing

The current system for funding vaccine services has achieved high levels of childhood immunization, but new challenges exist, including the increased number of recommended vaccines, high prices, disparities in coverage, low levels of adult immunization, the growing burden of vaccine practice on clinicians, shortages, and the increased costs of bringing new products to market. In 2009, after many years of study and with input from many stakeholders, NVAC released a report on vaccine financing.[44] Recommendations included expanding the VFC program to broaden access and cover administration fees, reducing barriers to vaccination in the medical home, gaining a better handle on the true costs of immunization services, and expanding 317 funding. 2

Supply

The early 2000s saw unprecedented shortages in the supply of many routinely used vaccines.[45] The impact of these shortages included frequent and sometimes confusing changes in the recommended immunization schedule, temporary revision of state school entry requirements, parental frustration, and a burden placed on providers to track interrupted schedules and recall patients when vaccine supplies returned to sufficiency. To date, there is no evidence that shortages caused disease outbreaks.

Shortages result from a convergence of factors, including the following[46,47]:

- *Fewer manufacturers*—Vaccines are low-profit products compared with other pharmaceuticals. The costs of development have skyrocketed, the time line from preclinical testing to market may be longer than a decade, and the risks are substantial—a licensed vaccine may or may not be recommended for use in large numbers of people. Moreover, the risk of failure persists for some time after marketing—the low tolerance for adverse events leaves manufacturers vulnerable to market failure after millions of doses have been distributed. In the late 1960s, there were >20 major vaccine manufacturers licensed in the United States; today, there are only six—GlaxoSmithKline, AstraZeneca (which acquired MedImmune in 2007), Merck, Novartis, Sanofi Pasteur, and Pfizer (which acquired Wyeth in 2009). Some of this decrease was due to mergers but some resulted from companies simply getting out of the business. With so few manufacturers, disruptions at one company can have a major effect on supply. The effect is magnified for single-source products.
- *Business decisions*—Some companies have chosen to pull products from the market rather than invest in costly changes in manufacturing processes or facilities. Such changes might be mandated in order to adhere to GMPs; others might be prompted by new recommendations. An example of the latter was the 1999 recommendation to remove thimerosal from childhood vaccines (see *Chapter 7: Addressing Concerns About Vaccines—Did the Thimerosal Used as a Preservative in Vaccines Cause Autism?*), which led some companies to pull out rather than retool their manufacturing and packaging processes (ie, to make single-dose vials or prefilled syringes) and demonstrate equivalency of the reformulated products in clinical trials.

- *Production problems*—Production problems may have a biologic basis. For example, the influenza A(H3N2) strain used for the 2000-2001 vaccine grew slowly in culture, delaying vaccine production. Similarly, a low yield of vaccine strain VZV in culture led to shortages of MMRV. Production problems can also result from routine physical plant maintenance activities.
- *Underestimated demand*—The recommendation in April 2000 to decrease the age for routine influenza vaccination from 65 to 50 years compounded production problems by increasing demand. Similarly, greater-than-expected demand for PCV7 and MCV4-D after each of these vaccines was licensed contributed to shortages.

When deferral of doses is recommended because of shortages, providers should keep lists of patients who will need to be recalled once supplies improve.

The CDC has maintained stockpiles of vaccines since 1983.[48] These might be more accurately termed *storage and rotation contracts* or *dynamic strategic inventories*—some portion of vaccine production lots enters the stockpile, and older vaccine with at least 12 months of shelf life left is released onto the market. Between 1983 and 2002, only single-source vaccines were stockpiled. Since 2002, the goal has been to stockpile 6 months' worth of each routine childhood vaccine (except for influenza vaccine, which changes in composition from year to year). The stockpile has been accessed on at least eight occasions because of supply issues.

In 2003, the NVAC suggested the following short-term measures to improve vaccine supply[49]:

- Increase funding for vaccine stockpiles that would include all routinely administered vaccines
- Increase support for CBER in order to enhance review of the scientific evidence supporting the safety, efficacy, and quality of vaccines
- Highlight the function of NVPO and NVAC in identifying vaccine priorities
- Maintain and strengthen the National Vaccine Injury Compensation Program, which removes liability concerns as a barrier to manufacturers; include coverage for injuries due to preservatives, additives, and excipients, not just the vaccine antigens
- Require manufacturers to warn HHS of intent to withdraw a product from the market
- Improve availability of accurate supply information for opinion leaders and consumers
- Enhance the valuation of vaccines through educational campaigns.

REFERENCES

1. Marshall V, et al. *Pediatrics*. 2011;127(suppl 1):S23-S30.
2. Light DW, et al. *Vaccine*. 2009;27:6627-6633.
3. International Conference on Harmonisation of Technical Requirements for Registration of Pharmaceuticals for Human Use Web site. http://www.ich.org. Accessed October 10, 2011.
4. Weinberg GA, et al. *J Infect Dis*. 2010;201:1607-1610.
5. FDA announces the Final Rule on the requirements for prescribing information for drug and biological products, January 18, 2006: Summary. FDA Web site. http://www.fda.gov/Drugs/GuidanceComplianceRegulatoryInformation/LawsActsandRules/ucm085169.htm. Accessed October 6, 2011.
6. Smith JC. *Vaccine*. 2010;28S:A68-A75.
7. Lieu T, Meltzer MI, Messonnier ML. Guidance for health economics studies presented to the Advisory Committee on Immunization Practices (ACIP). Centers for Disease Control and Prevention Web site. http://www.cdc.gov/vaccines/recs/acip/downloads/economics-studies-guidance.pdf. Accessed October 6, 2011.
8. Advisory Committee on Immunization Practices Workgroup on the Use of Vaccines During Pregnancy and Breastfeeding. http://www.cdc.gov/vaccines/recs/acip/downloads/preg-principles05-01-08.pdf. Accessed October 6, 2011.
9. Kroger AT, et al. *MMWR*. 2011;60(RR-2):1-61.
10. ACIP provisional recommendations. Centers for Disease Control and Prevention Web site. http://www.cdc.gov/vaccines/recs/provisional/default.htm. Accessed October 10, 2011.
11. Centers for Disease Control and Prevention. *Epidemiology and Prevention of Vaccine-Preventable Diseases*. 12th ed. Atkinson W, et al, eds. Washington, DC: Public Health Foundation, 2011.
12. Ahmed F, et al. *Vaccine*. 2011;29:9171-9176.
13. Pickering LK, Baker CJ, Kimberlin DW, Long SS, eds. *Red Book: 2009 Report of the Committee on Infectious Diseases*. 28th ed. Elk Grove Village, IL: American Academy of Pediatrics; 2009.
14. U.S. Department of Health & Human Services. 2010 National Vaccine Plan. http://www.hhs.gov/nvpo/vacc_plan/2010%20Plan/nationalvaccineplan.pdf. Accessed October 6, 2011.
15. Immunization Coverage in the U.S. Centers for Disease Control and Prevention Web site. http://www.cdc.gov/vaccines/stats-surv/imz-coverage.htm#nis. Accessed October 6, 2011.
16. Black CL, et al. M*MWR*. 2011;60:1157-1163.
17. Dorell C, et al. *MMWR*. 2011;60:1117-1123.
18. Dickerson JB, et al. *Hum Vaccines*. 2011;7:211-219.
19. Luman ET, et al. *JAMA*. 2005;293:1204-1211.
20. Final state-level influenza vaccination coverage estimates for the 2010–11 season—United States, National Immunization Survey and Behavioral Risk Factor Surveillance System, August 2010 through May 2011. CDC Web site. http://www.cdc.gov/flu/professionals/vaccination/coverage_1011estimates.htm. Accessed October 6, 2011.
21. Stokley S, et al. *MMWR*. 2011;60:700-704.

22. Manual for the Surveillance of Vaccine-Preventable Diseases. 4th Edition, 2008-2009 & 5th Edition, 2011. Centers for Disease Control and Prevention Web site. http://www.cdc.gov/vaccines/pubs/surv-manual/index.html. Accessed October 6, 2011.
23. Active bacterial core surveillance (ABCs). Centers for Disease Control and Prevention Web site. http://www.cdc.gov/abcs/index.html. Accessed October 6, 2011.
24. New vaccine surveillance network. Centers for Disease Control and Prevention Web site. http://www.cdc.gov/vaccines/stats-surv/nvsn/default.htm. Accessed October 6, 2011.
25. Kanesa-thasan N, et al. *Pediatrics*. 2011;127 (suppl 1):S16-S22.
26. Ball R, et al. *Pediatrics*. 2011;127(suppl 1):S31-S38.
27. Zhou W, et al. *MMWR*. 2003;52(SS-1):1-24.
28. Varricchio F, et al. *Pediatr Infect Dis J*. 2004;23:287-294.
29. Baggs J, et al. *Pediatrics*. 2011;127(suppl 1):S45-S53.
30. Yih WK, et al. *Pediatrics*. 2011;127(suppl 1):S54-S64.
31. LaRussa PS, et al. *Pediatrics*. 2011;127(suppl 1):S65-S73.
32. Bonhoeffer J, et al. *Vaccine*. 2002;21:298-302.
33. Available definitions. Brighton Collaboration Web site. https://brightoncollaboration.org/public/what-we-do/standards/case-definitions/available-definitions.html. Accessed October 7, 2011.
34. Bonhoeffer J, et al. *Vaccine*. 2009;27:2282-2288.
35. Bonhoeffer J, et al. *Vaccine*. 2009;27:2289-2297.
36. McNeil MM, et al. *Vaccine*. 2007;25:3428-3436.
37. Salmon DA, et al. *Pediatrics*. 2011;127(suppl 1):S78-S86.
38. National Institute of Allergy and Infectious Diseases; National Institutes of Health. Task Force on Safer Childhood Vaccines: Final Report and Recommendations (1998). http://permanent.access.gpo.gov/lps22576/safevacc.pdf. Accessed October 9, 2011.
39. Immunization Safety Review. Institute of Medicine of the National Academies Web site. http://www.iom.edu/Activities/PublicHealth/ImmunizationSafety.aspx. Accessed October 9, 2011.
40. Adverse effects of vaccines: evidence and causality. Institute of Medicine Web site. http://www.iom.edu/Reports/2011/Adverse-Effects-of-Vaccines-Evidence-and-Causality.aspx. Accessed October 6, 2011.
41. Affordable Care Act and Immunization. HealthCare.gov Web site. http://www.healthcare.gov/news/factsheets/affordable_care_act_immunization.html. Accessed October 10, 2011.
42. Lee GM, et al. *JAMA*. 2007;298:638-643.
43. Orenstein WA, et al. *Clin Pharmacol Ther*. 2007;82:764-768.
44. National Vaccine Advisory Committee. *Pediatrics*. 2009;124:S558-S562.
45. Hinman AR, et al. *Annu Rev Public Health*. 2006;27:235-259.
46. Klein JO, et al. *Pediatrics*. 2006;117:2269-2275.
47. Smith J, et al. *Lancet*. 2011;378:428-438.
48. Pediatric vaccine stockpiles. Centers for Disease Control and Prevention Web site. http://www.cdc.gov/ncird/progbriefs/downloads/pediatric-vacc-stkpl.pdf. Accessed October 10, 2011.
49. Santoli JM, et al. *JAMA*. 2003;290:3122-3128.

3 Standards, Principles, and Regulations

Healthy People 2020

The *Healthy People* initiative began in 1979 with *Healthy People: The Surgeon General's Report on Health Promotion and Disease Prevention*, an attempt to systematically identify the most significant preventable public health threats and to focus public and private efforts to address those threats.[1] Subsequent reports were published every 10 years, with the most recent, *Healthy People 2020*, published in late 2010. Each report, the work of many federal and state agencies, scientists, professional organizations, and members of the public, sets out a comprehensive set of health objectives for the subsequent decade. There are nearly 600 objectives in the 2020 report, each with a reliable data source, a baseline measure, and a specific target for improvement.

Healthy People 2020 contains ambitious goals with respect to vaccine-preventable diseases, not the least of which are maintaining the total elimination status of congenital rubella syndrome and polio, eliminating new cases of hepatitis B among persons 2 to 18 years of age, reducing the annual number of measles cases to 30 and mumps cases to 500, and keeping pertussis down to 2500 cases under 1 year of age and 2000 cases between 11 and 18 years of age.[2] Major immunization goals are summarized below:

- Routine childhood vaccines
  - 90% coverage for each vaccine by 19 to 35 months of age (exceptions: 85% for HepA and 80% for RV)
  - 95% coverage for all recommended vaccines by kindergarten entry
  - 95% of children through 5 years of age have records in a fully operational, population-based immunization information system
- Routine adolescent vaccines
  - 80% coverage for Tdap, MCV, and HPV (females only)
  - 90% coverage with 2 doses of VAR for those without a history of chickenpox
- Routine adult vaccines
  - 90% coverage for pneumococcal vaccine among adults ≥65 years of age
  - 60% coverage for pneumococcal vaccine among high-risk adults 18 to 64 years of age
  - 30% coverage for ZOS among adults ≥60 years of age
- Influenza vaccine
  - 80% coverage from 6 months to 64 years of age

– 90% coverage among high-risk adults 18 to 64 years of age, HCP, and adults ≥65 years of age
– 80% coverage among pregnant women.

Standards for Immunization Practices

Standards for both pediatric and adult immunization practices have been developed. Rather than setting a mark for the minimum standard of care, they represent the most desirable practices that pediatric health care professionals should strive to achieve. Providers also should be aware that extensive evidence-based guidelines on immunization, such as those from the Infectious Diseases Society of America (IDSA), have been published.[3]

■ Standards for Child and Adolescent Immunization Practices

In 1992, a working group convened by the National Vaccine Advisory Committee (NVAC) developed a set of standards for pediatric immunization practices, largely in response to the measles resurgence in the late 1980s. These standards were revised and updated in 2003 and have been endorsed by most professional organizations that deal with pediatric immunization.[4] The AAP offers guidance on implementing many of these standards.[5]

Key elements of each standard are listed below. The means to implement many of these standards are elaborated upon elsewhere in this book.

- ***Standard 1—Vaccination services are readily available.*** Routinely recommended vaccines should always be part of primary care. Vaccination status should be assessed at all points of contact with the health care system, including subspecialty practices, schools, and specialty clinics. If vaccines cannot be offered at these sites, patients should be referred elsewhere. Primary care providers should be notified about vaccines given outside the medical home.
- ***Standard 2—Vaccinations are coordinated with other health care services and provided in a medical home when possible.*** Vaccinations should be coordinated with routine well-child visits or other visits. Patients who receive vaccines outside the medical home should be encouraged to receive subsequent vaccines from their primary care provider. Those who do not have a primary care provider should receive assistance in finding one.
- ***Standard 3—Barriers to vaccination are identified and minimized.*** Vaccine visits should be scheduled promptly and, if necessary, independently of visits for other well-child services. Long waiting periods in the office should be avoided and culturally and age-appropriate educational materials should be available. A physical examination is not required for immunization—observation and screening are sufficient.

Providers should ask parents and patients how they could make vaccinations more accessible.

- ***Standard 4—Patient costs are minimized.*** Money should not be a barrier to vaccination. Free vaccines are available through public programs like the Vaccines for Children (VFC) Program, Public Health Service Section 317 grants to states, and state and local programs. Providers utilizing these resources should make it clear that even though the patient may be charged for administration of the vaccines, they will not be denied vaccination because of inability to pay. Health and insurance plans should cover all routinely recommended vaccines and reimbursement to providers should be enough to cover all expenses associated with delivering vaccines in practice.
- ***Standard 5—Health care professionals review the vaccination and health status of patients at every encounter to determine which vaccines are indicated.*** Any and all health care visits are an opportunity to review vaccination status and minimize missed opportunities. This might include, for example, emergency room visits, hospitalizations, and appointments with specialists. Undervaccination should be documented in the patient's chart. Providers who do not give vaccines should refer patients to a primary care provider who does.
- ***Standard 6—Health care professionals assess for and follow only medically accepted contraindications.*** There are very few true contraindications to vaccination. Decisions to withhold vaccination should be supported by published guidelines and should be documented in the medical record.
- ***Standard 7—Parents/guardians and patients are educated about the benefits and risks of vaccination in a culturally appropriate manner and in easy-to-understand language.*** Sufficient time should be allowed to discuss the benefits of vaccines, the diseases they prevent, and the known risks. The schedule should be reviewed and the importance of bringing the hand-held vaccination record should be emphasized. Parents should be told how to report adverse events. Vaccine Information Statements (VISs) should be provided and supplemented by oral or visual explanations when appropriate, and the parent's questions and concerns should be addressed. Reporting of adverse events should be encouraged.
- ***Standard 8—Health care professionals follow appropriate procedures for vaccine storage and handling.*** This is critical to maintaining potency and effectiveness.
- ***Standard 9—Up-to-date, written vaccination protocols are accessible at all locations where vaccines are administered.*** Protocols should detail vaccine storage and handling; the recommended schedule; contraindications; administration technique; treatment and reporting of adverse events; risk-benefit

communication; and record maintenance and accessibility.

- ***Standard 10—People who administer vaccines and staff who manage or support vaccine administration are knowledgeable and receive ongoing education.*** Vaccine recommendations change frequently, and all personnel involved in the process of vaccine delivery should remain abreast of these changes. Many resources are available for this purpose, including free e-mail listservs and distance-based training opportunities through the CDC.
- ***Standard 11—Health care professionals simultaneously administer as many indicated vaccine doses as possible.*** There are essentially no routine vaccines that cannot be administered at the same time at separate sites. When vaccines are not given simultaneously, arrangements should be made for the patient's earliest return to receive the needed vaccines. Although not specifically mentioned in the standard, combination vaccines allow delivery of multiple antigens with fewer shots and are generally preferred to separately administered components.
- ***Standard 12—Vaccination records for patients are accurate, complete, and easily accessible.*** This standard goes beyond the record keeping mandated by law. It calls for a permanent record that the parents carry with them and verification of vaccines received from other providers. All vaccinations should be reported to state or local immunization information systems (IISs or registries). Vaccine refusal also should be documented.
- ***Standard 13—Health care professionals report adverse events after vaccination promptly and accurately to the Vaccine Adverse Events Reporting System (VAERS) and are aware of a separate program, the National Vaccine Injury Compensation Program (VICP).*** These programs are described below. The law requires reporting of certain events, and reporting of all significant events is encouraged, even if causality is not established. Health care professionals should be aware that parents and patients could report adverse events to VAERS on their own.
- ***Standard 14—All personnel who have contact with patients are appropriately vaccinated.*** Offices and clinics should have policies to review and maintain the vaccination status of their staff.
- ***Standard 15—Systems are used to remind parents/guardians, patients, and health care professionals when vaccinations are due and to recall those who are overdue.*** Computerized or manual tracking, recall, and reminder systems should be in place.
- ***Standard 16—Office- or clinic-based patient record reviews and vaccination coverage assessments are performed annu-***

ally. A simple random survey of patient records can yield information about coverage rates, missed opportunities, and record quality; in general, physicians will find that they overestimate the proportion of their patients who are appropriately immunized. Systematic assessments should be conducted. Feedback and incentives are important elements of quality improvement.

- ***Standard 17—Health care professionals practice community-based approaches***. Providers should be responsive to the needs of their patients, but it should be recognized that high coverage rates protect the entire community. Partnering with other service providers, such as the US Department of Agriculture's Special Supplemental Nutrition Program for Women, Infants, and Children (WIC), advocacy groups, schools, and service organizations should be encouraged.

In 1996, the ACIP, AAP, AAFP, and AMA called for routine health care visits for all children at 11 to 12 years of age. Before 2005, vaccinations during adolescence consisted for the most part of catch-up, with the exception of the Td booster. Since then, new vaccines (MCV, Tdap, HPV, and seasonal influenza) have been recommended for adolescents, and since 2006, the National Immunization Survey has reported coverage rates for adolescents. In 2007, the routine schedule for the first time included a standalone chart for older children and adolescents. While there are as yet no adolescent standards per se, it is worth emphasizing that optimally immunizing adolescents represents a special set of challenges for providers, not the least of which is the fact that adolescents make infrequent visits for preventive health services.[6]

■ Standards for Adult Immunization Practices

The National Coalition for Adult Immunization first offered standards for adult immunization practices in 1990. In 2003, an NVAC working group revised these standards to reflect changes in the health care system and new information regarding adult vaccine coverage.[7] Many of the standards, shown in **Table 3.1**, parallel the pediatric standards.

Annual mortality from vaccine-preventable diseases among adults reaches into the tens of thousands; hospitalizations reach into the hundreds of thousands and societal costs into the billions of dollars. Yet historically, adult and adolescent immunization rates have lagged behind childhood rates.[8] In 2007, the IDSA published a set of principles—billed as a "call to action"—designed to rectify this situation.[9] Some of the principles reiterate the adult practice standards; others extend into the area of policy. In 2008, the IDSA and the American College of Physicians released a joint statement, endorsed by many other professional organizations, encouraging subspecialty physicians to take a more active role in keeping adults up-to-date.[10]

TABLE 3.1 — Standards for Adult Immunization Practices

Standard 1—	Adult vaccination services are readily available
Standard 2—	Barriers are identified and minimized
Standard 3—	"Out-of-pocket" costs are minimized
Standard 4—	Health care professionals routinely review the immunization status of patients
Standard 5—	Health care professionals assess for valid contraindications
Standard 6—	Patients are educated about risks and benefits in easy-to-understand language
Standard 7—	Written protocols are available at all locations where vaccines are administered
Standard 8—	Persons who administer vaccines are properly trained
Standard 9—	Health care professionals recommend simultaneous administration of indicated vaccine doses
Standard 10—	Immunization records are accurate and easily accessible
Standard 11—	All personnel who have contact with patients are appropriately immunized
Standard 12—	Systems are developed and used to remind patients and health care professionals when vaccinations are due and to recall patients who are overdue
Standard 13—	Standing orders are employed
Standard 14—	Regular assessments of coverage levels are conducted in providers' practices
Standard 15—	Patient-oriented and community-based approaches are used to reach target populations

Adapted from Poland GA, et al. *Am J Prev Med.* 2003;25:144-150.

Unfortunately, there remains much room for improvement in adult immunization. A 2009 survey indicated that only 27% of family physicians and internists stock all adult vaccines.[11] Among the reasons cited were difficulties getting reimbursed for the vaccines and administration costs, reluctance of patients to be vaccinated because of out-of-pocket costs, and the need to use vaccines before their expiration date.

National Childhood Vaccine Injury Act

In response to public concern about vaccine safety and the effects that liability issues were having on the pharmaceutical industry, threatening vaccine supply, Congress passed the National Childhood Vaccine Injury Act of 1986 (NCVIA). The NCVIA established two important programs with which providers need to be familiar, the VICP and VAERS. In addition, the NCVIA required providers to give adult vaccine recipients or the parents or guardians of minors receiving vaccines a VIS for each vaccine received.

■ National Vaccine Injury Compensation Program (VICP)

The VICP, which went into effect on October 1, 1988, is a no-fault alternative to the tort system for resolving claims that result from adverse reactions to mandated childhood vaccines.[12] It is administered jointly by the Health Resources and Services Administration of HHS, the US Court of Federal Claims (the Court), and the Department of Justice (DOJ), and is funded by an excise tax levied on every dose of vaccine that is purchased.

Anyone who feels they were injured by a covered vaccine must first pursue a remedy through the VICP. In order to receive compensation, petitioners must show that any one of the following occurred: 1) they incurred an injury found in the Vaccine Injury Table (VIT)[13]; 2) the vaccine caused the injury; or 3) the vaccine significantly aggravated a pre-existing condition. The VIT, which lists specific injuries or conditions and the timeframes in which they must have occurred, serves as a basis for presumption of causation. The listed events are similar to those in the Reportable Events Table (RET); see below and **Table 3.2**. Providers should be aware that some conditions listed on the VIT (eg, encephalopathy after pertussis vaccine) have remained there even though current assessments of the evidence show no evidence of causation (see *Chapter 7: Addressing Concerns About Vaccines—Does Pertussis Vaccine Cause Encephalopathy?*). Individuals can file claims for injuries not listed in the VIT, but *proof of causation* must be given. In recent years, the standard for proof seems to have shifted from a *preponderance of the evidence* to *biologic plausibility*.[14]

In order for a claim to be filed, the injury must have lasted for at least 6 months following vaccination, resulted in hospitalization and surgery, or resulted in death. In order to be compensated, the petitioners must prove that a) they received a vaccine listed on the VIT, and b) the first signs of injury occurred within the specified time frame, or the vaccine caused the injury or caused an existing illness to get worse (it must also be determined that the injury or death did not have another cause). When a claim is filed, HHS reviews the medical aspects and makes recommendations to a DOJ lawyer representing the Secretary of Health and Human Services, who reviews the legal aspects of the case. The HHS and DOJ reviews are then forwarded to the Court, wherein a Special Master (a lawyer appointed by the Court) decides if the claim will be paid and how much money will be offered. If the medical case is straightforward—for example, an individual develops chronic arthritis (not otherwise explained) within 7 to 42 days after receiving a rubella-containing vaccine—HHS may

TABLE 3.2 — Reportable Events Table (Effective November 10, 2008)

Vaccine	Event[a]	Interval From Vaccination When Event Occurs
Note: For all vaccines, events listed in the package insert as contraindications to additional doses are considered reportable events, even if they are not listed here. Reporting of any clinically significant or unexpected event for any vaccine is encouraged. Manufacturers are required to report all adverse events made known to them for any vaccine.		
Tetanus (in any combination)	Anaphylaxis or anaphylactic shock	7 days
	Brachial neuritis	28 days
Pertussis (in any combination)	Anaphylaxis or anaphylactic shock	7 days
	Encephalopathy or encephalitis	7 days
MMR (in any combination)	Anaphylaxis or anaphylactic shock	7 days
	Encephalopathy or encephalitis	15 days
Rubella (in any combination)	Chronic arthritis	42 days
Measles (in any combination)	Thrombocytopenic purpura	30 days
	Vaccine-strain measles virus infection in an immunodeficient recipient	6 months
OPV	Paralytic polio	Immunocompetent: 30 days Immunocompromised: 6 months
	Vaccine-strain poliovirus infection	Immunocompetent: 30 days Immunocompromised: 6 months
IPV	Anaphylaxis or anaphylactic shock	7 days

HepB	Anaphylaxis or anaphylactic shock	7 days
Hib	No specific event listed[b]	
VAR	No specific event listed[b]	
RV	No specific event listed[b]	
PCV	No specific event listed[b]	
HepA	No specific event listed[b]	
Influenza	No specific event listed[b]	
Meningococcal	No specific event listed[b]	
HPV	No specific event listed[b]	

[a] See reference below for event definitions. Any acute complications or sequelae of these events, including death, are also reportable, with no applicable interval from the date of vaccination.

[b] Where no specific event is listed, the general mandate to report any event listed in the package insert as a contraindication to additional doses still applies.

Adapted from VAERS Table of Reportable Events Following Vaccination. Vaccine Adverse Event Reporting System Web site. http://vaers.hhs.gov/resources/VAERS_Table_of_Reportable_Events_Following_Vaccination.pdf. Accessed October 10, 2011.

concede the case in its review, acknowledging that the injury fits the VIT definition (this is often referred to as a *Table injury*). In this instance, the Special Masters will usually pay the claim. If it is not a Table injury and HHS contests the claim, hearings may be held. The decision of the Special Masters can be appealed by either party (HHS or the petitioner) to a judge of the Court, then to the US Court of Appeals for the Federal Circuit, and ultimately to the US Supreme Court.

Vaccines recommended by the ACIP for routine use in children are automatically covered under the VICP. Advice regarding the VICP and recommended changes to the VIT comes from the Advisory Commission on Childhood Vaccines, which consists of 9 members (3 health care professionals, 3 members of the general public, and 3 attorneys) who meet at least quarterly. Nonvoting, ex-officio members include the Director of the National Institutes of Health, the Assistant Secretary for Health, the Director of the CDC, and the Commissioner of the FDA, or their designees.

Important points about the VICP include:

- Covered vaccines as of July 2011 are listed in footnote e in **Table 3.3**.
- Claims can be filed by individuals, parents, legal guardians, trustees, legal representatives of the estate of deceased persons, non-US citizens, and, under certain conditions, individuals vaccinated outside of the United States.
- Adults are covered under the program if they receive one of the covered vaccines.
- Petitioners are free to reject the decision of the Court and pursue civil litigation.
- Compensation is available for past and future nonreimbursable medical, custodial, and rehabilitation costs and lost earnings. There are no limits on compensation for attorney's fees; petitioners representing themselves can only recover legal costs, not fees. Compensation for pain and suffering, and compensation to the estate in the case of death, is capped at $250,000. As of January 2011, the VICP had awarded a total of $2.1 billion to more than 2500 families and individuals.[12]

Many people had not heard of the vaccine court or the VICP until 2009 and 2010, when landmark decisions regarding vaccines and autism were handed down—see *Chapter 7: Addressing Concerns About Vaccines—Did the Thimerosal Used as a Preservative in Vaccines Cause Autism?* Also, in a 2011 decision (Bruesewitz vs Wyeth[15]), the Supreme Court found that the NCVIA preempts all vaccine design defect claims where plaintiffs seek compensation for injury or death caused by a vaccine's adverse effects. This ruling acknowledges Congress' intent to set vaccines aside from other consumer goods, for which manufacturers can be held liable if harms result from design defects, regardless of how much care was exercised in their production and sale.[16] Vaccines may have unavoidable side effects that relate to how they function—for example, they may cause fever, which is indicative of the inflammatory response that drives the immune response that ultimately protects the person from disease. Fever, then, in a sense, is not a "design defect," and if it results in damage, the vaccine manufacturer cannot be held liable—as long as the vaccine was properly manufactured and was accompanied by proper directions and warnings. The Supreme Court decision should help to ensure that manufacturers are not driven away from the market for concerns about liability.

■ Vaccine Adverse Event Reporting System (VAERS)

VAERS, in operation since 1990, is a passive surveillance program that collects and analyzes postmarketing information about adverse vaccine events.[17] Any event following vaccination can be reported, with no restriction on the interval between vaccination and the onset of illness and no requirement for medical care having been rendered. Anyone can submit a report, including health care professionals, pharmaceutical companies, lawyers, parents, and patients. However, health care providers are *required* to report events that are listed by the manufacturer as a contraindication to subsequent doses as well as events listed in the RET (**Table 3.2**). Reports can be submitted directly on the Internet or forms can be downloaded and mailed. VAERS data are available to the public for analysis, although caveats regarding interpretation are offered (see *Chapter 2: Vaccine Infrastructure in the United States—Vaccine Adverse Event Reporting System*).

■ Vaccine Information Statements (VISs)

A VIS is a concise (1-page, 2-sided) description of the risks and benefits of a given vaccine, written for lay people and published by the CDC. **Table 3.3** summarizes the use of VISs and lists other obligations that are binding on vaccine providers. Keep in mind that there may be state laws that supplement these national requirements.

Public Readiness and Emergency Preparedness (PREP) Act

Just as the NCVIA protects companies from liability in the manufacture of routinely recommended vaccines, the PREP Act, enacted in 2005, provides legal immunity to manufacturers of pandemic vaccines.[18] It also protects those who distribute and administer pandemic vaccines and other "covered countermeasures," the only exception being willful misconduct. The PREP Act is invoked when the secretary of HHS declares a public health emergency, as happened in June 2009 with the influenza H1N1

TABLE 3.3 — Federal Requirements Regarding Vaccination

Requirement	Details
Give a VIS	Give a current, *take-home* copy of the relevant VIS before *each* dose of *each* vaccine[a]
	Children: give to the parent or legal representative[b]
	Adults: give to the patient or legal representative[c]
	Use the VIS published by the CDC[d]
	Mandatory for vaccines covered under the National Vaccine Injury Compensation Program (VICP)[e]
	Mandatory for any vaccines purchased under a federal (CDC) contract
	Encouraged for all other vaccines
	Provide VIS for each component of a combination vaccine if there is no VIS for the combination
	Use translations if necessary[f]
Document in the permanent medical record or office log	Name of the VIS, edition date, and date it was given to the recipient[g]
	Name, office address and title of the individual who administered the vaccine
	Date of administration
	Manufacturer
	Lot number
Report to VAERS	Any event listed by the manufacturer as a contraindication to subsequent doses of the vaccine
	Any event listed in the Reportable Events Table (**Table 3.2**) that occurs within the specified time period after vaccination

[a] VISs may be read *before* the immunization visit, but patients must still be given a copy *at* the immunization visit (they may choose not to take the VIS with them, but it must still be offered). The take-home copy can be an electronic version downloaded to a mobile device. The VIS should

be supplemented as needed with oral discussions, videotapes, other printed material, and whatever else is needed for the parent or patient to gain understanding. The information on the VIS must still be conveyed to the vaccinee even if he or she is blind, deaf, or cannot read.

[b] If immunizations are to be given when the parent is not present, for example during a school-based program, the following options can be exercised:
Consent prior to administration of each dose of a series. The VIS is mailed to the family or sent home with the student prior to each dose. A consent form is signed and returned before vaccination, and the form is placed in the medical record.
Single signature for series. Some states permit the parents to sign a single consent form for the entire vaccine series. They first receive a copy of the VIS and sign a statement acknowledging receipt of the VIS and authorizing the complete series. A VIS is still sent home prior to each dose in the series.

[c] For incompetent adults living in long-term care facilities, all relevant VISs may be provided at the time of admission or at the time of consent if later than admission.

[d] Available from Vaccine Information Statements. Centers for Disease Control and Prevention Web site. http://www.cdc.gov/vaccines/pubs/vis/default.htm. Accessed October 10, 2011. Providers may not alter a VIS or make their own version of a VIS, but they can add the practice's name, address, and phone number. In 2008, a multiple-vaccines-VIS was released that covers all of the vaccines in the first 6 months of life. Providers do not need to withhold a vaccine if a VIS for it does not yet exist. In this situation, the package insert or a homemade information sheet can be used until the official VIS is available. At that point, the VIS should be used.

[e] As of July 2011, the following vaccines are included: DT, DTaP, HepA, HepB, Hib, HPV, IIV, IPV, LAIV, MCV, MMR, MMRV, MPSV, PCV, RV, Td, Tdap, TT, VAR, and any component or combination of these. DTwP and OPV are covered but are no longer used in the United States.

[f] VISs have been translated into 39 different languages. These are considered de facto equivalents of the English versions and are available from the Immunization Action Coalition Web site (Vaccine information statements. Immunization Action Coalition Web site. http://www.immunize.org/vis. Accessed October 10, 2011).

[g] The patient's signature is not required and the VIS should not be construed as informed consent, which may be required in certain states.

Adapted from Instructions for the use of the vaccine information statements. Centers for Disease Control and Prevention Web site. http://www.cdc.gov/vaccines/pubs/vis/downloads/vis-instructions.pdf. Accessed October 10, 2011.

pandemic. Persons claiming to have been injured by a covered countermeasure may seek compensation from a fund administered by HRSA. However, unlike the NCVIA, the PREP Act does not allow for judicial review or civil litigation if such claims are denied.

Occupational Safety and Health Administration (OSHA)

Because most vaccines are injected percutaneously, vaccine providers and their employees are at risk for needlestick injuries. As such, all facilities where vaccinations are given, including doctor's offices, public health clinics, and hospitals, fall under OSHA regulations designed to minimize occupational exposure to bloodborne pathogens. Some states may have OSHA plans that exceed the federal requirements discussed below, but those plans cannot be less stringent.

In 1991, OSHA promulgated the Bloodborne Pathogens Standard, which mandated that employers establish and implement an exposure-control plan for their employees. This plan had to include work-practice controls, procedures for handling exposures, personal protective clothing and equipment, training, medical surveillance, HepB vaccination, signs, and labels. In addition, engineering controls designed to isolate or remove hazards, such as sharps-disposal containers, self-sheathing needles, and plastic capillary tubes, were mandated. In 2000, Congress passed the Needlestick Safety and Prevention Act, which directed OSHA to revise the blood-borne pathogens standard, including more detail in the requirements for engineered devices and adding new elements to the exposure-control plan. The revised standard went into effect in April 2001.[19]

The basic elements of the Standard are listed below. With respect to vaccinations, the most important element is the use of engineered sharps protections on needles and the proper disposal of sharps. However, most physicians' offices perform other procedures, such as phlebotomy, wound cleansing, and suturing, necessitating attention to many other aspects of the standard.

- *Exposure-control plan*—A *written* plan needs to be in place that details all of the elements listed below. In addition, the procedures and job classifications where exposure to blood might occur should be delineated. An annual review and update must be conducted that takes into account innovations in medical procedures and new technological developments that reduce the risk of exposure.
- *Sharps-injury log*—Employers must maintain a log of percutaneous injuries from contaminated sharps. It must include, at a minimum, the type and brand of device, department or work area where the incident occurred, and an explanation of how

the incident occurred (including, for example, the procedure being performed and the body part affected). In addition, it must protect the confidentiality of the injured employee. The log should serve as a tool to identify high-risk areas and evaluate devices.

3

- *Engineered sharps protections*—Devices with built-in safety features or mechanisms that effectively reduce the risk of exposure must be used for procedures that will have contact with blood. Such features should be an integral part of the device, allow the worker's hands to remain behind the needle at all times, remain in effect after the procedure and during disposal, and should be as simple as possible. Examples pertinent to immunizations include syringes with sheaths that slide forward by a single-handed operation to cover the attached needle after use, as well as retractable needles. Documentation must be provided in the exposure-control plan that appropriate, commercially available, engineered devices are evaluated each year, and justification must be provided for selecting a particular device (*not* selecting an engineered device is *not* an option). In addition, it must be documented that nonmanagerial, front-line employees with direct patient care responsibilities had input into the selection (this can take the form of meeting minutes or written evaluations filled out by employees). Selected devices must not jeopardize patient or employee safety or be medically inadvisable. Since sheaths and the like are considered temporary measures, even sharps with engineered protections must be disposed of in an approved container.
- *Universal precautions*—All blood and body fluids must be treated as if infectious for hepatitis B, hepatitis C, and HIV, even if they are from low-risk individuals. Facilities for hand-washing and personal protective equipment (eg, gloves, gowns, masks, mouthpieces, and resuscitation bags) must be available at no cost to employees. Employers must launder lab coats and scrubs, if used as protective equipment, at no cost; home laundering is not permitted. Gloves (hypoallergenic if necessary) must be available and hand washing is required after use. However, use of gloves is *not* required when administering intramuscular or subcutaneous injections as long as bleeding is not anticipated.
- *Procedures*—Detailed protocols must be given for all procedures with risk, including decontamination of equipment, handling of sharps-disposal containers and other regulated waste, broken glassware, and laundry. Routine cleaning of work sites should be described.
- *Sharps handling*—The exposure control plan must contain a protocol for handling of sharps. Recapping contaminated needles is prohibited but this should not be an issue since

needles will have engineered controls. If recapping is necessary for uncontaminated needles, such as those used to draw vaccine from a vial into a syringe, the cap should be scooped up from a flat surface using the hand that is holding the syringe and needle. Disposal containers should be closable, puncture resistant, leak proof, labeled appropriately, and located where procedures are performed. The protocol should specify how the containers are handled once they are filled.

- *Warning labels*—Orange or orange-red biohazard labels must be affixed to containers of regulated waste and refrigerators and freezers containing blood or infectious materials (labeled bags may also be used).
- *HepB vaccination*—Vaccination should be available at no cost to all employees with potential blood contact. The employee's health insurance cannot be used to pay this expense unless the employer routinely pays the entire premium. Employees must sign a declination form if they choose to opt out.
- *Postexposure evaluation*—Specific procedures should be outlined for the handling of exposures. Baseline and follow-up laboratory tests should be done after consent is obtained and must be provided free of charge. Provisions for confidential medical follow-up must be made. Postexposure HIV prophylaxis should be offered if indicated in accord with current guidelines. The source individual's blood should be tested for blood-borne pathogens after consent is obtained; if consent is not given, this needs to be documented. Medical records on employees must be kept for the duration of employment plus 30 years.
- *Training*—Training that includes background information and the exposure-control plan must be provided upon assignment and annually thereafter. Documentation of training sessions, including the dates, content, trainer, and attendees must be maintained.

Many vaccines are now available from manufacturers in prefilled syringes and needles with engineered protections. More information on implementing the Standard can be obtained from the International Healthcare Worker Safety Center at the University of Virginia.[20]

Mandates

There are no federal laws specifying which people, short of those entering military service and immigrants, must receive which vaccines. However, some states, employers, or institutions might require certain vaccines or proof of immunity for selected individuals. Examples include influenza vaccine, MMR, Tdap, and HepB for HCP, influenza and pneumococcal vaccines for residents and employees of long-term care facilities, vaccines for laboratory workers who work with specific pathogens, and RAB for animal handlers. There are, however, state laws specifying which vaccines must be received before attendance at day care, preschool, school, or college is allowed.

■ Schools

School requirements have been instrumental in the eradication or near-eradication of many diseases.[21] The courts have repeatedly upheld the legal basis for these statutes, which rests on three main concepts: 1) *beneficence*, or doing the right thing (protecting individuals and society from the harm of vaccine-preventable diseases; 2) *nonmaleficence*, or not doing harm (vaccines are among the safest medical products in use); and 3) *justice*, or equally protecting the rights of all people (including the right of children to be protected despite their parents' actions or inactions, the right of children who cannot be vaccinated to be protected, and the right of all people to benefit from herd immunity).[22]

The case for mandates that prevent the spread of highly contagious diseases (such as measles) in schools is relatively straightforward. The situation becomes complicated when considering infections such as human papillomavirus, which is arguably not spread in schools, can largely be prevented by avoidance of high-risk behaviors, and which represents a very complex political and ethical situation.[23] Some have argued that HPV should not be considered for school mandates;[24] others argue that there are moral grounds for compulsory vaccination with HPV.[22] In 2008, NVAC offered guidance for states considering adolescent vaccination mandates.[25]

In interpreting the validity of an immunization record, the CDC recommends a 4-day grace period for specific minimum age and interval requirements. For counting purposes, "Day 1" is the day before the day that marks the minimum age or interval. Thus, a child who receives MMR 3 days before his first birthday (the minimum age) is considered effectively immunized; one who receives MMR a week before his first birthday is not. Similarly, Dose 3 of DTaP is considered valid if given 26 days after Dose 2, even though the minimum interval is 28 days. One exception to the grace period is the minimum interval between certain live vaccines, which is 28 days, period (see *Chapter 5: General Recommendations—Rules by Which to Vaccinate*; another exception is the RAB series, which must be given exactly according to schedule). Thus, a dose of VAR given 26 days after LAIV is considered invalid.

The grace period should be used for interpreting the validity of vaccinations that have already been given, not for scheduling future ones. Some local school districts may not accept the 4-day grace period, so the best advice is to give vaccines at the recommended ages. Practitioners may have to balance the issues surrounding giving a vaccine before the exact specified age with the risk that the patient may not return to be vaccinated at the appropriate time.

All states allow exemption from school immunization requirements for medical reasons. As of 2011, 46 states plus the District of Columbia granted some form of religious exemption (the exceptions were Arizona, California, Mississippi, and West Virginia) and 19 states granted some form of philosophical or personal belief exemption.[26] In a 1997 policy statement, reaffirmed in 2009, the AAP emphasized the need for sensitivity and flexibility in dealing with parents' religious beliefs.[27] It was acknowledged that constitutional guarantees of freedom of religion do not permit children to be harmed through religious practices, and while the AAP called for the repeal of religious exemption laws, it also argued against the stringent application of medical-neglect laws when parents refuse the recommended childhood immunizations. Personal belief exemptions are more problematic because the level of proof can be minimal (it may be minimal for religious exemptions as well), amounting simply to parents being "opposed to immunization." In some cases, parents request personal belief exemptions as a matter of convenience when their children's immunizations are not up-to-date.

Any way you look at it, exemption from immunization requirements places others in harm's way, and society has a mandate to prevent this. As John Stuart Mill (1806-1873) wrote in his 1859 essay *On Liberty*, "the only purpose for which power can be rightfully exercised over any member of a civilized community, against his will, is to prevent harm to others." Put another way by Zachariah Chafee (1885-1957) in his 1919 essay *Freedom of Speech in Wartime*, "Your right to swing your arms ends just where the other man's nose begins."

Some professional organizations, including the Pediatric Infectious Diseases Society, have taken a stand against personal belief exemptions,[28] and the AAP has called upon pediatricians to work individually and collectively to make sure that all children without true contraindications are immunized on time.[29] Physicians, public health providers, and school officials should not grant philosophical exemptions out of convenience, and in general should work toward the repeal of philosophical exemption laws. Importantly, the risk of some vaccine-preventable diseases has been shown to increase with the availability of philosophical exemptions and the ease with which these are granted (see *Chapter 7: Addressing Concerns About Vaccines—The Costs of Public Concern*). For parents considering exemption, physicians should emphasize that disease rates among exemptors are higher than among vaccinated persons; in addition, large numbers of exemptors in a community put everyone at risk, including vaccinated children.

Contact your state health department (see *Appendix*) for the most up-to-date information about school mandates.

■ Hospitals and Other Institutions

Nationally, less than half of HCP receive influenza vaccine every year. In 2007, responding to this dismal statistic, the Joint Commission on Accreditation of Health Care Organizations approved a standard that requires accredited organizations to offer influenza vaccination to staff and even volunteers with close patient contact. Since then, many professional organizations, state and local health departments, and individual institutions and practices have adopted mandates.[30] The legal and ethical framework for mandatory HCP immunization continues to be debated, something that was brought to the forefront during the 2009 H1N1 pandemic.[31,32] Detractors cite deprivation of liberty without due process, guarantees against illegal search and seizure, violation of the establishment clause of the First Amendment, and freedom of contract between employee and employer. Proponents—including, by and large, the courts—cite precedents that uphold the state's authority to restrict privileges and personal economic, even religious, freedoms in the interest of preserving the public welfare.

Several things, however, are clear. First, HCP may be leery of mandates because of misperceptions about vaccine safety and their risk of acquiring influenza at work.[33] Second, when HCP do get vaccinated, they do so for their own benefit and not for the benefit of their patients.[34] Third, immunization rates may depend on how the issue is raised; for example, uptake is higher using opt-out rather than opt-in strategies.[35] Finally, influenza vaccine coverage rates among HCP should be followed as an integral part of all health care facility patient safety programs.

A survey of 808 acute care hospitals in 2011 found that 55.6% required influenza vaccination for HCP; fewer than half of these imposed any consequences for noncompliance.[36]

REFERENCES

1. HealthyPeople.gov. HealthyPeople.gov Web site. http://www.healthypeople.gov/2020/default.aspx. Accessed October 11, 2011.
2. Immunization and infectious diseases. HealthyPeople.gov Web site. http://www.healthypeople.gov/2020/topicsobjectives2020/objectiveslist.aspx?topicId=23. Accessed October 11, 2011.
3. Pickering LK, et al. *Clin Infect Dis*. 2009;49:817-840.
4. National Vaccine Advisory Committee. *Pediatrics*. 2003;112:958-963.
5. NVAC Standards of Excellence. American Academy of Pediatrics Web site. http://www.aap.org/immunization/pediatricians/nvacstandards.html. Accessed October 20, 2011.
6. National Vaccine Advisory Committee. *Am J Prev Med*. 2008;35:152-157.
7. Poland GA, et al. *Am J Prev Med*. 2003;25:144-150.
8. Hinman AR, et al. *Clin Infect Dis*. 2007;44:1532-1535.

9. Infectious Diseases Society of America. *Clin Infect Dis*. 2007;44: e104-e108.
10. ACP-IDSA Joint Statement of Medical Societies Regarding Adult Vaccination by Physicians. Infectious Diseases Society of American Web site. http://www.idsociety.org/Adult_and_Adolescent_Immunization/. Accessed October 11, 2011.
11. Freed GL, et al. *Vaccine*. 2011;29:1850-1854.
12. Cook KM, et al. *Pediatrics*. 2011;127(suppl 1):S74-S77.
13. Vaccine injury table. Health Resources and Services Administration Web site. http://www.hrsa.gov/vaccinecompensation/vaccinetable.html. Accessed October 11, 2011.
14. Offit PA. *N Engl J Med*. 2008;358:2089-2091.
15. Bruesewitz v Wyeth LLC. 562 US ___ (2011). Case No. 09-152.
16. Kesselheim A. *N Engl J Med*. 2011;364:1485-1487.
17. US Department of Health and Human Services. Vaccine Adverse Event Reporting System. http://vaers.hhs.gov/index. Accessed October 11, 2011.
18. Parmet WE. *N Engl J Med*. 2010;362:1949-1952.
19. Bloodborne pathogens and needlestick prevention. Occupational Safety & Health Administration Web site. http://www.osha.gov/SLTC/bloodbornepathogens/index.html. Accessed October 11, 2011.
20. International Healthcare Worker Safety Center. University of Virginia Health System Web site. http://www.healthsystem.virginia.edu/internet/epinet/home.cfm. Accessed October 11, 2011.
21. Hinman AR, et al. *J Law Med Ethics*. 2002;30:122-127.
22. Balog JE. *Am J Pub Health*. 2009;99:616-622.
23. Colgrove J, et al. *N Engl J Med*. 2010;363:785-791.
24. Opel DJ, et al. *Pediatrics*. 2008;122:e504-e510.
25. National Vaccine Advisory Committee. *Am J Prev Med*. 2008;35: 145-151.
26. School vaccination requirements, exemptions and Web links. Centers for Disease Control and Prevention Web site. http://www2a.cdc.gov/nip/schoolsurv/schImmRqmtReport.asp. Accessed October 12, 2011.
27. American Academy of Pediatrics Committee on Bioethics. *Pediatrics*. 1997;99:279-281.
28. Vaccine Advocacy Committee of the Pediatric Infectious Diseases Society. *Pediatr Infect Dis J*. 2011;30:606-607.
29. Committee on Practice and Ambulatory Medicine and Council on Community Pediatrics. *Pediatrics*. 2010.125:1295-1304.
30. Honor roll for patient safety. Immunization Action Coalition Web site. http://www.immunize.org/honor-roll. Accessed October 12, 2011.
31. Van Delden JJM, et al. *Vaccine*. 2008;26:5562-5566.
32. Stewart AM. *N Engl J Med*. 2009;361:2015-2017.
33. Douville LE, et al. *Arch Pediatr Adolesc Med*. 2010;164:33-37.
34. Hollmeyer HG, et al. *Vaccine*. 2009;27:3935-3944.
35. Chapman GB, et al. *JAMA*. 2010;304:43-44.
36. Miller BL, et al. *Clin Infect Dis*. 2011;53:1051-1059.

4 Vaccine Practice

Handling, Storage, and Transport

Mishandling of vaccines can reduce potency and leave vaccinated people susceptible to disease. Here are some general guidelines[1]:

- *Basics*
  - Designate one person (and a backup) to be in charge, but educate all staff about vaccine storage, handling, and inventory. Responsibilities of the Immunization Tsar or Tsarina are listed in **Table 4.1**.
  - Make sure deliveries are scheduled when the facility is open and knowledgeable staff are present, keeping in mind holidays, vacations, and changes in hours of operation.
  - Anticipate seasonal changes in vaccine needs (eg, influenza season and back-to-school time).
  - Know the demographics of the clinical population in order to anticipate particular vaccine needs, keeping in mind that each vaccine has particular age indications, formulations and presentations.
- *Inventory*
  - Maintain an inventory log, including product name, manufacturer, lot number, doses received, date received, condition on arrival, and expiration date.
  - Inspect products on delivery, including the integrity of containers and cold chain monitoring devices.
  - Store vaccines immediately under appropriate conditions.
  - If there are questions about a vaccine's condition at delivery, store the vaccine under the recommended conditions, label it "DO NOT USE," and contact the manufacturer's quality-control office or the state immunization program.
  - Discard mishandled and expired vaccines (vaccines can be used until the last day of the month indicated on the expiration date).
  - Rotate stock so that vaccine with the shortest expiration date is up front.
  - Keep vaccines purchased through VFC separate from privately purchased vaccines.
  - Keep vaccines in original boxes until ready for use.
  - Inspect stock every day.
  - Designate an alternate site where vaccines can be safely stored.
  - Discourage "brown bagging," where patients pick up their vaccines at a pharmacy and bring them to the provider for administration (this practice is popular for ZOS).

TABLE 4.1 — Responsibilities of the Immunization Tsar or Tsarina

- Order vaccines
- Oversee receipt and storage
- Organize refrigerator and freezer
- Monitor and record refrigerator and freezer temperature twice daily
- Inspect refrigerator and freezer daily
- Rotate stock
- Remove expired vaccine
- Respond to temperature excursions
- Oversee vaccine transport
- Maintain storage and handling documentation
- Maintain storage equipment and corresponding records
- Maintain VFC documentation
- Ensure training of designated staff
- Keep up with new recommendations
- Prepare talking points to address concerns
- Look for ways to improve coverage and timeliness
- Champion vaccine issues

Adapted from Centers for Disease Control and Prevention. *Epidemiology and Prevention of Vaccine-Preventable Diseases*. 12th ed. Atkinson W, et al, eds. Washington, DC: Public Health Foundation, 2011.

- *Administration*
  - Consider as invalid any doses that were inadvertently given with mishandled or expired vaccine.
  - Do not open more than one multidose vial at a time.
  - Be aware that for some multidose vials, there is a limited shelf life after the vial is first entered.
  - Do not prefill syringes with vaccines that are supplied in vials.
  - Use only the diluent supplied by the manufacturer to reconstitute lyophilized vaccines.
  - Dispose of all vaccine materials using medical waste disposal procedures, including sharps/biohazard containers (materials coming in contact with live vaccines carry the risk of contagion).
- *Storage*
  - Storage conditions for vaccines licensed in the United States are shown in **Table 4.2**.
  - The freezer should be a separate sealed unit and should have a separate external door; better yet, completely separate refrigerator and freezer units should be used. Dormitory style units that have a freezer compartment within the refrigerator should not be used. The only exception is temporary storage for the day's supply of *refrigerated* vaccines

(that do not contain VAR); at the end of the day the vaccines must be returned to the permanent refrigerator.

- Keep a logbook for each piece of equipment, including serial number, date of installation, maintenance and repair dates, and service contact information.
- Position the units ≥4 inches from any wall to ensure good air circulation.
- Use a duster to keep the coils clean.
- Do not store food in the vaccine refrigerator or freezer (frequent opening of the door can cause temperature fluctuations).
- Do not store vaccines on shelves in the refrigerator door.
- Vaccines that need to be refrigerated but protected from freezing should be stored in the middle of the refrigerator, away from the freezer portion of the unit.
- Use clearly labeled, color-coded, breathable plastic mesh trays for each product and include separate compartments for unopened and opened vials (record the date of opening or reconstitution directly on the label). Locate the trays 2 to 3 inches from the walls and away from cold air vents. For refrigerated vaccines that require reconstitution, the corresponding diluents should be stored with the vaccines (diluents should never be frozen).
- Arrange vaccines by age group (pediatric, adolescent, adult).
- Post a sign that specifies which vaccines are stored in the refrigerator and which are stored in the freezer.
- Keep a thermometer in the refrigerator and one in the freezer and record the temperatures on a log when the office opens in the morning and when it closes in the evening (the logs should be kept for ≥3 years). Alternatively, a recording thermometer can be used. All thermometers should have a *Certificate of Traceability and Calibration* (this certifies calibration *after* manufacturing). *Appropriate ranges are 35°F to 46°F (2°C to 8°C) for the refrigerator and ≤5°F (-15°C) for the freezer.*
- Keep jugs of water the floor of the refrigerator (after removal of vegetable/fruit bins and deli drawer) and on the shelves in the door (label "DO NOT DRINK"). Place ice packs in the freezer. These measures help maintain a steady temperature and provide some stability in the event of a power outage.
- Place a "DO NOT UNPLUG" sign near the outlet for the refrigerator and freezer units. Mark other points along the circuit (eg, fuses, circuit breakers) in a similar fashion.
- Do not use an outlet with a ground fault circuit interrupter (ie, one with test and reset buttons) or one connected to a wall switch.

TABLE 4.2 — Vaccine Storage[a]

Vaccine	Trade Name	Special Instructions
Store in Refrigerator		
Adenovirus	—	Store type 4 and type 7 vaccine together
Anthrax	BioThrax	—
DT	—	—
DTaP	Daptacel	—
	Infanrix	—
DTaP-HepB-IPV	Pediarix	—
DTaP-IPV	Kinrix	—
DTaP-IPV/Hib-T	Pentacel	Store lyophilized Hib-T and DTaP-IPV diluent together May store reconstituted vaccine in refrigerator for ≤30 minutes
HepA	Havrix	—
	Vaqta	—
HepA-HepB	Twinrix	—
HepB	Engerix-B	—
	Recombivax-HB	—
HepB-Hib-OMP	Comvax	—
Hib-OMP	PedvaxHIB	—
Hib-T	ActHIB	Store lyophilized Hib-T and diluent together May store reconstituted vaccine in refrigerator for ≤24 hours
	Hiberix	Store lyophilized Hib-T and diluent together[b]

		May store reconstituted vaccine in refrigerator for ≤24 hours Protect from light
HPV2	Cervarix	—
HPV4	Gardasil	May store vaccine at room temperature for ≤72 hours before administration Protect from light
IIV	See **Table 16.1**	Protect Afluria, Agriflu, Fluarix, FluLaval, and Fluvirin from light
IPV	IPOL	—
JE-VC	Ixiaro	—
LAIV	Flumist	—
MCV4-CRM	Menveo	Store lyophilized MenA and MenC/Y/W-135 diluent together May store reconstituted vaccine at room temperature or in refrigerator for ≤8 hours Protect from light
MCV4-D	Menactra	—
MMR	M-M-R_{II}	Store lyophilized MMR and diluent together[b,c] May store reconstituted vaccine in refrigerator for ≤8 hours Protect from light
MPSV4	Menomune	Store lyophilized MenA/C/Y/W-135 and diluent together May store reconstituted vaccine in refrigerator for ≤30 minutes May store reconstituted multidose vial in refrigerator for ≤35 days

Continued

TABLE 4.2 — *Continued*

Vaccine	Trade Name	Special Instructions
PCV13	Prevnar 13	—
PPSV23	Pneumovax 23	—
RAB-HDC	Imovax Rabies	Store lyophilized RAB and diluent together
RAB-PCEC	RabAvert	Store lyophilized RAB and diluent together
		Protect from light
RV1	Rotarix	Store diluent at room temperature
		May store reconstituted vaccine at room temperature or in refrigerator for ≤24 hours
		Protect from light
RV5	RotaTeq	Protect from light
Td	Decavac	—
Tdap	Adacel	—
	Boostrix	—
TT	—	—
TViPSV	Typhim Vi	—
Ty21a	Vivotif	—
YFV	YF-Vax	Store lyophilized YFV and diluent together
Store in Freezer		
MMRV	ProQuad	Store diluent at room temperature or in refrigerator

		May store vaccine in refrigerator for ≤72 hours before reconstitution May store reconstituted vaccine at room temperature for ≤30 minutes Protect from light
Smallpox	ACAM2000	Store diluent at room temperature May store reconstituted vaccine at room temperature for 6 to 8 hours May store reconstituted vaccine in refrigerator for ≤30 days
VAR	Varivax	Store diluent at room temperature or in refrigerator May store vaccine in refrigerator for ≤72 hours before reconstitution May store reconstituted vaccine at room temperature for ≤30 minutes Protect from light
ZOS	Zostavax	Store diluent at room temperature or in refrigerator May store vaccine in refrigerator for ≤72 hours before reconstitution May store reconstituted vaccine at room temperature for ≤30 minutes Protect from light

[a] Refrigerator temperature should be maintained at 35°F to 46°F (2°C to 8°C). Refrigerated vaccines and diluents should never be frozen (MMR is an exception since the lyophilized vaccine can be stored in the refrigerator or freezer). Freezer temperature should be maintained at -58°F to 5°F (-50°C to -15°C). Room temperature is 68°F to 77°F (20°C to 25°C).

[b] Diluent may be stored at room temperature but it is preferable to keep it with the lyophilized vaccine.

[c] MMR may be stored in the freezer but the diluent should never be frozen. Storing it in the freezer can free up refrigerator space and reduce the risk that MMRV, which *must* be frozen, will inadvertently be moved to the refrigerator.

Adapted from the respective package inserts and from Centers for Disease Control and Prevention. *Vaccine Storage & Handling Guide: October 2011*. http://www.cdc.gov/vaccines/recs/storage/guide/vaccine-storage-handling.pdf. Accessed October 17, 2011.

– Use plug guards to prevent accidental dislodging.
– If possible, use an outlet connected to an auxiliary power source.
– **Table 4.3** gives some suggestions for managing the vaccine inventory in the event of a power failure or weather emergency.

• *Off-site transportation*
– FDA regulations require that multidose vials be used only by the provider's office where they were first opened (partially used vials may be moved to other sites operated by the same provider as long as the cold chain is maintained).
– The following may be used to transport vaccines at 35°F to 46°F (2°C to 8°C): original shipping containers, hard-sided plastic insulated containers, and Styrofoam coolers with walls that are at least 2" thick (do not use the thin-walled coolers typically found in grocery stores).
– Use refrigerated or frozen gel packs, not loose or bagged ice (use enough of these to maintain the proper temperature and validate a stable temperature before using the cooler for vaccines).
– Keep the vaccines in their original boxes.
– Place bubble wrap, crumpled brown packing paper, or Styrofoam peanuts around the vaccines to prevent direct contact with the refrigerated or frozen gel packs; include a thermometer next to the vaccines.
– VAR-containing vaccines may be transported at 35°F to 46°F (2°C to 8°C) using the methods described above but must be used within 72 hours and should not be refrozen.
– Diluents should travel with their corresponding vaccines at all times. They can stay at room temperature. If packed inside coolers, they should be refrigerated ahead of time and should not come in direct contact with the refrigerated or frozen gel packs.

Improving Delivery

A large evidence base exists on strategies to improve pediatric immunization delivery (**Table 4.4**). Many of the following strategies, some of which are also applicable to adults, are emphasized in *Chapter 3: Standards, Principles, and Regulations—Standards for Pediatric Immunization Practices* and *Standards for Adult Immunization Practices*.

■ Reminder, Recall, and Tracking Systems

Reminders are messages that immunizations are due. They may be directed at parents in the form of telephone calls (by humans or computers) or mailings (simple postcards or letters), or they may be directed at physicians, nurses, or other staff members in the

TABLE 4.3 — Storage and Handling During Emergencies

Power Outages • Do not open refrigerators and freezers until power is restored • Record temperature after power is restored and note duration of outage (do not open to monitor temperature during outage) • Transfer to alternative storage with reliable power source if possible, maintaining cold chain and monitoring temperature • Contact state or local public health authorities or the vaccine manufacturer if there is *any* question about the potential potency of exposed vaccine • Label exposed vaccine and keep it separated from new stock • Remember that live vaccines are the most susceptible to inactivation by warming
Weather Emergencies • Suspend vaccination and implement emergency procedures in advance of the event • Identify alternative storage facilities with backup power • Ensure availability of staff to package and transport vaccine • Maintain appropriate packing materials • Ensure availability of transportation • Include the following in standard operating procedures: – Emergency phone numbers for power company, equipment repair, alarm monitoring companies, backup storage facility, dry ice vendor, generator repair company, National Weather Service, and vaccine manufacturers – Working agreements with hospitals, health departments, or other facilities to serve as emergency vaccine storage facilities – Procedures for entering facilities and storage areas during emergency or after hours, including location of emergency equipment and packing materials, as well as phone numbers for responsible persons – Procedures for packaging (including inventory documentation and cold-chain monitoring) and transporting vaccines (including preferred and alternative routes) – Priority list for vaccine rescue, aiming to minimize dollar loss but ensure ability to deliver the routine schedule in the short term

Adapted from Vaccine Storage and Handling Toolkit. Centers for Disease Control and Prevention Web site. http://www2a.cdc.gov/vaccines/ed/shtoolkit. Accessed October 17, 2011.

TABLE 4.4 — Strategies for Increasing Pediatric Immunization Coverage

Good Evidence of Effectiveness	Insufficient Evidence of Effectiveness
Client reminder/recall systems	Community education
Child care, school, and college requirements	Patient incentives
Multicomponent patient education	Patient-held medical records
Reduced out-of-pocket costs	Schools and child care centers as vaccination sites
Vaccination settings closer to patients' homes	Provider education
Expanded clinic hours	Standing orders
Use of emergency departments, subspecialty clinics, and WIC sites	
Drop-in vaccination services	
Home-visiting services	
Electronic records	
Office-based quality-improvement activities	

Adapted from AAP. *Pediatrics*. 2010;125:1295-1304.

form of chart or electronic medical record flags saying "vaccines are due." One recent study successfully used text messages (along the lines of "vaccines r do"!) to remind parents about HPV doses for their daughters.[2] Recall messages are notices to parents that vaccinations are overdue. Tracking systems, which can be manual or computerized, allow each child's immunization status to be followed precisely.

Studies have consistently shown improvements in immunization rates for both children and adults if tracking and messaging systems are used, in both public and private settings.[3,4] However, reminder and recall systems are particularly difficult to implement in practices with high patient turnover or in populations that change residence frequently. Keep in mind that in some areas, bilingual reminders may be necessary.

■ Missed Opportunities

Providers should utilize all clinical encounters, including acute care visits, to assess immunization status and administer all vaccines for which a person is eligible, as long as true contraindications do not exist. The idea is to prevent contacts with the health care system from becoming *missed opportunities* for vaccination.[5,6] In order to minimize missed opportunities, providers must be able to accurately determine immunization status "on the fly"—electronic health records and Immunization Information Systems (IISs) can facilitate this, as can attentive office staff. In the absence if IIs, written documentation of immunization status is required; the only exceptions are influenza vaccine and PPSV23, for which self-reported doses are considered valid. Erroneous contraindications (**Table 5.4**) must not stand in the way. Additional barriers may exist in emergency departments and other acute care facilities, including time constraints, concerns about insurance reimbursement, and the perception that by giving routine immunizations, the patient's relationship with his primary care provider will be disrupted.

■ Expanding Access

After-hours or weekend clinics may help boost coverage rates by making it more convenient for parents to bring their children in or for adults to stop by after work. In addition, access to vaccination once a patient enters the office can be facilitated through the use of "vaccination express lanes" and drop-in clinics. With proper vaccine storage and handling, there is no reason why home visits could not be used to vaccinate those persons who are receiving home health services for other reasons.

The medical home is the preferred place for vaccination. The problem is that as children get older they make fewer and fewer visits for preventive health care, especially in middle and late adolescence.[7] Schools are an attractive alternative site for vaccination when one considers that, well, that's where the kids are.

In addition, schools are located in communities and school nurses are trusted health care professionals.[8] Providers are generally not opposed to school-located vaccination (SLV), although they may have concerns about record-keeping and maintaining their relationship with the patient.[9] Parents may also be favorably inclined to having their kids vaccinated in school.[10,11]

Influenza vaccination programs lay the foundation for SLV.[12] However, there are many reasons why broadening SLV to include other vaccines may be difficult. For one, influenza campaigns are seasonal, focused, employ one vaccine, and target all children every year. In contrast, programs designed to address other childhood vaccines would require year-round implementation, would target only children who are behind or have no medical home, and would be highly dependent on accurate IISs. Successful programs require partnership between school personnel and governance, parent-teacher associations, providers, and local health departments. Among the issues to be addressed are methods of obtaining parental consent, screening for VFC eligibility, and obtaining reimbursement.

Expanding access for adults, which serves to protect them as well as their infant contacts, requires thinking outside the box in terms of where immunization could occur. For example, women could receive Tdap postpartum in the hospital through a standing order *(see below)*. This idea was successfully implemented at a hospital in Houston—over 90% of postpartum women, and many other family members who anticipated contact with the infant, were immunized.[13] The idea of surrounding infants in a sea of immune contacts, in essence erecting a barrier to disease transmission, is called "cocooning." This strategy is most germane to preventing pertussis, since older individuals are the source of infection for infants, and to preventing influenza, since immunization does not begin until 6 months of age. Parents of infants who are hospitalized could be immunized when they visit the hospital; this takes the concept one step further, since those parents, unlike postpartum women, are not themselves patients. Nevertheless, the strategy has been successfully employed for both influenza[14] and pertussis[15] immunization. One added value to this approach is that immunization rates among HCP tend to increase!

The pediatric office is also fair game as a venue for adult immunization.[16] **Table 4.5** lists some benefits of and concerns about this approach.

■ Standing Orders

Standing orders enable nonphysician personnel, such as nurses and pharmacists, to prescribe or deliver vaccinations by protocol at the time of the encounter; direct physician involvement is not required. This is one of the most effective interventions for increasing adult immunization rates, and recent studies even show

TABLE 4.5 — Immunizing Adults in the Pediatric Office

Benefits

- Convenient for parents and other household members
- Knowledge base of pediatricians facilitates education about vaccines
- Culture of pediatric practices encourages immunization
- Vaccines are available

Concerns

- Immunized adults may defer other preventive services available in their medical home
- Screening for contraindications may be suboptimal
- Facilities for handling emergencies may be inadequate
- Liability[a]
- A medical record of some sort should be maintained
- Vaccine doses should be communicated to the primary care physician and state IIS
- Adequate supplies must be maintained for both children and adults
- Payment needs to be assured[b]
- Staffing may need to be expanded
- The scope of eligible adults (eg, parents, grandparents, etc) needs to be defined
- The spectrum of vaccines offered needs to be defined[c]

[a] Providers are automatically covered for administering routine childhood vaccines, regardless of the age of the vaccince (see *Chapter 3: Standards, Principles, and Regulations—The National Childhood Vaccine Injury Act*).

[b] Providers may submit charges to the adult's insurer or ask for payment at the time of service. Some insurers may limit coverage for vaccinations that occur outside the medical home. In general, vaccines obtained through the VFC program cannot be used for adults.

[c] Influenza and Tdap would make the most sense.

Adapted from Lessin HR, et al. *Pediatrics*. 2012;129:e247-e253.

that the entire process can be computerized—that is, patients can be screened for eligibility electronically and the orders can be generated automatically, without investment of personnel time. Employing standing orders in nursing homes, hospitals, clinics, physicians' offices, and other institutional settings can increase coverage rates. In fact, standing orders for adult pneumococcal and influenza vaccination are recommended.[17] Standing orders are also applicable to pediatric patients. In fact, it is recommended that all birthing hospitals have standing orders in place for HepB immunization of newborns. Standing orders could be employed for influenza immunization of children ≥6 months of age who are hospitalized in the fall for any reason.

■ Immunization Information Systems (IISs)

IISs, formerly known as *registries*, are confidential, population-based, centralized computerized systems that maintain information about immunizations. The ideal IIS contains all persons in a geographic area and receives vaccination data from all regional providers. The need for IISs is easy to see—an increasingly complex vaccine schedule must be administered to children who frequently relocate and change health care providers, and the number of vaccines being recommended for adults is increasing. For both children and adults, vaccination histories are often incomplete and fragmented, leading to both missed opportunities and unnecessary duplication. For these reasons, one of the *Healthy People 2020* goals is for at least 95% of children <6 years of age to participate in a fully operational population-based IIS (see *Chapter 3: Standards, Principles, and Regulations—Healthy People 2020*). As of 2009, 77% of US children in this age group participated in an IIS.[18]

In a 2010 review of 71 published and 123 unpublished studies, the Task Force on Community Preventive Services concluded that there was strong evidence of the effectiveness of IISs in increasing vaccination rates.[19] IISs can provide recalls and reminders; ensure timely vaccination after changes in location or provider; reduce unnecessary immunization; provide accurate documentation of immunization history; assess coverage rates and provide feedback to providers; assist in pubic health responses to outbreaks; facilitate vaccine management and accountability; allow surveillance on issues such as missed opportunities, invalid doses, and disparities in coverage; and facilitate monitoring of adverse events, among other benefits. There are also potential downsides, including the costs of data entry and retrieval; difficulties integrating into existing business practices; problems interfacing with other medical records and billing systems; concerns about confidentiality; and the perception of minimum value-added for participation.[20] Organizations such as the American Immunization Registry Association, in collaboration with the CDC, have worked on defining best practices to help overcome these barriers and ensure that IISs can support required core program activities at the state and local levels.[21]

The CDC has supported the development of state IISs since 1993 through Section 317 Public Health Service grants.[22] Additional support has come from organizations such as the Robert Wood Johnson Foundation. In 1998, the National Vaccine Advisory Committee launched the Initiative on Immunization Registries to facilitate community- and state-based registries.[23] Four major challenges were identified:

- *Protecting confidentiality*—The need to gather and share information must be balanced with the family's right to privacy. Minimum specifications include executing written confidentiality policies, notifying parents of the existence of the registry and allowing them to opt out, and defining who has access and what can be done with the information.

- *Participation by providers and recipients*—Because the majority of vaccine delivery has shifted to the private sector, efforts to recruit private providers are essential. Part of what makes a registry attractive to providers is simplicity, minimization of administrative burden, high quality of data, and functionality (eg, ability to generate reminders).
- *Operational challenges*—The functional capabilities of registry hardware and software differ from community to community; this is not conducive to the overall goal of seamless information exchange. For this reason, the CDC developed minimum operational standards.[24]
- *Resources to maintain registries*—Registries are likely to result in cost savings by reducing the manual labor involved in pulling medical records for provider visits, managed care reporting, and school system review. However, accurate cost assessments are difficult to come by because of rapid changes in technology, participation rates, and functionality.

The AAP has strongly supported the development of IISs and has suggested that research be done into their cost-effectiveness in increasing immunization rates.[25] In addition, it has called for a critical examination of the cost and benefits for the practicing physician and has suggested that physicians be reimbursed for entering historical information into databases. Finally, the AAP has cautioned that the data in IISs be used to improve quality, not to penalize poor performers.

■ Other Strategies

Parent and community education regarding the importance of immunizations may play some role in improving coverage rates by increasing demand. Physician and staff education is also important, and this can be facilitated by the Immunization Tsar or Tsarina (**Table 4.1**). Regular, systematic assessment and feedback can identify problem areas and evaluate the effectiveness of new interventions.

Along these lines, the CDC has developed a quality improvement methodology called AFIX, for **A**ssessment (of a provider's vaccination coverage levels and practices), **F**eedback (of results to the provider along with suggestions for improvement), **I**ncentives (to reward improved performance), and e**X**change (of information and resources to facilitate improvement).[26] Traditionally used to evaluate immunization delivery systems for children, AFIX can be generalized to apply to any age group. The data used in AFIX assessments come from IISs or from chart reviews. A software application called CoCASA, for Comprehensive Clinic

Assessment Software Application, is available from the CDC to assess immunization practices in clinics, private practices, or other sites where immunizations are given.[27]

Screening

Screening patients for contraindications, precautions, and other problems before every dose of a vaccine is an important part of preventing adverse events and ensuring vaccine "take." This can be effectively accomplished by asking the simple questions shown in **Table 4.6**, which are applicable to both children and adults. The issues addressed by these questions are also indicated in the table. Standardized forms for screening can be downloaded from the Immunization Action Coalition web site free of charge.[28]

Administration

■ General Issues

During well care visits, it is probably most efficient to bring the vaccines to the examination room rather than have the patient move to a designated shot area. If reconstitution is needed, it should be done for each individual patient, rather than in batches, in order to reduce the risk of confusion and wastage. Young infants may do better if held on the parent's lap, while older children may prefer to sit on the edge of the examining table and hug their parent. Adolescents who are at risk for syncope should probably sit or lie down. HCP should wash their hands or use antiseptic hand gel before each patient.

Here are some additional administration pearls:

- Gloves are not routinely needed to administer vaccines, but should be worn if the vaccinator may come in contact with body fluids or has open lesions on his or her hands.
- The rubber stopper on vaccine vials is not sterile and should be cleaned with a *sterile* alcohol pad (yes, there are *nonsterile* alcohol pads!) after the protective cap is removed.
- It is not necessary to change the needle after withdrawing a vaccine from the vial and before administering it to the patient. This only increases the risk of sharps injury and bacterial contamination.
- The injection site should also be swabbed with a sterile alcohol prep and allowed to dry.
- Aspirating back on the syringe after insertion but before injection is not necessary. There are no large vessels in the anatomic areas that are recommended for vaccine administration.
- The British call vaccinations "jabs" for a reason: the best technique involves a direct, rapid plunge of the needle through

the skin, followed by a rapid withdrawal after delivering the vaccine.

- Multiple vaccines can be given in the same limb but should be separated by 1″ to 2″. Simultaneous administration by different personnel may minimize anticipatory anxiety.

■ Routes

For *intramuscular* administration, the needle enters the skin at a 90° angle, penetrating deep enough to hit the muscle (**Figure 4.1**). Traction can be applied to the skin and subcutaneous tissue before injection and released after injection. Preferred sites, which differ by age, include the anterolateral aspect of the upper thigh (vastus lateralis muscle) and the upper, outer part of the arm above the armpit and below the acromion (deltoid muscle); the required needle length varies by patient age (**Table 4.7**). The buttocks should not be used because the fat layer is too thick and damage to the sciatic nerve is possible.

For *subcutaneous* injections, the skin and subcutaneous tissue are pinched-up, and the needle directed at a 45° angle (**Figure 4.1**). The preferred sites and needle length again vary with age (**Table 4.7**).

For infants, *oral* administration of RV is best accomplished with the child lying in the feeding position in the parent's arms. The tip of the applicator is placed in the infant's mouth toward the inner cheek and slowly emptied until all of the liquid is dispensed. If the infant spits or regurgitates, the dose is counted and not repeated.

LAIV is supplied in a syringe-like sprayer for *intranasal* administration. The recipient should be in the upright position. The tip of the sprayer is inserted just inside the nose and the plunger is rapidly depressed until the dose-divider clip stops the plunger. The clip is then removed and the remainder of the dose is given in the other nostril. Sneezing or leakage of some of the liquid from the nose is not a reason to repeat the dose.

Two vaccines are given *intradermally*. For smallpox, a bifurcated needle is used to puncture the skin, drawing a small amount of blood. As such, gloves should be worn and the site should be covered with gauze and a semipermeable dressing. Skin preparation is not required unless there is gross contamination, in which case soap and water should be used for cleansing. If alcohol is used, the skin must dry thoroughly before inoculation to prevent inactivation of the vaccine virus. Intradermal IIV is given using a unique microinjection system that is supplied with the product. After removing the needle cap, the syringe is held between the thumb and the middle finger and the needle is inserted perpendicular to the skin in the deltoid region (the vaccine is not labeled for administration in other regions, such as the forearm, which is where a tuberculin skin test is given). The index finger is then

TABLE 4.6 — Screening Questions

Question	Issues Addressed
Is the patient sick today?	Moderate-to-severe illness is a precaution for all vaccines
Does the patient have severe allergies to drugs, foods, vaccine components, or latex?	Severe allergy to vaccine components or previous doses is a contraindication for future doses Severe egg allergy is a contraindication for influenza and YFV Severe allergy to drugs (eg, neomycin) or other food ingredients (eg, gelatin, baker's yeast) may contraindicate certain vaccines
Has the patient had serious reactions to previous vaccinations?	Various contraindications and precautions for further doses
Is the patient on long-term aspirin therapy?	LAIV is contraindicated because of the theoretical risk of Reye syndrome
Has the patient or a close family member had a seizure or a brain or neurologic problem?	Evolving neurologic disorder is a precaution for pertussis-containing vaccines Patients who are susceptible to febrile seizures may benefit from fever prophylaxis Guillain-Barré syndrome within 6 weeks of previous influenza vaccine or tetanus-containing vaccine is a precaution for further doses MMR plus VAR is preferred to MMRV for toddlers with personal, sibling, or parental history of febrile seizures (this applies to the first dose only)
Does the patient have a history of bowel obstruction?	RV is contraindicated if there is a history of intussusception

Does the patient have asthma or another chronic medical condition (eg, lung, heart, kidney, or metabolic)?	LAIV may be contraindicated Certain nonroutine vacines may be recommended
If the patient is a child between 2 and 4 years of age, has a health care provider diagnosed wheezing or asthma in the past year?	LAIV may be contraindicated
Does the patient have cancer, leukemia, a blood disorder, HIV infection, AIDS, tuberculosis, or any problem with the immune system?	Live vaccines are generally contraindicated in patients with immune impairment MMR can cause thrombocytopenia Active untreated tuberculosis is a precaution for MMR, VAR, and ZOS
In the last 3 months, has the patient received any treatment that might weaken his or her immune system, such as steroids, cancer chemotherapy, or radiation?	Live vaccines are generally contraindicated in patients with immune impairment Patient may respond poorly to vaccination
Are there any family members who have problems with their immune system?	The patient might be at risk for a heritable immune deficiency that would contraindicate live vaccines
Has the patient received blood transfusions or immune globulin in the past year?	Antibody-containing blood products can interfere with response to MMR and VAR The patient may have an undisclosed serious underlying illness
Is the patient pregnant or is there a chance she could become pregnant in the next 3 months?	Live vaccines are generally contraindicated during pregnancy Pregnancy is an indication for influenza vaccine and Tdap

Continued

TABLE 4.6 — *Continued*

Question	Issues Addressed
Has the patient received any other vaccines in the last 4 weeks?	Certain live vaccines not given on the same day need to be separated by ≥4 weeks The AAP (but not the ACIP) recommends that if Tdap and MCV4-D are not given on the same day, they need to be separated by ≥4 weeks MCV4-D and PCV13 need to be separated by ≥4 weeks in functionally and anatomically asplenic children Violating the minimum interval between doses in a series may invalidate doses

Adapted from Screening for contraindications. Immunization Action Coalition Web site. http://www.immunize.org/clinic/screening-contraindications.asp. Accessed October 17, 2011.

FIGURE 4.1 — Injection Technique

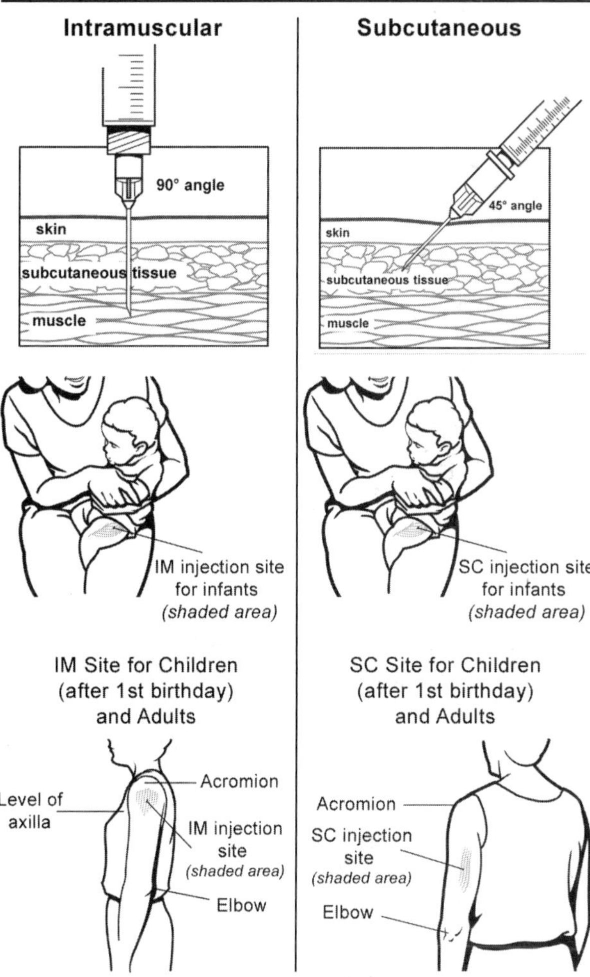

Adapted from Administering vaccines. Immunization Action Coalition Web site. http://www.immunize.org/catg.d/p2020.pdf. Accessed October 15, 2011.

4

TABLE 4.7 — Needle Type and Injection Site

	Intramuscular[a] (22- to 25-gauge)		Subcutaneous[b] (23- to 25-gauge)	
Age	Site	Needle (inch)	Site	Needle (inch)
0 to 28 days[c]	Anterolateral upper thigh	⅝	Anterolateral upper thigh	⅝
1 to 12 months	Anterolateral upper thigh	1	Anterolateral upper thigh	⅝
1 to 2 years	Anterolateral upper thigh[d]	1 to 1¼	Anterolateral upper thigh or upper outer triceps	⅝
	Deltoid	⅝ to 1		
3 to 18 years	Deltoid[d]	⅝ to 1	Anterolateral upper thigh or upper outer triceps	⅝
	Anterolateral upper thigh	1 to 1¼		
≥19 years	Deltoid	Male or female <130 lbs (<60 kg): ⅝ to 1 Male or female 130 to 152 lbs (60 to 70 kg): 1 Female 152 to 200 lbs (70 to 90 kg): 1 to 1½ Male 152 to 260 lbs (70 to 118 kg): 1 to 1½ Female >200 lbs (90 kg): 1½ Male >260 lbs (118 kg): 1½	Anterolateral upper thigh or upper outer triceps	⅝

[a] The needle is inserted at a 90° angle. When using a ⅝-inch needle, the skin should be stretched tight to ensure that the muscle is reached.
[b] Skin and fatty subcutaneous tissue are bunched up and the needle is inserted at a 45° angle.
[c] Includes premature infants.
[d] Preferred site.

Adapted from Kroger AT, et al. *MMWR*. 2011;60(RR-2):1-61.

used to push down the plunger and inject the vaccine. After injection, a needle shield is activated by pressing the plunger further down with the thumb until a click is heard.

Jet injectors produce a narrow stream of liquid under high pressure, penetrating the epidermis and delivering vaccines into the subcutaneous tissue or muscle. They eliminate the threat of needlestick injury and are particularly amenable to mass vaccination campaigns. Whereas there are jet injection devices that have been cleared by the FDA, the only vaccine that is licensed to be delivered in this fashion is MMR.[29] IIV should not be given by jet injection in the United States.

■ Anxiety, Pain, and Fever

For infants, pain can be reduced by oral sucrose solution (50%) given directly into the mouth with a small syringe or administered on a pacifier; breastfeeding, non-nutritive sucking, and simply holding the baby also work well. For older children, stress and anxiety can be ameliorated by truthfully informing them what to expect before the visit occurs and by parental endorsement of vaccination as being valuable.[30] Parents should be allowed to comfort young children (rather than assist in restraining them) and should try to distract them by telling stories, playing music, or having them blow into pinwheels or imaginary candles. Technique is important: a quick "jab" into and out of the muscle is less painful than a slow injection with aspiration.[31] Stroking the adjacent skin before and during the injection may help, as may pressure applied to the site after withdrawal. For sequential injections, the least painful one should be given first.

Topical anesthetics, such as eutectic mixture of local anesthetic (EMLA cream) or vapocoolant sprays, should be considered for patients who are phobic or extremely anxious about the injection.[32] Acetaminophen may be considered as needed for analgesia or antipyresis after immunization, but there is no role for prophylactic use, even in children with a history of febrile seizures.[33] In fact, whereas prophylactic acetaminophen does reduce fever, there is some evidence that it interferes with antibody responses (one possible mechanism is decreased inflammation at the injection site, which could interfere with innate immunity; see *Chapter 1: Introduction to Vaccinology—Basic Vaccine Immunology*).[34] Fortunately, high fevers and medical attention for fever or other symptoms after vaccination are rare.

Emergencies

■ Preparation

Acute emergencies after vaccine administration are rare—the risk for children and adolescents is estimated at less than one episode per million doses.[35] The AAP suggests that when possible, patients should be observed in the office for 15 to 20 minutes after vaccination; the ACIP has recommended this for HPV, where syncope appears to be a particular problem. Life-threatening emergencies such as anaphylaxis usually occur within minutes, when the patient is still likely to be within reach of medical personnel. The benefits of rapid, mass vaccination programs, such as "drive-by" influenza vaccine clinics, probably far outweigh the risks of curtailing any medical observation period.

Standing orders for the medical management of vaccine reactions, including anaphylaxis, in children and adults should be available in the office. Exemplary standing orders and equipment lists are available from the Immunization Action Coalition.[36,37]

■ Syncope

Vasovagal reactions are most common in adolescents and young adults, particularly females. About 60% occur within 5 minutes of vaccination and approximately 90% occur within 15 minutes. Between 1990 and 2001, slightly over 2200 reports of syncope were made to VAERS. Approximately 12% of cases resulted in hospitalization, and there are some reports of serious injury such as skull fracture. Since the advent of the adolescent vaccine platform—Tdap and MCV4 in 2005 and especially HPV in 2006—there has been a sharp increase in reported syncopal episodes related to vaccination.[38] However, the absolute number of reported episodes remains low—463 VAERS reports between 2005 and 2007, most of them in female adolescents. HCP should be aware of predisposing conditions (eg, needle phobia) and presyncopal symptoms (eg, light-headedness, dizziness, pallor, diaphoresis, cold extremities, nausea, weakness, visual disturbance). At-risk individuals should be encouraged to sit or lie down; a cool, damp cloth to the face and neck may help. If syncope does occur, the patient should be protected as much as possible from fall injury and should be placed supine with the legs raised until symptoms abate.

■ Anaphylaxis

Anaphylaxis occurs rapidly and is a medical emergency. Signs and symptoms include:

- Flushing, warmth, urticaria, erythema, soft tissue edema, pruritus
- Dry mouth, swelling of the lips, tongue and throat, sneezing, congestion, rhinorrhea
- Hoarseness, stridor, cough, dyspnea, chest tightness, wheezing, cyanosis
- Tachycardia, hypotension, weak pulse, dizziness, shock, cardiovascular collapse
- Crampy abdominal pain, nausea, vomiting, diarrhea

For patients with signs of anaphylaxis, the emergency medical system should be activated. Vital signs should be monitored. If the blood pressure is low, elevate the legs; if breathing is difficult, elevate the head and monitor the airway. Administer epinephrine 1:1000 (aqueous) at a dose of 0.01 mL/kg intramuscularly (the maximum dose is 0.3 mL in children and 0.5 mL in adolescents and adults) in the lateral thigh. A dose can be repeated every 5 to 15 minutes if necessary for up to 3 total doses. In addition, an antihistamine such as diphenhydramine can be given at a dose of 1-2 mg/kg (maximum 30 mg in children, 50 mg in adolescents and adults) PO, IM, or IV. Patients should be observed for several hours and may require intensive care, including airway maintenance, oxygen, and blood pressure support with isotonic intravenous fluids and vasopressors. Biphasic reactions may account for up to 50% of fatal cases. Asymptomatic intervals vary widely and can be as long as 24 hours. All patients with mild or severe anaphylaxis reactions should be referred to an allergist prior to future vaccinations and at a minimum should carry an epinephrine autoinjector.

Coding, Billing, and Costs

Billing third-party payers for immunization services (and all other health services) is complex, which is why there are coding professionals. There are basically 3 systems of which providers should be aware[39]:

- *Current Procedural Terminology (CPT) Codes*—These codes, which are published each year,[40] describe the *procedures* or *services* performed during a visit. The *visit itself* usually falls under evaluation and management codes for preventive medicine services performed in the outpatient setting, provided the immunization occurs in the context of a comprehensive "checkup." There are corresponding codes for the *vaccines themselves*. There are also codes for the *administration* of the vaccines. If the visit is *only* for immunization (eg, before travel), most offices bill only for the vaccine and the administration, using the vaccine product CPT codes and the administration codes. If evaluation and management services unrelated to vaccination are performed during the vaccine visit, those services receive separate codes.
- *International Classification of Diseases, Ninth Revision, Clinical Modification (ICD-9-CM) Codes*—These codes, also published each year,[41] describe the *reason* for the service. For example, the ICD-9-CM code that accompanies DTaP-HepB-IPV vaccination is V06.8, "need for prophylactic vaccination and inoculation against other combinations of diseases." In some cases, the diagnosis codes are sufficiently ambiguous as to allow several options. For example, although the code V05.8 ("need for prophylactic vaccination and inoculation against other specified disease") could be used for ZOS, the

code V04.89 ("need for prophylactic vaccination and inoculation against other viral diseases") might also be appropriate. The *visit itself* usually falls under V20.2 (routine infant or child health check beyond the first month of life) or V70.0 (routine adult general medical examination). If the visit is for a school physical, V70.3 (general medical examination for adoption, camp, school admission, etc) may be used. The tenth revision of these codes (ICD-10-CM) should be out by October 2013.[42]

- *National Drug Codes (NDCs)*—Many payers are now requiring that National Drug Codes (NDCs) for vaccines be submitted along with CPT and ICD-9-CM codes. The NDC is a unique 10-digit, 3-segment number. The first segment identifies the company that makes, repacks, or distributes the product. The second segment identifies the product, strength, dosage form, and formulation. The third segment identifies the package size and type. Sometimes an asterisk appears as a placeholder. NDCs can easily be found by searching the National Drug Code Directory[43] by proprietary name, active ingredient, or company name. It is also found on the package insert in the "How Supplied" section.

A routine visit for a 6-month-old infant might be coded as shown in **Table 4.8**. Remember, all components of all services should be clearly documented in the medical record. If the practice receives vaccines free-of-charge through the VFC Program, it cannot bill for the *vaccine itself*, but it can bill for *administration of the vaccine* and for the *visit itself*.

The vaccine tables in *Section B* contain information on the purchase price for commonly used vaccines. The public sector cost is the contracted price between the CDC and the manufacturer, which changes from year to year.[44] The listed private sector cost is based on the direct purchase price from the manufacturer and is most useful for highlighting relative differences between products. However, these data can be misleading. In a study conducted in 2007, 76 private practices in five states supplied data on their purchase price for vaccines for privately insured children.[45] Significant variation was seen—for example, some practices paid $8.77 per dose for Infanrix while others paid $21.60. Variables associated with the price paid included the size of the practice, its location, use of purchasing cooperatives or buying groups, and the availability of discounts and rebates. Large variation was also seen in reimbursement—for example, some practices were reimbursed $45.32 per dose of ActHIB, others $15.33. Reimbursement for first-dose vaccine administration ranged from $0 to $26.55. In negotiating contract prices with private payers, physicians must consider all of the costs involved in providing vaccines, some of which are listed in **Table 4.9**.

TABLE 4.8 — Typical Coding for a Routine Visit at 6 Months of Age, 2011[a]

	Visit		Vaccine		Vaccine Administration	
Procedure	**CPT[b]**	**ICD-9-CM[c]**	**CPT[b]**	**ICD-9-CM[c]**	**CPT[b]**	**ICD-9-CM[c]**
Checkup	99391	V20.2	—	—	—	—
DTaP-HepB-IPV	—	—	90723	V20.2/V06.8	90460[d]	V06.8
					90461[e]	
					90461	
					90461	
					90461	
Hib-T	—	—	90648	V20.2/V03.81	90460	V03.81
PCV13	—	—	90670	V20.2/V03.82	90460	V03.82
IIV	—	—	90655	V20.2/V04.81	90460	V04.81
RV5	—	—	90680	V20.2/V04.89	90460	V04.89

[a] Billing rules may vary by insurance company.

[b] CPT codes denote *what was done*. In this case, there was a periodic comprehensive preventive medicine visit for an established patient <1 year of age ("Visit" CPT code 99391), particular vaccine products were given (eg, DTaP-HepB-IPV, CPT code 90723), and the administration of these vaccines was performed (eg, "Vaccine Administration" CPT code 90460). The CPT code for the vaccines might need to be accompanied by the appropriate National Drug Code.

[c] ICD-9-CM codes denote *why a procedure was done*. In this case, the reason for the periodic comprehensive preventive medicine visit (CPT code 99391) was to perform a routine infant health check-up (ICD-9-CM code V20.2). The reason for giving Hib-T (CPT code 90648) was "part of the routine health check-up" (ICD-9-CM code V20.2 [primary]) and "to prevent *H influenzae* disease" (ICD-9-CM code V03.81 [secondary]);

the reason for administration of the vaccine (CPT code 90460) was, well, to prevent *H influenzae* disease (ICD-9-CM code V03.81). The codes V03 through V06 denote specific diseases being prevented; they may be reported as secondary codes or may be required by certain insurance companies.

[d] 90460 denotes the first component of each vaccine administered (in this case, diphtheria).

[e] 90461 denotes each additional component that is part of a combination vaccine (in this case, one code each is submitted for tetanus, pertussis, HepB, and IPV). For monovalent vaccines like Hib-T, only one code (90460) is submitted. Some vaccines are multivalent (like PCV13, which contains 13 different pneumococcal polysaccharides) but are considered monovalent (ie, "prevents one disease") for billing purposes.

TABLE 4.9 — Provider Costs for Vaccination Services

Direct Costs

- Vaccine purchase (includes excise tax)
- Sales or usage tax

Overhead

- Personnel time: order and inventory vaccines; negotiate prices, delivery, and payment terms; monitor stock; track unpaid claims
- Storage: refrigerator; freezer; locks; temperature monitoring devices and alarm systems; electricity; generators; associated monitoring and maintenance costs (some of these costs are depreciated)
- Insurance against vaccine loss
- Wastage: spills; expiration; damage; drawing up vaccine but not giving it
- Nonpayment despite collection efforts
- Lost opportunity costs: occupied rooms that could have been used for other income-generating activities; money tied up in inventory that could have been gaining interest

Administration Expenses

- Physician work: time; technical skill and physical effort; mental effort and judgment; psychological stress associated with concerns about risks
- Staff work: time; technical skill and physical effort; mental effort and judgment; data entry into IISs
- Medical supplies: gloves; exam tables and paper; OSHA-compliant syringes with needles; sterile alcohol swabs; adhesive bandages; emergency response items; token patient rewards
- Professional liability insurance

Adapted from The Business Case for Pricing Vaccines and Immunization Administration. American Academy of Pediatrics Web site. http://practice.aap.org/content.aspx?aid=1808. Accessed October 20, 2011.

REFERENCES

1. Vaccine Storage and Handling Guide (October 2011). Centers for Disease Control and Prevention Web site. http://www.cdc.gov/vaccines/recs/storage/guide/vaccine-storage-handling.pdf. Accessed October 16, 2011.
2. Kharbanda EO, et al. *Vaccine*. 2011;29:2537-2541.
3. Szilagyi PG, et al. *JAMA*. 2000;284:1820-1827.
4. Jacobson VJC, Szilagyi P. Patient reminder and recall systems to improve immunization rates. Cochrane Review Web site. http://www.cochrane.org/reviews/en/ab003941.html. Accessed October 30, 2011.
5. CDC. *MMWR.* 1994;43:709-718.
6. Walton S, et al. *Arch Dis Child.* 2007;92:620-622.
7. Rand CM, et al. *Arch Pediatr Adolesc Med.* 2007;161:252-259.
8. Mazyck D. *J Sch Nursing*. 2010;26:3S-6S.
9. Schaffer SJ, et al. *Arch Pediatr Adolesc Med.* 2001;155:566-571.
10. Allison MA, et al. *Pediatr Infect Dis J.* 2010;29:751-755.
11. Middleman AB, et al. *Vaccine*. 2011;29:3513-3516.
12. Hull HF, et al. *Hum Vaccines*. 2011;7:153-160.
13. Healy CM, et al. *Clin Infect Dis*. 2011;52:157-162.
14. Shah SI, et al. *Pediatrics*. 2007;120:e617-e621.
15. Dylag AM, et al. *Pediatrics*. 2008;122:e550-e555.
16. Walter EB, et al. *Academic Pediatr*. 2009;9:344-347.
17. McKibben LJ, et al. *MMWR*. 2000;49(RR-1):15-16.
18. Brand W, et al. *MMWR.* 2011;60:10-12.
19. Universally recommended vaccinations: Immunization information systems. The Community Guide Web site. http://www.thecommunityguide.org/vaccines/universally/RRimminfosystems.html. Accessed October 30, 2011.
20. Turning barriers into opportunities: survey and best practice report. American Immunization Registry Association Web site. http://www.immregistries.org/pdf/Provider_Participation_Final_2005.pdf. Accessed October 30, 2011.
21. American Immunization Registry Association. Registry standards of excellence in support of an immunization program. http://www.immregistries.org/pdf/PROWstandardscomp1.pdf. Accessed October 30, 2011.
22. CDC. *MMWR.* 2008;57:289-291.
23. National Vaccine Advisory Committee. Development of community and state-based immunization registries: report of the National Vaccine Advisory Committee (NVAC). Atlanta, GA: US Department of Health and Human Services, CDC; 1999. Available at http://www.cdc.gov/vaccines/programs/iis/pubs/nvac.htm. Accessed October 30, 2011.
24. IIS: 2001 minimum functional standards for registries. Centers for Disease Control and Prevention Web site. http://www.cdc.gov/vac

cines/programs/iis/stds/min-funct-std-2001.htm. Updated May 26, 2009. Accessed October 30, 2011.

25. Committee on Practice and Ambulatory Medicine, et al. *Pediatrics*. 2006;118:1293-1295.
26. Assessment, Feedback, Incentives, and Exchange (AFIX). Centers for Disease Control and Prevention Web site. http://www.cdc.gov/vaccines/programs/afix/index.html. Accessed October 30, 2011.
27. Comprehensive Clinic Assessment Software Application (CoCASA). http://www.cdc.gov/vaccines/programs/cocasa/index.html. Accessed October 30, 2011.
28. Screening questionnaires. Immunization Action Coalition Web site. http://www.immunize.org/printmaterials/topic_screening.asp. Accessed October 30, 2011.
29. FDA updated communication on use of jet injectors with inactivated influenza vaccines. FDA Web site. http://www.fda.gov/BiologicsBloodVaccines/Vaccines/QuestionsaboutVaccines/ucm276773.htm. Accessed October 30, 2011.
30. Schechter NL, et al. *Pediatrics*. 2007;119:e1184-e1198.
31. Taddio A, et al. *Clin Ther*. 2009;31(suppl B):S48-S76.
32. Shah V, et al. *Clin Ther*. 2009;31(suppl B):S104-S151.
33. Kroger AT, et al. *MMWR*. 2011;60(RR-2):1-61.
34. Prymula R, et al. *Lancet*. 2009;374:1339-1350.
35. Bohlke K, et al. *Pediatrics*. 2003;112:815-820.
36. Medical management of vaccine reactions in children and teens. Immunization Action Coalition Web site. http://www.immunize.org/catg.d/p3082a.pdf. Accessed October 30, 2011.
37. Medical management of vaccine reactions in adult patients. Immunization Action Coalition Web site. http://www.immunize.org/catg.d/p3082.pdf. Accessed October 30, 2011.
38. CDC. *MMWR*. 2008;57:457-460.
39. Tuck RH. *Pediatr Ann*. 2006;35:507-512.
40. American Medical Association. CPT 2012 Professional Edition. Chicago, IL: AMA Press; 2012.
41. Buck CJ. 2012 ICD-9-CM for Physicians, Professional Edition. Philadelphia, PA: W.B. Saunders; 2012.
42. Office of the Secretary, Department of Health and Human Services. Federal Register. 2009;74:3328-3362 (45 CFR Part 162).
43. National Drug Code Directory. US Food and Drug Administration Web site. http://www.accessdata.fda.gov/scripts/cder/ndc/default.cfm. Accessed October 30, 2011.
44. CDC Vaccine Price List. Centers for Disease Control and Prevention Web site. http://www.cdc.gov/vaccines/programs/vfc/cdc-vac-price-list.htm. Accessed October 30, 2011.
45. Freed GL, et al. *Pediatrics*. 2009;124:S459-S465.

5 General Recommendations

Rules by Which to Vaccinate

5

Vaccine recommendations are complex. The following general rules, derived from the CDC's *General Recommendations on Immunization*,[1] are offered as guidance for day-to-day practice. Just remember—there are exceptions to every rule.

■ Any Vaccines Can Be Given at the Same Time

EXCEPTIONS: ***1) VAR and smallpox vaccine; 2) MCV4-D and PCV13 in anatomically or functionally asplenic children.***

Simultaneous administration of all vaccines for which a person is eligible at a given visit is encouraged for two reasons: achievement of optimal protection is not delayed and completion of all recommended vaccine series is more likely. There are no vaccines that cannot be given at the same time, considering both reactogenicity and immunogenicity, except for 1) VAR and smallpox, where the concern is increased complications of smallpox vaccination, and 2) MCV4-D and PCV13 in asplenic children, where the data suggest the possibility of decreased responses to pneumococcal antigens (MCV4-D should not routinely be given to asplenic children 9 to 23 months of age; if given to asplenic children ≥2 years of age, it should be separated from PCV13 by ≥4 weeks). Vaccines given on the same day must be given at separate sites and should never be mixed in the same syringe unless the products are specifically labeled for that purpose. Licensed combination vaccines can reduce the high number of shots that are now unavoidable at certain visits during childhood.

Package inserts may warn against concomitant use of certain vaccines. For example, the ZOS package insert (June 2011) says to consider separating the vaccine and PPSV23 by ≥4 weeks because the antibody response to VZV might be impaired after simultaneous administration. However, the ACIP considers simultaneous administration acceptable, because lower antibody levels do not necessarily mean reduced protection.

■ Live Vaccines Not Given at the Same Time Should Be Separated by ≥28 Days

EXCEPTIONS: ***1) YFV may be given at any time after single-antigen measles vaccine; 2) Live oral vaccines (RV, typhoid Ty21a, and adenovirus) may be given at any time in relation to any other live vaccines.***

If live vaccines are to be given sequentially, they should be separated by ≥4 weeks so that replication of the first vaccine does not interfere with replication of the second. LAIV, even though it replicates at a mucosal surface (as do oral vaccines, which *are* an exception to this rule), is *not* an exception—if not given on the same day, LAIV and live parenteral vaccines should be administered ≥28 days apart. The 4-day grace period (*Chapter 3: Standards, Principles, and Regulations—Mandates*) does not apply to minimum intervals between live vaccines.

■ **Any Timing Sequence Between Different Inactivated Vaccines, or Between Live and Inactivated Vaccines, is Acceptable**

EXCEPTIONS: ***MCV4-D and PCV13 in anatomically or functionally asplenic children.***

Simultaneous administration, or better yet the use of combination vaccines, is preferred because of improved compliance. However, there is no evidence that sequential administration of *different* inactivated vaccines, or live and inactivated vaccines, at any time interval interferes with immunogenicity or increases reactogenicity. The case of simultaneous administration of MCV4-D and PCV13 is discussed above. The case of sequential administration of Tdap and MCV4-D is a little tricky. While these are ostensibly *different* vaccines, they both contain diphtheria toxoid (it is the carrier protein for the polysaccharide in MCV4-D). The AAP suggests a minimum interval of 1 month between Tdap and MCV4-D if the vaccines are not given on the same day—the concern is that too many doses of diphtheria toxoid in sequence can cause increased reactogenicity. The ACIP, however, does not recommend a minimum interval.

■ **There Are Minimum Acceptable Intervals Between Doses of the Same Vaccine**

EXCEPTIONS: ***1) The 4-day grace period for inactivated vaccines; 2) Early, accelerated, or compressed schedules in certain situations.***

Proper spacing of doses within a given vaccine series is essential for optimal immune responses. For this reason, doses of the same vaccine administered sooner than the specified minimum interval are considered invalid. The 4-day grace period (*Chapter 3: Standards, Principles, and Regulations—Mandates*) applies to inactivated vaccines (except RAB) but does not apply to most live vaccines *(see above)*. Invalid doses should be repeated, but the minimum interval should elapse between the invalid dose and the repeat dose. There are circumstances where early, accelerated, or compressed schedules can be used, such as for catch-up immunization or impending international travel. However, even here the minimum intervals should be followed. **Table 5.1** shows the recommended minimum intervals for routinely used vaccines.

One caveat: a minimum interval is a minimum interval except when it is not. Here are some examples:

- The minimum interval between doses 3 and 4 of DTaP is 6 months. However, if Dose 4 is given ≥4 months after Dose 3, it is considered valid.
- Under 13 years of age, the minimum interval between doses of VAR is 12 weeks, but if Dose 1 is given ≥28 days after Dose 2, it is considered valid (except for immunocompromised persons, for whom doses given <12 weeks apart are considered invalid).
- Dose 3 of HPV should be given ≥24 weeks after Dose 1, but if the interval is ≥16 weeks the dose is considered valid.

5

One could ask why, then, are the respective minimum intervals not 4 months, 28 days, and 16 weeks? One explanation might be that the studies leading to licensure of these vaccines used the longer intervals, but that subsequent studies attest to the safety and immunogenicity of the shorter intervals.

The minimum interval between doses of modern combination vaccines is determined by the component antigen with the longest minimum interval.

■ There Are Minimum Ages for Administration of All Vaccines

EXCEPTIONS: ***HepB and RAB***.

Live parenteral vaccines can be inactivated by circulating maternal antibody, which can persist for as long as a year. Maternal antibody can also interfere with responses to inactivated vaccines.[2,3] Live oral vaccines such as RV have not been studied in children <6 weeks of age. For other vaccines such as Hib, the issue is that administration in the first 6 weeks of life might induce immunologic tolerance. HepB may be given at birth. During measles outbreaks when cases are occurring in infants <1 year of age, and for impending travel outside the United States, measles vaccine can be given before the recommended minimum age of 12 months (and as early as 6 months). Doses given <12 months of age, however, are not counted as part of the routine series. BCG may be given at birth but is not licensed in the United States.

The 4-day grace period *(see above)* applies to minimum ages for both live and inactivated vaccines. The minimum age for modern combination vaccines is determined by the component antigen with the oldest minimum age. **Table 5.1** shows the recommended minimum ages for routinely used vaccines.

■ Partial or Fractional Doses of a Vaccine Should Never Be Used

EXCEPTION: ***None***.

In the past, some practitioners gave "split" doses of vaccines (particularly DTwP) in order to minimize potential reactions. There is no support for this practice, even in premature infants. Less than full doses of vaccines are not valid.

TABLE 5.1 — Minimum Ages and Intervals for Routine Vaccines

		Age		Interval to Next Dose	
Vaccine	Dose Number	Recommended	Minimum	Recommended	Minimum
DTaP	1	2 months	6 weeks	8 weeks	4 weeks
	2	4 months	10 weeks	8 weeks	4 weeks
	3	6 months	14 weeks	6 to 12 months	6 months[a]
	4	15 to 18 months	12 months	3 years	6 months
	5	4 to 6 years	4 years	—	—
HepA	1	12 to 23 months	12 months	6 to 18 months	6 months
	2	≥18 months	18 months	—	—
HepB	1	Birth[b]	Birth[b]	4 weeks to 4 months	4 weeks
	2	1 to 2 months	4 weeks	8 weeks to 17 months	8 weeks[c]
	3	6 to 18 months	24 weeks	—	—
Hib	1[d]	2 months	6 weeks	8 weeks	4 weeks
	2	4 months	10 weeks	8 weeks	4 weeks
	(3)[e]	6 months	14 weeks	6 to 9 months	8 weeks
	4	12 to 15 months	12 months	—	—
HPV	1	11 to 12 years	9 years	8 weeks	4 weeks
	2	11 to 12 years (plus 2 months)	9 years (plus 4 weeks)	4 months	12 weeks[f]

	3	11 to 12 years (plus 6 months)	9 years (plus 24 weeks)	—	—
IIV	1[g]	Annual	6 months[h]	4 weeks	4 weeks
IPV	1	2 months	6 weeks[i]	8 weeks	4 weeks[i]
	2	4 months	10 weeks	8 weeks to 14 months	4 weeks
	3	6 to 18 months	14 weeks	3 to 5 years	6 months
	4[j]	4 to 6 years	4 years	—	(6 months)[j]
LAIV	1[g]	Annual	2 years	4 weeks	4 weeks
MCV[k]	1	11 to 12 years	2 years	5 years	8 weeks
	2	16 years	11 years (plus 8 weeks)		
MMR	1	12 to 15 months	12 months	3 to 5 years	4 weeks[l]
	2	4 to 6 years	13 months	—	—
MPSV[m]	1	—	2 years	5 years	5 years
	2	—	7 years	—	—
PCV	1[d]	2 months	6 weeks	8 weeks	4 weeks[n]
	2	4 months	10 weeks	8 weeks	4 weeks[n]
	3	6 months	14 weeks	6 months	8 weeks[n]
	4	12 to 15 months	12 months	—	(8 weeks)[o]
	(5)[o]	14 to 59 months	14 months	—	—
PPSV[p]	1	—	2 years	5 years	5 years
	2	—	7 years	—	—

Continued

TABLE 5.1 — *Continued*

Vaccine	Dose Number	Age		Interval to Next Dose	
		Recommended	**Minimum**	**Recommended**	**Minimum**
RV[q]	1	2 months	6 weeks	8 weeks	4 weeks
	2	4 months	10 weeks	(8 weeks)	(4 weeks)
	(3)	6 months	14 weeks	—	—
Td	1	11 to 12 years[r]	7 years	10 years	5 years
Tdap	1	≥11 years	7 years[h,s]	—	—
VAR	1	12 to 15 months	12 months	3 to 5 years	12 weeks[l,t]
	2	4 to 6 years	15 months	—	—
Zoster	1	≥60 years	60 years	—	—

Age means that the individual has passed one mark in time but has not yet reached the next relevant mark (see *Front Matter—Conventions Used in This Book*). For example, "2 months of age" means at or beyond the 2-month birthday but not yet at the 3-month birthday. Age intervals are indicated by the word *to*; thus, *4 to 6 years of age* means *from the 4th birthday until the day before the 7th birthday*. *Weeks* are 7 days. Under 4 months, *months* are 28 days; at 4 months and beyond, *months* are *calendar months*, in which case the interval is to the same date in the appropriate month. For example, for an infant vaccinated on January 6, an interval of 6 months would be on July 6.

[a] Dose 4 need not be repeated if given ≥4 months after Dose 3.
[b] Combination products cannot be used for the birth dose.
[c] Dose 3 should be given ≥16 weeks after Dose 1.
[d] Children receiving Dose 1 after 6 months of age require fewer doses.
[e] A dose at 6 months of age is not necessary if Hib-OMP (PedvaxHIB; Merck) is used for Doses 1 and 2.
[f] Dose 3 should be given ≥24 weeks after Dose 1 but need not be repeated if given ≥16 weeks after Dose 1.

[g] Two doses separated by ≥4 weeks are required for children <9 years of age who are being immunized for the first time (if a child turns 9 before the second dose is given, that dose becomes unnecessary). For the 2011-2012 season, children <9 years of age who received ≥1 dose in the prior year only need one dose, even if last year was the first time they were immunized. In past seasons, children <9 years of age who were immunized for the first time in the prior year and received only one dose would have required two doses in the current season. The reason for this is the fact that the vaccine strains did not change from the 2010-2011 to the 2011-2012 seasons.

[h] The minimum age differs by product.

[i] Minimum age and minimum intervals during the first 6 months of life should only be used if the child is at risk of imminent exposure to poliovirus.

[j] Dose 4 is not necessary if Dose 3 was given at ≥4 years of age and ≥6 months after the previous dose. A 5th dose is needed if all previous doses were given before 4 years of age (the final dose of IPV should be given at ≥4 years of age regardless of the number of previous doses). This would apply, for example, if a child received 4 doses of IPV as DTaP-IPV/Hib-T by 18 months of age.

[k] Routine (one-time) revaccination is recommended at 16 years of age for adolescents who received Dose 1 at 11 to 12 years of age. For those who received Dose 1 at 13 to 15 years of age, routine (one-time) revaccination is recommended 5 years later, up to 21 years of age. Persons who are at high risk for meningococcal disease because of immunocompromise (eg, complement deficiency, asplenia, HIV infection) should receive a primary series consisting of 2 doses of MCV given 8 weeks apart, followed by routine revaccination every 5 years (if immunization was initiated at 2 to 6 years of age, the first revaccination should occur in 3 years). MCV4-D is labeled for high-risk infants as young as 9 months of age. Persons at high risk because of prolonged exposure (eg, laboratory workers) should receive a single dose followed by revaccination every 5 years. MPSV should be used instead of MCV for high-risk persons ≥56 years of age. Recommendations for revaccination are off-label, except for 2 doses of MCV4-D at 9 to 23 months of age and a second dose of MCV4-CRM at 2 to 5 years of age.

[l] The minimum interval is 12 weeks if MMRV is used.

[m] MCV is recommended for routine vaccination of adolescents and is preferred for high-risk persons 2 to 55 years of age. MCV4-D is the only product licensed for infants 9 to 23 months of age. MPSV should be used instead of MCV for high-risk persons ≥56 years of age.

[n] At <12 months of age, the minimum interval between doses of PCV is 4 weeks. At ≥12 months of age, the minimum interval is 8 weeks.

[o] PCV7 was used from 2000 through 2009. PCV13 was licensed in February 2010 and replaced PCV7 in the routine schedule. Children who started with PCV7 should have completed the series with PCV13. Those who have received 4 doses of PCV7 and are ≤59 months of age should receive a single supplemental dose of PCV13 (for high-risk children, the single supplemental dose may be given up to 71 months of age). High-risk children between 6 and 18 years of age should receive a single dose of PCV13 (off-label recommendation).

Continued

TABLE 5.1 — *Continued*

[p] PPSV is recommended for children with high-risk conditions after the PCV series is completed. Dose 2 is recommended for children at highest risk. Adults ≥65 years of age should receive a dose of PPSV23. High-risk adults <65 years of age should be vaccinated, with one-time revaccination in 5 years for those at highest risk.

[q] RV1 is given as a 2-dose and RV5 as a 3-dose series. The labeled schedules differ from the ACIP recommendations (ACIP recommendations are usually followed in practice). According to the RV1 package insert (February 2011), Dose 1 may be given between 6 and 20 weeks of age, and no dose should be given beyond 24 weeks. According to the RV5 package insert (July 2011), Dose 1 should be given at 6 to 12 weeks of age, and no dose should be given beyond 32 weeks. ACIP recommends that Dose 1 of either vaccine be given between 6 weeks and 14 weeks 6 days of age and all doses be given by 8 months 0 days. If any dose in the series is RV5 or unknown, a total of 3 doses should be given.

[r] Tdap should be used routinely at 11 to 12 years of age rather than Td.

[s] The minimum labeled age for Boostrix is 10 years and for Adacel 11 years, but either product may be used beginning at 7 years of age (off-label recommendation).

[t] If the second dose is given ≥28 days after the first dose, this should be considered valid and should not be repeated. The minimum interval is 4 weeks if the series is initiated ≥13 years of age. For immunocompromised persons such as those with HIV infection, doses given <12 weeks apart are considered invalid.

Adapted from Kroger AT, et al. *MMWR*. 2011;60(RR-2):1-61.

■ A Multidose Vaccine Series Should Not Be Restarted if the Recommended Dosing Interval Is Exceeded

EXCEPTION: ***Oral typhoid Ty21a.***

If there is a lapse in the administration of sequential doses of a given series, simply begin where the series was suspended, keeping in mind the minimum intervals between doses. The only exception to this rule is the oral typhoid Ty21a vaccine, for which some experts recommend repeating the series if all 4 doses are not given within 3 weeks.

■ Similar Vaccines Made by Different Manufacturers Are Interchangeable

EXCEPTION: ***There is a preference for using the same DTaP, HPV and RV products for the entire series.***

Vaccines from different manufacturers differ in composition, formulation, and content. However, sufficient data exist to consider many of the vaccines made by different manufacturers interchangeable in a given series, including diphtheria toxoid, tetanus toxoid, HepA, HepB, and IPV. Hib vaccines are also interchangeable, but if Hib-T (ActHIB) is used as Dose 1 or Dose 2, the primary series should include 3 doses (an all-Hib-OMP [PedvaxHIB] schedule requires only 2 doses for the primary series). When 2 doses of influenza vaccine are needed in the same season, all brands of IIV are considered interchangeable, provided they are used in the appropriate age groups. There is a preference for using the same *type* of vaccine for 2 doses in the same season (eg, 2 doses of IIV *or* 2 doses of LAIV). However, if the particular type of influenza vaccine that is called for is not available, *use what you have* rather than deferring the dose. Similarly, there is a preference for the same DTaP product for the entire series, but vaccination *should not be deferred* if the same product is not available or if the previous products are not known. Same thing with RV; however, if any one of the doses in the series was RV5 or unknown, 3 total doses should be given (an all-RV1 schedule requires only 2 doses).

Keep in mind that different vaccines for the same disease are not strictly interchangeable. For example, both MCV and MPSV protect against meningococcal disease. However, the former is a protein-polysaccharide conjugate and the latter is a pure polysaccharide, and the recommendations for each differ. The same is true for PCV and PPSV. VAR and ZOS contain the exact same live-attenuated VZV strain (in differing amounts), but the two vaccines are used for entirely different purposes (respectively, prevention of varicella and prevention of herpes zoster). Likewise, DTaP and Tdap may contain the same antigens (in differing amounts) but are used for different purposes (respectively, primary immunization and booster immunization). Finally, whereas both HPV2 and HPV4 protect against cervical cancer, only HPV4 prevents genital warts.

■ There Is No Harm in Vaccinating a Person Who Has Already Had the Disease or the Vaccine

EXCEPTIONS*: 1) Administering too many doses of PPSV, tetanus toxoid, or diphtheria toxoid can cause increased reactogenicity; 2) Anthrax vaccine in persons who have had anthrax disease.*

For some diseases, vaccination is *indicated* even if the person has had the disease. For example, infants <2 years of age who had invasive *H influenzae* infection should still be vaccinated because infection at that age does not confer immunity. ZOS is *specifically designed* to be given to people who have had VZV infection. For *S pneumoniae*, the vaccine protects against multiple serotypes, so prior infection with a particular serotype does not obviate the need for vaccination; similarly, completion of the 4-dose PCV7 schedule does not obviate the need for a dose of PCV13 in children ≤59 months of age, since this confers immunity to 6 additional serotypes. Along similar lines, HPV *should be given* to women who have had cervical dysplasia or other evidence of human papillomavirus infection, not to alter the course of infection (which it does not do) but to protect against other serotypes. Influenza vaccine *must* be given each year whether or not the person has had influenza in the past. Some experts recommend pertussis vaccine for children who have had well-documented pertussis (culture positive or epidemiologically linked to a culture-positive case) because the duration of natural immunity is not known. Clinicians often wonder if a child with a questionable history of chickenpox or varicella vaccination should receive the vaccine. The motto here is—*when in doubt, vaccinate*! With chickenpox, as with most other diseases, there is no evidence of harm if a person who has had the disease or adequate immunization receives another dose of the vaccine (except for anthrax, where there is some evidence that vaccine adverse events are more severe in persons who have had the disease).

■ Live Vaccines Should be Deferred After Receipt of Antibody-Containing Blood Products

EXCEPTIONS*: 1) YFV, oral typhoid Ty21a, LAIV, RV, adenovirus, and ZOS; 2) MMR and VAR should not be deferred in postpartum women who received antibody-containing blood products during pregnancy, including anti-Rho(D) globulin*

Antibodies contained in blood products can inactivate live vaccines and reduce effectiveness or "take." Several factors play into whether or not deferral is recommended and determine the time interval after which a vaccine can be given. One factor is the product itself—immune globulin intravenous is likely to contain more antibody than packed red cells, hence necessitating a longer delay. Another factor is the specific antibody content of the product; for example, blood products in the United States are unlikely to contain antibodies to YF virus and *S typhi*, so these vaccines can be given at any time with respect to blood products. ZOS does not need to be delayed because it is *designed* to be given to persons with antibody to VZV. Finally, passively transferred antibodies are unlikely to inactivate vaccines delivered at mucosal surfaces—hence the exceptions for LAIV, adenovirus, and RV.

Table 5.2 shows the recommended intervals between blood product administration and MMR, VAR, and MMRV. In general, the antibodies in blood products do not interfere with inactivated vaccines. Here are a few other things to know:

- If a child has already received MMR, VAR, or MMRV, 14 days should elapse before an antibody-containing blood product is given, because the vaccine viruses must still replicate in order to induce immunity.
- If a pregnant woman receives a blood product, that should not result in deferral of her infant's first dose of RV.
- Monoclonal antibody products such as RSV-mAB (Synagis) do not interfere with live vaccines.

■ Administration Errors

Sometimes, despite the best of intentions, mistakes are made in vaccine administration. **Table 5.3** lists some common administration errors and gives recommendations to remedy the situation. Some common themes apply. For example, vaccine doses given by the wrong route (IM instead of SC or vice versa) are generally valid—except in the case of HepB and RAB, for which doses given SC are invalid.

■ More Vaccination Pearls

Here are some additional vaccination pearls (more can be found in *Chapter 4: Vaccine Practice—Administration*):

- Serology is of limited utility in vaccine practice. Testing for varicella antibodies before vaccination might be cost-effective in adults who do not have a personal history of chickenpox. However, in most other circumstances vaccines should be given without testing for immunity. This would include internationally adopted children with a questionable vaccination history—it is probably better just to reimmunize than to test for immunity to multiple antigens, some of which do not have known serological correlates of protection.

  For the most part, immunity is presumed to result from appropriate vaccine schedules and doses. With measles, for example, immunity is presumed if the person received 2 valid doses of MMR at the right ages and with appropriate minimum intervals—even if serological results are negative and even for HCP. Testing for seroconversion is indicated only rarely, such as in high-risk HCP or dialysis patients given HepB, laboratory workers receiving pre-exposure

TABLE 5.2 — Interval Between Receipt of Antibody-Containing Products and Administration of MMR, VAR, or MMRV[a]

Product (Route)	Indication	Usual Dose	Duration of Deferral
RSVmAB (IM)	Prevention of RSV disease	15 mg/kg	None[b]
IGIM	Hepatitis A prophylaxis:		
	Postexposure and short-term travel	0.02 (3.3 mg/kg)	3 months
	Long-term travel	0.06 mL/kg (10 mg/kg)	3 months
	Measles prophylaxis:		
	Standard	0.25 mL/kg (40 mg/kg)	5 months
	Immunocompromised[c]	0.5 mL/kg (80 mg/kg)	6 months
IGIV	Replacement therapy for immune deficiency[c]	400 mg/kg	8 months
	Postexposure prophylaxis for varicella	400 mg/kg	8 months
	Immune thrombocytopenic purpura	400 mg/kg	8 months
		1 g/kg	10 months
	Kawasaki disease	2 g/kg	11 months
Blood transfusion (IV)	Red blood cells:		
	Washed	—	None
	Adenine-saline added	10 mL/kg	3 months
	Packed	10 mL/kg	6 months
	Whole blood	10 mL/kg	6 months
	Plasma or platelet products	10 mL/kg	7 months

CMV-IGIV	Prevention of CMV disease in transplant patients[c]	150 mg/kg	6 months
HBIG (IM)	Postexposure prophylaxis for hepatitis B	0.06 mL/kg (10 mg/kg)	3 months
HRIG (IM and intrawound)	Postexposure prophylaxis for rabies	20 IU/kg (22 mg/kg)	4 months
RhoGAM (IM)	Prevention of maternal Rh isoimmunization	300 mcg	None[d]
TIG (IM)	Postexposure prophylaxis for tetanus	250 units (10 mg/kg)	3 months
VariZIG (IM)[e]	Postexposure prophylaxis for varicella	125 units/10 kg	5 months

[a] Other live vaccines (LAIV, RV, adenovirus, Ty21a, YFV, and ZOS) do not need to be deferred after receipt of antibody-containing blood products. Passively acquired antibodies would be unlikely to inactivate vaccines given at mucosal surfaces, like RV, adenovirus, LAIV, and Ty21a. In addition, blood products in the United States are unlikely to contain substantial amounts of antibody to *Salmonella typhi* and YF virus, and antibody to last year's influenza viruses might not be effective against this year's strains. ZOS is normally given to people who already have circulating antibodies to VZV.

[b] This is a monoclonal product that contains no antibody to the vaccine viruses.

[c] Live viral vaccines may be contraindicated in these patients.

[d] Administration of live vaccines, if indicated, to postpartum women should not be delayed if antibody-containing products were given during the last trimester (this includes RhoGAM). Likewise, the infant's immunization with rotavirus vaccine should not be delayed.

[e] This product is licensed in Canada and is available in the United States under an investigational new-drug application expanded-access protocol.

Adapted from Kroger AT, et al. *MMWR*. 2011;60(RR-2):1-61.

TABLE 5.3 — Administration Errors and Corrective Actions

Vaccine Involved	Administration Error	Why This Is Incorrect	Corrective Action to be Taken
Any	Expired or damaged inactivated vaccine given	Vaccines should be used before expiration date; damaged vaccines should not be used	Give nonexpired or undamaged vaccine as soon as error is discovered
	Expired or damaged live vaccine given	Vaccines should be used before expiration date; damaged vaccines should not be used	Give nonexpired or undamaged vaccine on same day or 4 weeks later
	Less-than-full dose of inactivated vaccine given	Correct dose should be used	Give correct dose of vaccine as soon as error is discovered
	Less-than-full dose of live vaccine given[a]	Correct dose should be used	Give correct dose of vaccine on same day or 4 weeks later
	More-than-full dose of vaccine given	Correct dose should be used	None—dose is valid
	Subcutaneously-administered vaccine (VAR, ZOS, MMR, MMRV, YFV, MPSV4) given intramuscularly	These vaccines should be given subcutaneously	None—dose is valid
DTaP	Dose given to adolescent or adult	Tdap should be used	None—dose is valid[b]
DTaP-IPV (Kinrix)	Dose given to child 15 to 18 months of age as Dose 4 of DTaP	DTaP-IPV only indicated for Dose 5 of DTaP and Dose 4 of IPV in children 4 to 6 years of age	None—DTaP dose is valid

DTaP-IPV (liquid component of Pentacel)	Dose given to child as any dose of DTaP or IPV	DTaP-IPV liquid component should only be used as part of Pentacel (after reconstitution of lyophilized Hib component)[c]	None—dose is valid
HepB	Dose given subcutaneously	Should be given intramuscularly	Give HepB intramuscularly as soon as error is discovered
	Dose given to an adult in the gluteal muscle	Should be given in deltoid muscle	Give HepB in deltoid muscle as soon as error is discovered
Hib-T (Hiberix)	Dose given as part of primary Hib series	Hiberix licensed only for the booster dose	None—dose is valid
LAIV	Dose given to person receiving influenza antivirals within 48 hours before or 2 weeks after dose	Antivirals can inhibit immune response	Give IIV as soon as error is discovered, or give LAIV 4 weeks later (if person is not on antivirals at that time)
	Dose given <4 weeks after dose of MMR, VAR, or MMRV	Replication of first vaccine viruses could interfere with immune response to LAIV	Give IIV as soon as error is discovered, or give LAIV 4 weeks later
MCV4-D or MCV4-CRM	Dose given subcutaneously	Should be given intramuscularly	None—dose is valid

Continued

TABLE 5.3 — *Continued*

Vaccine Involved	Administration Error	Why This Is Incorrect	Corrective Action to be Taken
MCV4-CRM	Liquid component (serogroups C, W-135, Y) given alone	Product licensed only as a 4-valent vaccine wherein liquid component is used to reconstitute lyophilized serogroup A component	Discard remaining vial of lyophilized vaccine Dose is valid if recipient does not plan to travel outside U.S. (not protected against serogroup A) If travel planned, give MCV4-D or correctly reconstituted MCV4-CRM as soon as error is discovered
PPSV	Dose given to child <2 years of age	PCV should be used	Give PCV as soon as error is discovered
RAB	Dose given to adult or child in gluteal muscle	Should be given in anterolateral thigh (infant) or deltoid (older child and adult)	Give RAB in appropriate muscle as soon as error is discovered
	Dose given subcutaneously	RAB should only be given intramuscularly	Give dose in the appropriate muscle as soon as error is discovered
Tdap	Dose given to infant or child as part of primary series	DTaP should be used	Give DTaP as soon as error is discovered
	Dose given to infant or child as Dose 4 or 5 in series	DTaP should be used	None—dose is valid

VAR	Dose given to adult ≥60 years of age for prevention of shingles	ZOS should be used	Give ZOS at same visit or 4 weeks later
ZOS	Dose given to a child for prevention of varicella	VAR should be used	None—dose is valid

[a] Exceptions: sneezing or blowing nose after LAIV administration, and vomiting, spitting up, or regurgitating after RV administration.
[b] Counts as the one-time dose of Tdap.
[c] The remaining lyophilized Hib component of Pentacel can only be used if reconstituted with the DTaP-IPV liquid component of Pentacel or the 0.4% saline diluent for ActHIB.

rabies vaccination, and in some cases where individuals received invalid doses. In fact, testing for antibody may give you information you did not want in the first place! For example, healthy persons who receive 3 doses of HepB are presumed to be immune, and serological testing is not recommended except in high-risk groups. What should you do about a (usual-risk) child who is (for some reason) found to be HBsAb-negative, despite 3 doses of HepB at appropriate ages and intervals? Options include 1) doing nothing and assuming protection based on adequate immunization history (antibody may have waned, but the person is probably still protected), and 2) giving a dose of HepB and looking for an anemnestic response in 4 to 6 weeks. If this occurs, the child likely responded to the initial series and at this point is protected. If it does not occur, you should make sure the person is HBsAg-negative (chronic carriage can lead to low levels of HBsAb), then give the remaining 2 doses of the second HepB series. If he remains negative after this, he is a non-responder and should be managed accordingly if there is an exposure to hepatitis B.

- A physical examination is not required for vaccination of healthy persons.
- There is no maximum number of vaccinations that can be given on a single day.
- Syringes should not be prefilled by the end user. This increases the risk of administration error and raises stability and storage issues. The one exception is mass influenza immunization campaigns where only one vaccine type is being used. In this situation, a small number of syringes can be prepared and labeled in advance; they should be used soon after filling, and unused syringes should be discarded. Many vaccines are now supplied in single-use, prefilled syringes.

Contraindications and Precautions

A *contraindication* is a condition that *increases the likelihood of a serious adverse event*; when present, the vaccine in question should not be given. The only permanent contraindication for all routine vaccines is severe allergy or anaphylaxis to the vaccine or any of its components. Severe allergy is IgE-mediated, occurs in minutes to hours, and requires medical attention. Examples include generalized urticaria, facial swelling, airway obstruction, wheezing, anaphylaxis, hypotension, and shock. Delayed-type hypersensitivity occurs by a different mechanism and is generally not a contraindication to vaccination. Most vaccines contain buffers as well as excipients, which are substances other than the vaccine that are included in the manufacturing process or added to the final product (excipients are listed in the relevant vaccine tables in *Section B*, and the more common relevant allergies are listed as contraindications). In addition, there may be contaminating substances that carry over from early steps in processing, and some vial stoppers and syringes contain latex, which can carry over to the patient during injection. Both excipients and contaminants can be triggers for allergic reactions in sensitized patients.

Acute encephalopathy within 7 days of receipt of a pertussis-containing vaccine is a permanent contraindication for DTaP and Tdap, based on the theoretical possibility of exacerbation or recurrence of encephalopathy. Pregnancy is a contraindication for live vaccines based on theoretical risks to the fetus and the possibility that naturally occurring birth defects might be attributed to the vaccine (see *Chapter 6: Vaccination in Special Circumstances—Pregnancy and Breast-Feeding*). However, there is no definitive evidence of fetal damage from any live vaccine except smallpox. In addition, in some circumstances, the benefits may outweigh the risks; for example, YFV can be considered for pregnant women traveling to high-risk areas. Although live vaccines are generally contraindicated in immunocompromised persons, there may be situations where the benefits outweigh the risks. For example, natural varicella probably represents a greater risk to a DiGeorge syndrome patient with mildly impaired cellular immunity than does the live-attenuated vaccine.

A *precaution* is a condition that *might increase the risk of a serious adverse event, compromise the immunogenicity* of the vaccine, or *be mistaken for a vaccine reaction*. Moderate-to-severe acute illness with or without fever is a precaution for all vaccines because of the difficulty distinguishing natural illnesses from vaccine reactions. Understanding what to do when a precaution is noted is sometimes difficult. In general, vaccination should be deferred. However, the risks of deferral (susceptibility to disease) must be weighed against the risks of vaccination (largely theoretical). In making these judgments, the provider must take into account the prevailing epidemiology of the disease, the patient's personal circumstances, and the possibility that an opportunity for vaccination will be missed. Here is an example. A 2-month-old experiences 4 hours of inconsolable crying immediately after Dose 1 of DTaP. This would constitute a precaution to the administration of Dose 2 at 4 months of age. However, because the risk of a recurrence of inconsolable crying is low, the consequences of crying are not permanent, and the risk of pertussis is appreciable, the provider may elect to give Dose 2. Here is another example. A provider may elect to give the 6-month shots to an infant with a moderate febrile illness (a precaution for all vaccines) *if* there is substantial risk that the child will not return for vaccination after the illness resolves.

Sometimes it is difficult to know when a condition is a "contraindication" or a "precaution" (package inserts also contain "warnings," but it is not clear how these differ from "precautions" in terms of actions to be taken). Here's an example: the ACIP states that HPV is "not recommended for use in pregnancy,"[4] and the HPV2 (July 2011) and HPV4 (April 2011) package inserts state that the vaccines are "not recommended for use in pregnant women." However, pregnancy is listed as a *precaution* (not *contraindication*) in the *General Recommendations*[1] and does not even appear in the *Contraindications* or *Warnings and Precautions* sections of either package insert (it is in the *Patient Counseling Information* section). Moreover, both vaccines are registered under Pregnancy Category B, as opposed to the much more ominous Category D (see *Chapter 6: Vaccination in Special Circumstances—Pregnancy and Breast-Feeding*).

Here is another example: based on recent study results, in June 2010[5] the ACIP removed a personal history of GBS as a precaution to administration of MCV. However, the MCV4-D package insert (November 2011) still lists GBS in *Warnings and Precautions* section. The MCV4-CRM package insert (March 2011) lists GBS under *Warnings and Precautions* but states that data are not available to evaluate the potential risk of GBS following vaccine administration. All of this can be very confusing! In *Section B*, each vaccine table lists contraindications and precautions, to be interpreted, respectively, as "do not vaccinate in these situations" and "defer vaccination in these situations, unless the benefits outweigh the risks."

Misconceptions about vaccine contraindications can result in missed opportunities. **Table 5.4** lists some erroneous contraindications; if present, vaccines can and should be given.

TABLE 5.4 — Erroneous Contraindications to Vaccination

- Mild acute illness, with or without fever
- Mild respiratory illness (including most cases of otitis media)
- Mild gastroenteritis
- Antibiotic or antiviral therapy[a]
- Low-grade or moderate fever and/or local redness, pain, and swelling after a previous dose
- Prematurity[b]
- Pregnant or immunosuppressed household contact[c]
- Unimmunized household contact
- Breast-feeding[c]
- Convalescent phase of illness
- Exposure to an infectious disease
- Positive tuberculin skin test without active disease[d]
- Simultaneous tuberculin skin test (TST) or interferon-gamma release assay (IGRA)[e]
- Allergy to penicillin, duck meat or feathers, or environmental allergens
- Fainting after a previous dose
- Seizures, sudden infant death syndrome, allergies, or vaccine adverse events in family members
- Malnutrition
- Lack of previous physical examination in a well-appearing individual
- Stable neurologic condition (eg, cerebral palsy, well-controlled seizure disorder, developmental delay)
- Allergy shots
- Extensive limb swelling after DTwP, DTaP, or Td that is not an Arthus-type reaction
- Brachial neuritis after previous dose of tetanus toxoid-containing vaccine
- Autoimmune disease
- Having had the disease that the vaccine is designed to prevent[f]

[a] Antibiotics could interfere with live bacterial vaccines (eg, Ty21a), and antivirals could interfere with live viral vaccines (eg, VAR).

[b] The birth dose of HepB should be delayed (because of poor immunogenicity) in infants weighing <2000 g whose mothers are HBsAg-negative.

[c] Pre-event smallpox vaccination is an exception.

[d] MMR, VAR and ZOS should not be given to patients with active, untreated tuberculosis.

[e] Measles vaccine can temporarily suppress the response to a TST and may cause false negative IGRA results. If testing for tuberculosis is warranted, the preferred option is to place a TST or perform an IGRA on the same day as measles vaccination. Otherwise, the tuberculosis test should be delayed ≥4 weeks.

Continued

TABLE 5.4 — *Continued*

[f] Immunity from natural infection may wane with time, as in the case of pertussis. Alternatively, the vaccine (eg, HPV, MCV, PCV, RV) might protect against serotypes to which the individual has not been previously exposed. Anthrax is an exception.

Adapted from Kroger AT, et al. *MMWR*. 2011;60(RR-2):1-61. *More detail can be found in individual vaccine sections.*

REFERENCES

1. Kroger AT, et al. *MMWR*. 2011;60(RR-2):1-61.
2. Sarvas H, et al. *J Infect Dis*. 1992;165:977-979.
3. Jones CE, et al. *JAMA*. 2011;305:576-584.
4. CDC. *MMWR*. 2010;59:626-630.
5. ACIP Summary Report, June 23-24, 2010. Centers for Disease Control and Prevention Web site. http://www.cdc.gov/vaccines/recs/acip/downloads/min-jun10.pdf. Accessed October 15, 2011.

6 Vaccination in Special Circumstances

General Considerations for Patients With Impaired Immunity

Vaccination of patients with impaired immunity requires special consideration for a number of reasons:

- *The balance between risks and benefits is complex*—Immunocompromised persons are at greater risk for complications and death from vaccine-preventable diseases. At the same time, they may be at increased risk for complications from live vaccines, and the response to all vaccines may be suboptimal. Decisions regarding vaccination are therefore more complicated than for healthy persons and must take into account the prevalence of disease and probability of exposure, the nature and degree of immunodeficiency, the type of vaccine and the likelihood of adverse events, the efficacy of the vaccine when immunity is impaired, and the confounding effects of other interventions. Unfortunately, in many situations there are few data available to provide guidance.
- *Immunocompromised states differ qualitatively*—Qualitative differences dictate not only which vaccines are indicated but which vaccines represent a danger to the patient. Congenital immunodeficiencies may affect humoral immunity, cell-mediated immunity, phagocyte function, or complement function in different and interconnected ways. Humoral immune defects place patients at higher risk for invasive infection with encapsulated bacteria, demanding special consideration for vaccination against *H influenzae* type b, *S pneumoniae*, and *N meningitidis*. Whereas isolated humoral defects do not increase the risk of serious varicella per se, they may predispose the patient to bacterial complications of varicella. Therefore, VAR is indicated in patients with isolated humoral defects—as long as they are not receiving immune globulin intravenous (IGIV), in which case the vaccine is unlikely to be effective because antibodies in the IGIV will inactivate the vaccine virus. Similarly, phagocyte dysfunction per se does not substantially weaken defenses against influenza virus, but it does increase the risk of bacterial superinfection. Thus patients with chronic granulomatous disease, whose neutrophils fail to undergo oxidative burst, should be on the high priority list for influenza vaccine in order to prevent bacterial pneumonia. Complement deficiencies put patients at risk for

bacterial infections but carry no implications for the safety of live or inactivated vaccines. Secondary immune deficiency states, such as those resulting from immunosuppressive medications, nephrotic syndrome, malnutrition, splenectomy, or bone marrow transplantation, also differ qualitatively from one another.

- *Immunocompromised states differ quantitatively*—In general, patients with cell-mediated immune defects should not receive live vaccines because of the risk of dissemination. However, cellular defects may range from mild to profound, and these differences affect the risk-benefit assessment for vaccination. For example, whereas VAR *should be avoided* in an HIV-infected person with very low CD4 count, poor T-cell function, and a history of opportunistic infections, it *should be given* to a mildly symptomatic HIV-infected child whose CD4 percentages are consistently ≥15%. In the former situation, the risk of vaccination is too great; in the latter, the risk of vaccination is small and is outweighed by the potential consequences of natural disease. Similarly, MMR may be given to HIV-infected children without severe immunosuppression as determined by CD4 counts. DiGeorge syndrome, a quantitative T-cell deficiency resulting from thymic dysplasia, is quite variable in expression. Whereas those patients with low CD4 and CD8 counts and abnormal T-cell function should not receive live vaccines, live vaccines are probably safe in those patients with normal T-cell studies.
- *Immune responses may be suboptimal*—Some patients with immune deficiencies are not expected to respond at all to vaccination. Patients with X-linked agammaglobulinemia (XLA), for example, do not make antibody, so administration of inactivated vaccines would seem to be futile. Live vaccines such as MMR and VAR would theoretically be useful in XLA patients because these vaccines engender T-cell responses (of which XLA patients are fully capable), were it not for the fact that XLA patients receive IGIV infusions that would inactivate the vaccines. Fortunately, the very same antibodies in IGIV that prevent the "take" of MMR and VAR also protect XLA patients from natural measles, mumps, rubella, and varicella. An outstanding question is whether there might be enough of a T-cell response to some inactivated vaccines—IIV, for example—to justify their use in these patients. Patients with common variable immunodeficiency may or may not respond to vaccination, so in general it is worth a try. Some patients who have normal concentrations of immune globulin may *still* not respond appropriately to certain vaccines. In fact, this constitutes an operational definition of *antibody deficiency with normal immunoglobulins*

or *antibody dysfunction syndrome*, most often diagnosed by failure to respond to PPSV23. In some cases, more intensive immunization regimens are necessary to achieve protective immunity.

- *Immunization of close contacts is important*—Immunocompromised patients can be protected by ensuring that close contacts, especially other household members, are appropriately immunized. For example, AIDS patients may not respond well to influenza vaccine but can be protected from influenza by immunizing family members. Likewise, HepA should be given to contacts of immunosuppressed persons if the family resides in a high-incidence area. Live vaccines carry the theoretical risk of transmission from vaccinees to immunocompromised contacts, in which they could cause disease. A historical example of this is vaccine-associated poliomyelitis resulting from transmission of OPV within the home. However, the risk of transmission varies by vaccine, and some live vaccines carry no risk of transmission at all. Likewise, the consequences of transmission range from demonstrably serious (eg, smallpox vaccine) to only theoretical (eg, RV). **Table 6.1** summarizes recommendations for use of live vaccines in household contacts of immunocompromised persons.

TABLE 6.1 — Use of Live Vaccines in Household Contacts of Immunocompromised Persons

Vaccine	Recommendation
Adenovirus	May be used (good hand hygiene around vaccinee)
LAIV	Contraindicated if the household contact is profoundly immunosuppressed[a]
MMR	May be used
MMRV	May be used (avoid direct contact if vaccinee develops skin lesions, until the lesions resolve)
RV	May be used (use good hand hygiene around vaccinee)
Smallpox	Contraindicated
Ty21a	May be used (use good hand hygiene around vaccinee)
VAR	May be used (avoid direct contact if vaccinee develops skin lesions, until the lesions resolve)
YFV	May be used
ZOS	May be used (avoid direct contact if vaccinee develops skin lesions, until the lesions resolve)

[a] One of the few examples of this is a bone marrow transplant patient who requires a special protective environment.

- *Official recommendations may differ from product labels*—Many package inserts list immunodeficiency states as contraindications to vaccination. This labeling derives from studies on file with the FDA at the time of licensure, which generally do not include data in immunocompromised persons. Subsequent recommendations may be discordant with product labeling because of the availability of new data or reasoned re-evaluations of the pertinent risks and benefits. Practitioners should be aware of these discrepancies. For example, the VAR package insert lists primary and acquired immunodeficiency states as contraindications to vaccination (it even lists a family history of congenital or hereditary immunodeficiency, unless the patient's immune competence has been demonstrated). The official recommendations, however, allow for vaccination of certain persons in these circumstances.
- *Passive immunoprophylaxis may be indicated*—Even though persons who receive IGIV on a monthly basis are probably protected against measles and varicella, in the case of exposure consideration should be given to shortening the interval to the next dose by 1 or 2 weeks.[1] Other immunocompromised persons at risk for serious measles should receive intramuscular immune globulin (IGIM; 0.5 mL/kg, maximum 15 mL) within 6 days of exposure. The AAP recommends immune globulin prophylaxis for *all* HIV-infected children and adolescents exposed to measles, regardless of vaccination status, degree of symptoms, and level of immunosuppression (the dose for asymptomatic HIV-infected persons is 0.25 mL/kg);[2] the ACIP specifies prophylaxis only for *symptomatic* HIV infection.[3]

  Varicella zoster immune globulin (VariZIG) should be given within 96 hours of exposure to immunosuppressed persons who are not immune to chickenpox (see **Table 26.2** for definition of immunity; persons with immunity who later become immunosuppressed are considered immune). The only product available in the United States is VariZIG, but this must be obtained under an investigational new drug protocol (FFF Enterprises, phone number 800-843-7477). IGIV can be used if VariZIG is not available. Chemoprophylaxis with acyclovir (20 mg/kg/dose given 4 times per day, maximum dose 800 mg) is another option. If used, it should be given for 7 days beginning about a week after exposure—this is intended to limit the primary viremia. Susceptible HIV-infected persons without evidence of immunosuppression do not need immunoprophylaxis.

  Tetanus immune globulin should be administered to HIV-infected children with tetanus-prone wounds, regardless of their immunization status.

Immune Deficiency States Other Than HIV Infection

Here are some general guidelines for vaccination of persons with impaired immunity other than that due to HIV infection.[1,4] In general, universally recommended vaccines should be given unless contraindicated for safety reasons or likely to be ineffective.

6

■ B-cell (Humoral) Deficiencies

- *Typical syndromes*:[5] XLA, common variable immunodeficiency, IgA deficiency, IgG subclass deficiency, antibody deficiency with normal immunoglobulins (vaccine nonresponder state or antibody dysfunction syndrome), transient hypogammaglobulinemia of infancy
- *Safety issues*: YFV is contraindicated. LAIV, smallpox vaccine, and Ty21a are contraindicated in severe deficiencies but may be considered in less severe conditions. VAR and MMR may be considered in patients who are not receiving IGIV. Patients with selective IgA deficiency can receive all vaccines safely. RV is probably safe to use in humoral deficiencies, but these conditions are seldom diagnosed before children become age-ineligible for vaccination.
- *Special considerations*: Optimizing immunity to *S pneumoniae* (**Table 6.2**) is important, but vaccine response may be impaired. Inactivated vaccines are not effective in patients with severe deficiencies of immune globulin synthesis. Since many of these patients receive monthly IGIV, live viral vaccines are unlikely to be effective as they are neutralized by passively acquired antibodies. Less severely affected persons who are not receiving IGIV may benefit from vaccination, including MMR and VAR; in these cases, postvaccination antibody titers may be used to confirm responses.

■ T-cell (Combined Humoral and Cell-Mediated) Deficiencies

- *Typical syndromes*:[5] severe combined immunodeficiency, DiGeorge syndrome, hyper-IgM syndrome (CD40 or CD40 ligand deficiency), bare lymphocyte syndrome, autoimmune polyendocrinopathy-candidiasis-ectodermal dystrophy (chronic mucocutaneous candidiasis), Wiskott-Aldrich syndrome, ataxia-telangiectasia
- *Safety issues*: Live vaccines are contraindicated in complete deficiencies but may be considered in partial deficiencies (for example, VAR may be considered in DiGeorge syndrome patients with minimal T-cell dysfunction).
- *Special considerations*: Optimizing immunity to *H influenzae* (completing the primary series of Hib plus the booster in young children and giving one dose for persons ≥6 years

TABLE 6.2 — Optimizing Immunity to *S pneumoniae* Among Persons at High Risk[a]

Current Age	PCV13 History	Vaccine Regimen
<2 years	Infant series incomplete[b]	Complete PCV13 series[b]
2 to 5 years	<3 doses before 24 months of age	2 doses of PCV13[c] then PPSV23[d,e]
	3 doses before 24 months of age	1 dose of PCV13[c] then PPSV23[d,e]
	4 doses before 24 months of age	PPSV23[d,e]
6 to 18 years	0 doses[f]	1 dose of PCV13[c] then PPSV23[d,e]
	1 dose[f]	PPSV23[d,e]
19 to 64 years	—	PPSV23[e,g]
≥65 years	—	PPSV23[e,g,h]

[a] High-risk conditions are categorized as follows:
Underlying medical conditions: chronic heart disease (including cyanotic congenital heart disease; heart failure; cardiomyopathies [but not including hypertension alone]); chronic lung disease (including adults ≥19 years of age with asthma); children with asthma who are on high-dose oral steroids; adults ≥19 years of age who smoke; chronic obstructive pulmonary disease; emphysema; diabetes; cerebrospinal fluid leaks; cochlear implants; alcoholism; chronic liver disease (including cirrhosis).
Anatomic or functional asplenia: sickle cell disease and other hemoglobinopathies; congenital or acquired asplenia; splenic dysfunction.
Immunocompromise: HIV infection; chronic renal failure; nephrotic syndrome; treatment with immunosuppressive medications (including cancer chemotherapy); immunosuppressive radiation therapy; hematologic malignancies (including lymphoma and Hodgkin's disease); metastatic cancer; solid organ transplantation; primary immunodeficiency (including humoral, combined humoral and cellular, complement, and phagocyte defects [except for chronic granulomatous disease]).

[b] What constitutes a complete series in infants and young children is dependent on age and the presence of underlying conditions. The schedule for healthy infants is a dose at 2, 4, 6, and 12 to 15 months of age (4 total doses); those who initiate the series between 7 and 11 months of age need 2 doses followed by a booster at 12 to 15 months (3 total doses), and those who initiate the series between 12 and 23 months of age need only

2 doses. For children <2 years of age with high-risk conditions, any series of <4 doses is considered incomplete; at ≥2 years of age, <2 doses is considered incomplete.

[c] The minimum interval between doses of PCV13 is 4 weeks <1 year of age and 8 weeks ≥1 year of age. PCV13 should be given even if the patient has previously received PPSV23. Use of PCV13 at 6 to 49 years of age is off-label.

[d] PPSV23 should be given ≥8 weeks after the last dose of PCV13.

[e] One-time revaccination with PPSV23 in 5 years is indicated for persons with anatomic or functional asplenia or immunocompromise (keep in mind that no one should receive more than 2 lifetime doses of PPSV23).

[f] Includes patients who previously received PCV7.

[g] PCV13 is labeled for use in persons ≥50 years of age.

[h] PPSV23 is recommended for all persons ≥65 years of age. Those who received a dose before 65 years of age should receive a second dose ≥5 years after the first dose. No more than 2 lifetime doses are recommended.

Adapted from Nuorti JP, et al. *MMWR*. 2010;59:1102-1106 and Nuorti JP, et al. *MMWR*. 2010;59(RR-11):1-19.

of age [off-label recommendation]), *N meningitidis* (**Table 6.3**), and *S pneumoniae* (**Table 6.2**) is important, but vaccine responses may be impaired.

Phagocyte Disorders

- *Typical syndromes*:[6] chronic granulomatous disease, leukocyte adhesion deficiency, Chédiak-Higashi syndrome, myeloperoxidase deficiency, hyper-IgE/recurrent infection syndrome (Job's syndrome), secondary granule deficiency
- *Safety issues*: Live bacterial vaccines (eg, Ty21a) are contraindicated.
- *Special considerations*: Optimizing immunity to *S pneumoniae* (**Table 6.2**) is important, but vaccine response may be impaired (patients with chronic granulomatous disease are an exception because they are not at increased risk). Effective responses to all routine vaccines probably occur. Influenza vaccine helps reduce the risk of secondary bacterial infection.

Complement Deficiencies

- *Typical syndromes*:[7] deficiency of individual early (C1-C4) or late (C5-C9) components, properdin, mannose-binding lectin, Factor D, or Factor I, secondary deficiency due to complement consumption, iatrogenic deficiency induced by eculizumab (a monoclonal antibody to C5 that is used to treat paroxysmal nocturnal hemoglobinuria and atypical hemolytic uremic syndrome)
- *Safety issues*: All vaccines can be used.
- *Special considerations*: Optimizing immunity to *N meningitidis* (**Table 6.3**) and *S pneumoniae* (**Table 6.2**) is important, but vaccine responses may be impaired. Patients with late component deficiencies are uniquely susceptible to infection with *N meningitidis*. Influenza vaccine helps reduce the risk of secondary bacterial infection.

Anatomic and Functional Asplenia

- *Typical syndromes*:[8] congenital, traumatic, or surgical asplenia, sickle cell disease, polysplenia syndrome, chronic graft-versus-host disease (GVHD), celiac disease, alcoholic liver disease
- *Safety issues*: All vaccines can be used.
- *Special considerations*: Because of impaired clearance of opsonized bacteria, coordination of lymphocyte responses, and synthesis of IgM and phagocytosis-enhancing factors, these patients are at risk for life-threatening infection with encapsulated organisms, particularly *S pneumoniae*. Optimizing immunity to *H influenzae* (completing the primary series of Hib plus the booster in young children and giving one dose for persons ≥6 years of age [off-label recommendation]), *N meningitidis* (**Table 6.3**), and *S pneumoniae* (**Table**

6.2) is important, but vaccine responses may be impaired. In addition, yearly IIV should be given, beginning at 6 months of age, to prevent secondary bacterial infection. Family members should be immunized as well. Live vaccines may be given, but keep in mind that LAIV is contraindicated in persons who have chronic pulmonary, cardiovascular (except hypertension), renal, hepatic, neurologic, neuromuscular, hematologic, or metabolic disorders. Prophylactic antibiotics are indicated in certain individuals.

6

Immunity to encapsulated bacteria should be optimized at least 2 weeks before *elective splenectomy*. For children <2 years of age, accelerated schedules for PCV13 and Hib should be used, based on the minimum allowable ages and intervals (**Table 5.1**); in addition, a 2-dose series of MCV4-D may be given at 9 to 23 months of age. For adults, and for children who have already received 4 doses of PCV13, a dose of PPSV23 should be given. Children up to 18 years of age who have not had 4 doses of PCV13 should receive a dose of PCV13 (use of PCV13 at 6 to 49 years of age is off-label). Adults should receive a dose of Hib (off-label recommendation). A dose of MCV4 (2 to 55 years of age) or MPSV4 (≥56 years of age) should be given. After splenectomy, one-time revaccination with PPSV23 in 5 years and revaccination with MCV4 every 5 years (off-label recommendation) is indicated (at ≥56 years of age, MPSV4 should be used).

HIV Infection

Vaccine practice in HIV-infected persons depends on the degree of immunosuppression[9,10]:

- *Perinatally exposed infants whose HIV status is indeterminate*—These patients should receive all routine vaccines, including RV. With appropriate testing *(see below)*, infants will generally be discovered to be HIV-infected or not infected by 4 months of age.
- *Perinatally exposed infants who are presumptively or definitively not infected with HIV*—HIV infection is presumptively excluded in nonbreastfed infants with negative virologic tests (eg, PCR) at ≥14 days and ≥1 month of age, or one negative virologic test at ≥2 months of age, or one negative HIV antibody test at ≥6 months of age; definitive exclusion requires negative virologic tests at ≥1 month and ≥4 months of age, or 2 negative antibody tests at ≥6 months of age.[11] Infants in this category should receive all routine vaccines. It should be mentioned that infants of HIV-infected mothers may have lower antibody levels to vaccine-preventable diseases during the first few weeks of life, even if they themselves are not infected.[12]

TABLE 6.3 — Optimizing Immunity to *N meningitidis* Among Persons at High Risk

	High-Risk Category	
Current Age	**Immunocompromise**[a]	**Exposure**[b]
9 to 23 months	2 doses of MCV4-D 3 months apart[c] Revaccinate 3 years later, then revaccinate every 5 years[d]	2 doses of MCV4-D 3 months apart
2 to 6 years	2 doses of MCV4 ≥8 weeks apart[c,d] Revaccinate 3 years later, then revaccinate every 5 years[d]	1 dose of MCV4[e]
7 to 55 years	2 doses of MCV4 ≥8 weeks apart[c,d] Revaccinate every 5 years[d]	1 dose of MCV4[e]
≥56 years	1 dose of MPSV4 Revaccinate every 5 years[d]	1 dose of MPSV4[e]

[a] The classic high-risk conditions are persistent complement component deficiency (C5 through C9, properdin, factor H, factor D) and anatomic or functional asplenia. Vaccination may be considered in other conditions where humoral immunity is defective.

[b] Includes persons traveling to or residents of countries where meningococcal disease is hyperendemic or epidemic, as well as members of a defined risk group during community or institutional outbreaks.

[c] Children with anatomic or functional asplenia should not receive MCV4-D under 2 years of age because of possible interference with PCV13 (pneumococcal disease is considered a bigger risk than meningococcal disease). Beyond 2 years of age, asplenic children who need MCV4-D and PCV13 should receive them ≥4 weeks apart. This precaution does not apply to MCV4-CRM.

[d] Use of multiple doses of MCV is off-label except for 2 doses of MCV4-D at 9 to 23 months of age and 2 doses of MCV4-CRM at 2 to 5 years of age.

[e] Whereas HIV infection per se is not a risk factor for meningococcal disease, it is a risk factor for suboptimal response to vaccination. Therefore, HIV-infected persons who are being vaccinated for other reasons (eg, pre-adolescents receiving routine meningococcal vaccination at 11 to 12 years of age) should receive 2 doses instead of one (in this example, one-time routine revaccination would still occur at 16 years of age). The same might apply to patients with other conditions where humoral immunity is defective.

Adapted from CDC. *MMWR*. 2011;60:72-76; CDC. *MMWR*. 2011;60:1018-1019; CDC. *MMWR*. 2011;60:1391-1392.

- *HIV-infected infants and children*—Many children with HIV infection who receive highly active antiretroviral therapy or are natural long-term nonprogressors (also called "elite controllers") are relatively healthy and can be immunized according to the routine childhood schedule. In general, immune responses are expected to be good, although there is concern about persistence of immunity and memory responses among children who were vaccinated before HAART was instituted.[13]

  The RV recommendations are permissive for young infants who are HIV-infected and still age-eligible, essentially saying that the risks of giving this live vaccine should be weighed against the benefits (the risks would appear to be very low in HIV-infected infants who are not severely immunosuppressed).[14] Special attention should be paid to influenza immunization, not only to protect the child, but also to prevent spread of influenza to HIV-infected household members; remember that LAIV is contraindicated in immunosuppressed persons and those with medical conditions that predispose to complicated influenza.

  MMR and VAR should be given to HIV-infected children who do not have evidence of *severe* immunosuppression, regardless of whether symptoms are present.[3,15] Up to 8 years of age, severe immunosuppression is indicated by a CD4 count <15%; beyond 8 years of age, severe immunosuppression is indicated by a CD4 count <200 cells/mcL. It is prudent to give the 2 required doses of each vaccine as early as possible, as immune function may deteriorate before 4 to 6 years of age when the second doses are routinely administered. Given the minimum intervals of 1 month for MMR and 3 months for VAR (doses given <3 months apart to immunocompromised persons are invalid), a simple approach would be to give both vaccines at 12 to 15 months of age and then again 3 months later. Remember that MMRV should not be used in HIV-infected persons.

  HIV-infected children are at increased risk for invasive *S pneumoniae* disease; optimizing immunity to *S pneumoniae* (**Table 6.2**) is important, but vaccine response may be impaired. HIV infection is not considered a risk factor for invasive *N meningitidis* disease per se, but it is a risk for not responding optimally to one dose of vaccine. Therefore, if being vaccinated for other reasons (eg, travel), HIV-infected infants and children should receive 2 doses separated by 8 weeks (**Table 6.3**).
- *HIV-infected adolescents and adults*—Optimizing immunity to *S pneumoniae* (**Table 6.2**) is important, but vaccine responses may be impaired. As discussed above, HIV infection is a risk factor for suboptimal response to vaccination.

Therefore, HIV-infected pre-adolescents receiving routine meningococcal vaccination at 11 to 12 years of age should receive 2 doses instead of one, with one-time revaccination at 16 years of age, as is recommended for children who are not HIV-infected (**Table 6.3**). **Figure 8.7** summarizes vaccination recommendations for older persons with HIV infection. Note that if the CD4 count is ≥200 cells/mcL, the schedule is the same as for healthy adults, with three exceptions: 1) IIV should be used instead of LAIV; 2) all nonimmune persons (not just high-risk) should be immunized with HepB; and 3) PPSV23 should be given soon after diagnosis (rather than waiting for routine vaccination at 65 years of age). If the CD4 count is ≥200 cells/mcL and there is no evidence of immunosuppression, ZOS may be given. For those with CD4 counts <200 cells/mcL, the same caveats hold true, but in addition MMR, VAR, and ZOS are contraindicated. Meningococcal vaccination is indicated only if other risk factors are present.

Medication-Induced Immunosuppression

Solid Organ Transplantation and Cancer Chemotherapy

- *Typical syndromes*[16]: renal, heart, or liver transplant, leukemia, lymphoma, breast cancer, lung cancer, colon cancer
- *Safety issues*: Live vaccines are generally contraindicated during active therapy, but may be considered before and after treatment.
- *Special considerations*: Solid organ transplantation is usually a scheduled event—this affords the opportunity to optimize immunizations before patients receive immunosuppressive medications to prevent rejection. Once transplanted, patients are likely to be chronically immunosuppressed, contraindicating live vaccines and increasing the risk of poor responses to inactivated ones. To complicate matters, some conditions that lead to transplant—end stage renal disease, for instance—can themselves lead to poor immune responses.

  As a general rule, patients should be caught-up on all age-appropriate immunizations in advance of transplantation. Serologic tests for IgG antibody against measles, mumps, rubella, and varicella can identify those patients who may need immunization; susceptible patients ≥12 months of age should be immunized with MMR and/or VAR (MMRV should not be used) at least 1 month before transplantation. Antibody titers should be measured 1 year after transplantation, as seronegative patients are candidates for passive immunization if exposed to disease. Routine yearly IIV can resume ≥6 months after transplantation; vaccination with other inactivated vaccines can resume about 1 year after transplantation, in order to ensure immunogenicity. Optimizing immunity to *S pneu-*

moniae (**Table 6.2**) is important, but vaccine response may be impaired. Meningococcal vaccine is not indicated unless the patient is eligible for routine adolescent vaccination or if splenectomy has occurred (if given, a 2-dose primary series is warranted because these patients are at risk for suboptimal response; **Table 6.3**). One dose of Hib should be considered for adolescents and adults (off-label recommendation).

In cancer patients, live vaccines are usually withheld for ≥3 months after immunosuppressive chemotherapy has been discontinued. This interval may vary with the type and intensity of immunosuppressive therapy, radiation therapy, underlying disease, and other factors. There is no harm in continuing routine inactivated vaccine schedules while on chemotherapy, although there is the risk of suboptimal responses. As above, pneumococcal vaccine and Hib should be considered.

■ Steroids

- *Typical syndromes*[17]: asthma, inflammatory bowel disease, rheumatoid arthritis, spondyloarthropathies, systemic lupus erythematosis, other autoimmune disorders
- *Safety issues*: Live vaccines may be contraindicated in some patients.
- *Special considerations*: Because steroids may be immunosuppressive, they represent a potential problem in the use of live vaccines. Any patient receiving steroids in any form who has clinical or laboratory evidence of immunosuppression should not receive live vaccines. In addition, patients whose underlying disease itself is immunosuppressive should not receive live vaccines, except under special circumstances. Here are some guidelines for live vaccines in other situations:
  - *Topical, inhaled, and compartmental depot injections*: Vaccination is acceptable.
  - *Physiologic replacement*: Vaccination is acceptable.
  - *Less than 2 mg/kg/day (<20 mg if >10 kg; daily or alternating days) of prednisone or equivalent*: Vaccination is acceptable.
  - *Greater than or equal to 2 mg/kg/day (≥20 mg if >10 kg; daily or alternating days) of prednisone or equivalent for <14 days*: Vaccinate right after stopping steroid therapy. Do not vaccinate if steroid therapy will extend to 14 days or more.
  - *Greater than or equal to 2 mg/kg/day (≥20 mg if >10 kg; daily or alternating days) of prednisone or equivalent for ≥14 days*: Vaccinate 1 month after stopping therapy.

■ Disease-Modifying Antirheumatic Drugs (DMARDs)

- *Typical syndromes*[17]: inflammatory bowel disease, rheumatoid arthritis, spondyloarthropathies, systemic lupus erythematosis, other autoimmune disorders

- *Safety issues*: Live vaccines are generally contraindicated, although some patients may be able to receive ZOS.
- *Special considerations*: This class of drugs includes methotrexate, hydroxychloroquine, sulfasalazine, azathioprine, leflunomide, cyclosporine, tumor necrosis factor inhibitors (eg, etanercept, infliximab, adalimumab), interleukin-1 receptor antagonists (eg, anakinra), selective costimulation modulators (eg, abatacept), and anti-B-cell monoclonal antibodies (eg, rituximab). Inactivated vaccines may be given, but responses are variable. Optimizing immunity to *S pneumoniae* (**Table 6.2**) is important, but vaccine response may be impaired. Patients are high-priority for yearly IIV. There are no specific recommendations regarding the interval between dosing of these drugs and vaccination. Patients receiving low doses of methotrexate (≤0.4 mg/kg/week), azathioprine (≤3 mg/kg/day), or 6-mercaptopurine (≤1.5 mg/kg/day) may receive ZOS (this is considered safe because patients receiving ZOS have pre-existing immunity to varicella; patients on DMARDs should not receive MMR, VAR, or MMRV).

Hematopoietic Stem-Cell Transplantation (HSCT) and Leukemia

Allogeneic HSCT presents a complicated vaccination paradigm. The underlying disease itself may be immunosuppressive, the therapy used to prepare for transplantation ablates existing immunity, immunosuppressive therapy may be given after the procedure (sometimes for life), patients may receive passive immunization with immune globulin preparations, and GVHD may further compromise immune function and lead to end-organ failure, including splenic dysfunction. Moreover, the adopted immune system of the donor provides unreliable immunity of uncertain duration; fortunately, immune memory can be recalled by immunization after engraftment (it is not clear whether lasting benefits accrue from immunization of the donor prior to transplant, but there is evidence of benefit from donor immunization with Hib, tetanus and diphtheria toxoids, PCV and HepB). Although GVHD is not an issue with autologous transplantation and the conditioning regimens may be less severe, studies show that vaccine-induced immunity may be lost after transplantation. Guidelines for vaccination of HSCT patients were published in 2000[18] and updated in 2009;[19] continued updates are provided in the *General Recommendations*.[1] **Table 6.4** provides a summary protocol.

There are studies demonstrating loss of immunity to some vaccine antigens after successful treatment for acute leukemia.[20,21] However, official guidelines for revaccination are hard to come by.[22] Some centers favor testing for antibodies once chemotherapy

TABLE 6.4 — Revaccination[a] of Hematopoietic Stem-Cell Transplant (HSCT) Recipients

		Timeframe After Transplantation and Number of Doses[b]	
Vaccine	**Age**	**6-23 Months**	**≥24 Months**
DTaP	<7 years	3 to 5	—
DTaP/Tdap[c]	≥7 years	3 DTaP then 1 Tdap	—
HepA[d,e]	≥1 year	2	—
HepB[f]	All ages	3	—
Hib[g]	≥6 weeks	3	—
HPV[e]	Females: 11 to 26 years[h]	3	—
	Males: 11 to 21 years[i]	3	—
IIV[j]	≥6 months	1 yearly	—
MMR[k]	≥1 year	Contraindicated	2 if immunocompetent[l,m]
MCV4	≥9 months[n]	1	Consider revaccination[o]
RV[p]	—	—	—
PCV13/PPSV23[q]	≥6 weeks	3 PCV13 then 1 PPSV23[r]	—
IPV	≥6 weeks	3	—
VAR[k]	≥1 year	Contraindicated	2 if immunocompetent[l,m]
ZOS	≥60 years	Contraindicated	—

HSCT patients should be revaccinated with routine vaccines regardless of the source of stem cells. HSCT patients are considered high-risk for complicated vaccine-preventable diseases, including those due to encapsulated bacteria like *N meningitidis*, *H influenzae*, and *S pneumoniae*. Chronic liver disease due to GVHD places patients at higher risk of serious hepatitis A and B. Routine penicillin prophylaxis is recommended for patients with chronic GVHD, as if they were asplenic. Practice varies from one transplantation center to another.

[a] This table gives recommendations for *re*vaccination, in other words repeat vaccinations in patients who already had them before transplant. New age-appropriate vaccinations could be given beginning 6 months (inactivated vaccines) or 24 months (live vaccines) post-transplant. For example, an adolescent who was transplanted before 11 years of age and never received HPV can begin the HPV series 6 months post-transplant. Likewise, a 60-year-old adult who is >24 months post-transplant, has never before received ZOS, and is considered immunocompetent could receive ZOS.

[b] **Table 5.1** gives the usual minimum ages and intervals between doses and **Tables 8.4** (4 months to 6 years of age) and **8.5** (7 to 18 years of age) give catch-up schedules. In the case of *re*vaccination of HSCT patients, a 4-week interval between doses of the same vaccine is reasonable.

[c] Use of DTaP >6 years of age, Adacel <11 and ≥65 years of age, and Boostrix <10 years of age is off-label.

[d] IGIM is recommended in addition to vaccine for immunocompromised persons who are traveling.

[e] Revaccination with HepA and HPV are considered optional.

[f] Test for HBsAb 1 to 3 months after the third dose; if negative, repeat the 3-dose series one time.

[g] Use of ActHIB >18 months, PedvaxHIB >5 years, and Hiberix >4 years of age is off-label.

[h] Either HPV2 or HPV4 may be used; the former is labeled for prevention of cervical cancer and the latter for prevention of cervical cancer, genital warts, and anal cancer.

[i] HPV4 may be given to males 22 to 26 years of age for prevention of genital warts and anal cancer, but is not routinely recommended.

[j] IIV may be given as early as 4 months after transplantation, but a second dose 4 weeks later should be considered in this situation. Children 6 months to 8 years of age who are receiving influenza vaccine for the first time post-transplant need 2 doses. Chemoprophylaxis should be considered for all patients regardless of vaccination status. LAIV is contraindicated.

[k] Passive immunoprophylaxis should be given to all measles- and varicella-exposed patients regardless of personal history of disease or vaccination.

[l] MMRV should not be used.

[m] Patients who have chronic GVHD should not receive VAR or ZOS. Use of MMR and VAR in immunocompromised persons is off-label.

[n] MCV4-D is labeled for use as early as 9 months of age; MCV4-CRM is labeled for use as early as 2 years of age. MCV4-D should not be used concomitantly with PCV13 in children who are functionally or anatomically asplenic, including those with chronic GVHD.

[o] Revaccination is recommended every 5 years for those who remain at high risk for invasive meningococcal disease (see **Table 6.3**). Use of multiple doses of MCV is off-label except for 2 doses of MCV4-D at 9 to 23 months of age and 2 doses of MCV4-CRM at 2 to 5 years of age.

Continued

TABLE 6.4 — *Continued*

[p] The RV series cannot be initiated beyond infancy.
[q] PCV13 may be given as soon as 3 months after transplantation. Use of PCV13 at 6 to 49 years of age is off-label.
[r] For patients with chronic GVHD, PCV13 may be substituted for the dose of PPSV23.

Adapted from Tomblyn M, et al. *Biol Blood Marrow Transplant*. 2009;15:1143-1238 and Kroger AT, et al. *MMWR*. 2011;60(RR-2):1-61.

is completed, with selective revaccination using those antigens for which the patient's antibody levels have fallen below protective levels. The problem is that serological correlates of protection are not known for all diseases. Another approach is to routinely revaccinate with some or all antigens, using guidelines like those in **Table 6.4**.

Predisposing Conditions Other Than Immune Deficiency

6

Persons with chronic underlying conditions may be unusually susceptible to infectious diseases, whether or not they have immune deficiency in the classic sense. As a general rule, all routine vaccines should be given unless they are specifically contraindicated. Most of these patients are on the high priority list for yearly IIV; LAIV should not be used in patients whose conditions predispose them to complications of influenza, including those with chronic cardiac (eg, congenital heart disease), respiratory (eg, cystic fibrosis), allergic (eg, asthma), hematologic (eg, sickle cell disease), metabolic (eg, diabetes), neuromuscular (eg, muscular dystrophy), hepatic (eg, cirrhosis), and renal (eg, chronic renal failure) disorders. HepB is recommended for diabetics <60 years of age and should be considered for those ≥60 years of age.[23] Patients with chronic liver disease are at risk for severe hepatitis and should receive HepA[24] and HepB.[25]

Some conditions place patients at particular risk for invasive *S pneumoniae* infection.[26] For example, patients with nephrotic syndrome are susceptible, due in part to loss of IgG in the urine—in this sense they are considered immunocompromised. Diabetes, chronic heart disease, and chronic lung disease also place patients at higher risk. In adults, asthma and smoking are considered risk factors (asthma is a risk factor for children who are treated with high-dose steroids).[27] Patients with CSF leaks and cochlear implants are at increased risk for pneumococcal meningitis. Optimizing immunity to *S pneumoniae* (**Table 6.2**) is important, but vaccine response may be impaired.

Pregnancy and Breast-Feeding

Whereas vaccination during pregnancy poses *theoretical* risks to the developing fetus, there is no evidence directly linking any routine vaccines, even live ones, to birth defects. Current thinking is that pregnant women should be vaccinated only when the risk for exposure to disease is high and the infection would pose a significant risk to the mother or fetus[28]; some have argued, however, for a universal *maternal immunization platform*, analogous to the childhood and adolescent platforms.[29] Delaying vaccination until the second or third trimester, when possible, is reasonable in order to minimize concerns about teratogenicity, despite the evidence against this—an exception is IIV, which should be given regardless of trimester to women who are or will be pregnant during influenza season.[30]

Pregnancy is an indication for influenza immunization—it is safe,[31] cost-effective,[32] and over 90% effective in preventing hospitalization of infants due to influenza in the first 6 months of life.[33] Likewise, pregnancy (beyond 20 weeks) is an indication for administration of Tdap—it is safe, likely to protect the infant against pertussis in the first few months of life, and unlikely to interfere with the infant DTap series.[34]

In considering vaccination during pregnancy, clinicians should be aware of the following:

- Approximately 2% of all newborns have a major congenital malformation; it follows that some women who are vaccinated during pregnancy will have infants with birth defects. While a causal relationship with the vaccine may be lacking, there may be a tendency to attribute the birth defect to the vaccine. Pregnant women should be counseled about this before being vaccinated. Along the same lines, it stands that some children of women who receive thimerosal-containing vaccines (eg, some brands of IIV) during pregnancy will develop autism, even though thimerosal (which contains mercury) does not cause autism (see *Chapter 7: Addressing Concerns About Vaccines—Did the Thimerosal Used as a Preservative in Vaccines Cause Autism?*). Unfortunately, some states have banned the use of thimerosal-containing vaccines, which could jeopardize the supply of IIV for pregnant women.
- Very few vaccines have been tested for safety and efficacy in large numbers of pregnant women. For this reason, the FDA classifies most vaccines as Pregnancy Category C (defined as: animal studies show adverse effects or have not been done *and* there are no adequate studies in pregnant women). Practically speaking, the official pregnancy classification has little impact on use. For example, Td is recommended during pregnancy if indicated, despite its category C designation. IIV is recommended during pregnancy, without brand preference, even though some brands are Pregnancy Category B and some are C (Pregnancy Category B is defined as: animal studies show no adverse effects but there are no adequate studies in pregnant women, *or* animal studies show adverse effects but adequate studies in pregnant women fail to demonstrate harm to the fetus). On the other hand, HPV is not recommended (albeit not specifically contraindicated) during pregnancy, despite the fact that both HPV2 and HPV4 are Pregnancy Category B. The only vaccines that carry a Pregnancy

Category D designation (evidence of risk to the fetus but benefits might outweigh risks) are anthrax and smallpox.

- Live vaccines are generally contraindicated during pregnancy, with the exceptions noted in **Table 6.5**. However, inadvertent receipt of live vaccines is not a reason to terminate the pregnancy. In the case of VAR, if a pregnant woman is known to be susceptible to varicella and a close contact develops a rash after vaccination, exposure should be avoided until the vaccinee's lesions are crusted. Some manufacturers maintain registries of women inadvertently vaccinated during pregnancy in order to gather data on outcomes; the phone numbers for reporting are usually given in the package insert.
- The only live vaccine that is contraindicated in household contacts of pregnant women is smallpox.
- Theoretical concerns include the possibilities that the immune response in pregnant women will be suboptimal; that transplacental antibodies might interfere with the infant's ability to respond to vaccines; and that in-utero antigen exposure could lead to immune tolerance in the baby.
- There are no known risks of passive immunization during pregnancy. In fact, VariZIG is *recommended* for susceptible pregnant women who are exposed to varicella because the risk of complicated disease in the mother is high (it is not know whether passive immunization protects the fetus).[15]
- Breast-feeding per se is not a contraindication to the use of any vaccines, including live ones, except for pre-event use of smallpox vaccine.

In 2008, an ACIP working group offered guidance on the drafting of recommendations for vaccination during pregnancy and breast-feeding.[35] This should lead to more uniformity in future recommendations.

Newborns

Newborn immunity is complex.[36] De-novo humoral responses are impaired, and protection during the first few months of life largely derives from transplacentally acquired maternal IgG—this is in part the rationale for immunizing pregnant women with IIV and Tdap *(see above)*. Newborns also have increased regulatory T-cells and decreased Th1-cells, presumably to prevent in-utero cellular responses to maternal tissues.

Nevertheless, newborns can respond well to some vaccines. In the United States, the only vaccine routinely given at birth is HepB (BCG and OPV are given elsewhere). HepB is immunogenic in infants and protection persists at least into young adulthood.[25] Other advantages of the birth dose include potentially

TABLE 6.5 — Vaccine Use During Pregnancy

Administer Because of Pregnancy[a]	Administer if Indicated for Other Reasons[b]	Consider Administration in Certain Situations[c]	Contraindicated or Not Recommended[d]
IIV	HepB	Anthrax vaccine	Adenovirus vaccine
Td or Tdap	MPSV4	HepA	HPV[e]
	RAB	IPV	LAIV
		JEV	MMR
		MCV4	VAR
		PPSV23	ZOS
		Smallpox vaccine[f]	
		Typhoid (TViPSV and Ty21a)	
		YFV	

[a] Pregnancy is a specific reason to give these vaccines. Because pregnancy increases the risk of complicated influenza, IIV should be given regardless of trimester to women who are or will be pregnant during influenza season. This also protects the infants during the first few months of life. Tdap should be given to pregnant women unless they have already had a dose. This not only protects the babies against neonatal tetanus, but also protects the mothers from getting pertussis and transmitting it to their infants.

[b] Examples include HepB for an unvaccinated pregnant injecting drug user; RAB for a pregnant woman who is bitten by a bat; and MPSV4 for an unvaccinated pregnant woman who has been diagnosed with a terminal complement component deficiency (MCV4 is probably preferred in this situation, but, because of a lack of data, is listed in the "Consider Administration" column).

[c] The language surrounding use of these vaccines in pregnant women is ultimately permissive. For example, the IPV recommendation reads as follows: "Although no adverse effects of IPV have been documented among pregnant women or their fetuses, vaccination of pregnant women should be avoided on theoretical grounds. However, if a pregnant woman is at increased risk for infection and requires immediate protection against polio, IPV can be administered…" As another example, the MCV4 recommendation reads: "MCV4 is safe and immunogenic among

nonpregnant persons aged 11-55 years, but no data are available on the safety of MCV4 during pregnancy" (the recommendation does not say *don't use* the vaccine in pregnant women). For all of the vaccines in this column, providers should use their best judgment in balancing the risks and benefits.

[d] Adenovirus vaccine, LAIV, MMR, VAR, and ZOS are contraindicated because they are live and there is the theoretical risk of harm to the fetus. Inadvertent administration of these vaccines during pregnancy is not a reason to terminate the pregnancy. Pregnancy should be avoided for 1 month following MMR or VAR administration and 6 weeks following adenovirus vaccine. ZOS is only recommended at ≥60 years of age and would therefore be unlikely to be used during pregnancy.

[e] ACIP recommends against routine use of HPV in pregnant women, although this is an inactivated vaccine that theoretically carries little risk of fetal harm.

[f] Smallpox is the only vaccine known to cause fetal harm. It should only be used as prophylaxis in pregnant women who have been exposed to smallpox.

Adapted from Guidelines for vaccinating pregnant women. Centers for Disease Control and Prevention Web site. http://www.cdc.gov/vaccines/pubs/preg-guide.htm#hpv. Accessed November 15, 2011.

reducing the number of concurrent injections that must be given at the 2-month visit, increasing the likelihood that the entire 3-dose series (and other vaccine series) will be completed.[37] The birth dose also emphasizes the importance of immunization for new parents, laying the groundwork for the routine schedule in infancy.

Newborn immunization can potentially lead to problems. For example, administration of DTaP at birth may result in decreased antibody responses later in infancy.[38] Similarly, giving Hib before 6 weeks of age can induce immune tolerance, although not all studies have demonstrated this to be the case.[39]

Preterm and Low Birth Weight Infants

Preterm (<37 weeks' gestation) and low birth weight (<2500 g) infants are at particular risk for vaccine-preventable diseases because of immune system immaturity and the possibility of decreased maternal antibody levels (robust transport of maternal IgG does not occur until the third trimester). Comorbidities contribute to risk and cause delays in immunization. Initiating the immunization series in the nursery not only protects the child but also improves coverage rates later on.[40] Preterm and low birth weight infants should be vaccinated according to the routine schedule, using the routine doses, at the appropriate chronologic age. The only vaccine for which weight is relevant is HepB. Infants weighing <2000 g at birth whose mothers are HBsAg-negative should receive the first dose of vaccine at 1 month of age (rather than at birth) or at hospital discharge.[25] Infants weighing <2000 g at birth whose mothers are HBsAg-positive or HBsAg-unknown should receive the first dose of vaccine within 12 hours of birth and should also receive HBIG 0.5 mL intramuscularly at a separate site from the vaccine. In these cases, the birth dose of vaccine does not count toward completion of the HepB series; 3 additional doses should be given as follows:

- *Mother HBsAg-positive*: doses at 1, 2, and 6 months of age. Test for HBsAg and HBsAb at 9 to 18 months of age. If HBsAg is negative and HBsAb is <10 mIU/mL, repeat the 3-dose vaccine series.
- *Mother HBsAg-unknown*: doses at 1, 2, and 6 months of age and test the mother; if she is HBsAg-positive, proceed as above.
- *Mother HBsAg-negative*: doses at 1, 2, and 6 to 18 months of age.

RV should be given to preterm infants who are clinically stable and are being discharged from the nursery or who are already home, keeping in mind that the first dose should be given between 6 weeks and 14 weeks 6 days of age.[14] Those who are remaining in the hospital should not receive RV—the vaccine virus strains are shed in the stool and there is the theoretical risk of transmission to other infants who may be acutely ill or ineligible for vaccination.

Preterm infants can experience cardiorespiratory events, such as apnea, bradycardia, and oxygen desaturation following vaccination and should be closely observed for at least 48 hours.[41]

International Adoptees, Refugees, and Immigrants

6

The Immigration and Nationality Act requires all immigrants entering the United States to show proof of having received all ACIP-recommended vaccines before a visa is granted. In 2009, CDC adopted the following criteria to determine which ACIP-recommended vaccines should be required: the vaccine must be age-appropriate and must either protect against a disease that has the potential to cause an outbreak or protect against a disease that has been eliminated or is in the process of being eliminated in the United States.[42] Based on these criteria, HPV and ZOS are not required. International adoptees <11 years of age can be exempted from this requirement but the adoptive parents must sign an affidavit indicating their intention to comply with immunization requirements within 30 days after the child arrives (children coming from Hague Convention countries such as China and the Philippines cannot be exempted). Refugees are exempted from immunization requirements at the time of entry, but must show proof of immunization at the time they apply for permanent residency.

The following issues are germane to the immunization management of persons from other countries, particularly international adoptees:

- Vaccination records are considered valid only if they are in written form and contain the vaccines, dates of administration, proper intervals between doses, and age at the time of immunization.
- Written records must be translated and interpreted correctly, and even then may be inaccurate or fraudulent.
- Even written records indicating adequate vaccination do not necessarily predict immunity.[43]
- Many immigrant adults are susceptible to vaccine-preventable diseases.[44]
- The immunization schedule in many countries differs from that in the United States. Some children will need additional vaccines to comply with the US schedule.
- Vaccines in some countries may have inadequate potency, especially because of improper handling. Country of origin predicts seroprotection, with the highest rates in children from Eastern Europe, then, in descending order, India, Latin America, China and Africa.[45]

- Serologic correlates of protection exist for some diseases but not for others. Testing may be expensive and the results require interpretation.
- There is no harm in revaccinating individuals who have already been vaccinated, although reactogenicity to DTaP and PPSV23 may increase if too many doses are given within a short time frame.
- International adoptees may have subclinical vaccine-preventable diseases that are a risk to close contacts in the United States. For example, children from endemic countries may have hepatitis A without jaundice when they arrive. This is the basis for HepA vaccination of persons who will be in close contact with them during the first 60 days after arrival (the first dose should be given at least 2 weeks before arrival).[46]

It is desirable for all persons entering the United States permanently to receive all routinely recommended vaccines. For reasons mentioned, the simplest (and possibly least expensive) approach is to start over and revaccinate.[47] An alternative, although somewhat less practical, approach is to test for antibodies to the major vaccine antigens and administer those vaccines to which the child has no immunity. Young infants can be vaccinated according to the routine childhood schedule (**Table 8.1**); older children can be vaccinated according to catch-up schedules (**Tables 8.4** and **8.5**), with attention paid to the minimum allowable intervals between doses (**Table 5.1**). For adults who immigrate to the United States, consideration should be given to vaccination with MMR, Tdap, HepB, and VAR. Individuals from hepatitis B-endemic areas should be screened for HBsAg; if positive, vaccination is not necessary.

Adults ≥65 Years of Age

Older persons are at increased risk for vaccine-preventable diseases because of immune senescence, or waning of immune responses.[48] Of particular importance is influenza, where deaths among those ≥65 years of age account for approximately 90% of all influenza-associated deaths.[49] Yearly administration of IIV is critical; high-dose IIV produces higher antibody titers among persons 65 years of age than standard-dose IIV,[50] but at this time there is no preference for use. Similarly, *S pneumoniae* is responsible for approximately 1.5 million annual hospital days due to pneumonia alone,[51] highlighting the importance of immunization with PPSV23. Vaccination with both IIV and PPSV23 is effective in preventing death from other causes such as myocardial infarction and stroke.[52] Despite this, only about 70% of persons ≥65 years of age in the United States receive yearly influenza vaccine or have ever received PPSV23.[53]

The term "HCP" refers to all paid and unpaid persons who work in health care settings (including residential institutions) and have the potential to be exposed to patients or infectious materials. The list of people who fall into this category is long, and includes physicians, nurses, nursing assistants, therapists, technicians, pharmacists, students, trainees, contractual staff, volunteers, and those who work in clerical, dietary, housekeeping, laundry, security, maintenance, administrative, billing, emergency medical, dental, laboratory, and autopsy capacities. HCP are at risk for acquiring vaccine-preventable diseases and transmitting them to their patients and their own families. The risk of infection might be particularly high for people working in emergency departments or ambulatory care settings, especially if the facility serves underimmunized populations. The consequences of transmission to patients might be particularly high wherever there are vulnerable patients, such as intensive care units, newborn nurseries, obstetric wards, chronic care facilities, and oncology or transplant units.

Health care facilities should develop vaccination policies for all HCP, and these should be part of comprehensive occupational health and patient safety programs. Immunizations should be provided at no cost to the worker. Whereas vaccination cannot be forced upon HCP, some institutions have developed strategies wherein individuals must sign a release form in order to opt out, acknowledging that exposure to a vaccine-preventable disease may result in leave without pay and that worker's compensation benefits would not apply unless the disease actually developed. Other institutions have dismissed workers who refuse to be vaccinated (see *Chapter 3: Standards, Principles, and Regulations—Mandates*).

Comprehensive immunization recommendations for HCP were published in 1997[54] and were updated in 2011.[55] HCP should receive all routinely recommended vaccines. Those that deserve particular attention are discussed below.

■ HepB

Cases of hepatitis B among HCP decreased dramatically in the 1980s and 1990s, due largely to routine vaccination and improved infection-control precautions; however, ≥3-dose coverage for HepB among HCP hovers just under 70%.[56]

HepB is recommended for all HCP who are likely to be exposed to blood or blood-containing body fluids. In fact, the Bloodborne Pathogens Standard (see *Chapter 3: Standards, Principles, and Regulations—Occupational Safety and Health Administration [OSHA]*) mandates that vaccination be made available at no cost to all employees with potential blood contact.

Prevaccination testing for immunity is indicated only for high-risk populations. Testing for HBsAb 1 to 2 months after Dose 3 is recommended for all HCP at high risk for percutaneous or mucosal exposure to blood or body fluids; such testing is not routinely recommended for HCP at low risk, such as those without direct patient contact. Persons who test negative (<10 mIU/mL) should receive another 3-dose series (one time only). Those who remain seronegative after a total of 6 doses should be tested for HBsAg (chronic carriage can explain failure to respond to the vaccine) and HBcAb (antibody to the core antigen indicates prior natural infection). Those who are not previously infected (HBcAb-negative) and not immune (HBsAb-negative) should be counseled about precautions to prevent hepatitis B infection and the need for HBIG if there is an exposure. Those who are chronically-infected (HBsAg-positive) should not be excluded from work but should be counseled about which exposure-prone procedures they may perform safely. Those who are previously (HBcAb-positive) but not chronically (HBsAg-positive) infected are considered immune and do not need vaccination.

Individuals who received the HepB series in the past need not be tested for HBsAb when they enter a health care–related job, but they should be tested at the time of an exposure and, if they are seronegative, managed accordingly. Guidelines for the management of potential occupational exposure to hepatitis B are given in **Table 14.2**.

■ IIV and LAIV

HCP are at high risk of acquiring influenza at work and transmitting it to their patients, many of whom are at high risk for complicated disease. Moreover, hospital outbreaks have been associated with low HCP vaccination rates.[57] All HCP should be immunized against influenza in the fall of each year; despite this longstanding recommendation, the coverage rate among HCP for the 2010-2011 season was only 63.5%.[58] HCP who are in close contact with severely immunosuppressed patients (the equivalent of HSCT patients who are in protective environments) should only receive IIV; HCP who receive LAIV should avoid contact with such patients for 7 days postvaccination. HCP who work in the neonatal intensive care unit may receive LAIV. HCP who themselves are too old to receive LAIV or have medical contraindications may nevertheless administer LAIV to others.

■ MMR

HCP are at high risk for acquiring measles,[59] and medical settings play a prominent role in perpetuating outbreaks.[60] Mumps transmission also occurs in medical settings.[61] Moreover, responding to hospital-associated measles and mumps outbreaks is expensive. Rubella was eliminated from the United States in

2004, but in the pre-elimination era, transmission in medical settings was well documented.[62]

For these reasons, all HCP should be immune to measles, mumps, and rubella (see **Table 18.2** for criteria for evidence of immunity). Prevaccination serology is not necessary for HCP without presumptive evidence of immunity. Likewise, testing for antibody after appropriate vaccination is not recommended; in fact, a person who has received 2 properly administered doses of MMR is presumed to be immune to measles, mumps, and rubella regardless of the results of serologic tests (technically, only one dose of rubella vaccine is necessary, but most people get 2 in the context of MMR). Even though MMR contains live viruses, there is no risk of horizontal transmission.

■ Tdap

Pertussis is transmitted in hospitals[63] and serological studies show that exposure of HCP is common.[64] To boost pertussis immunity, all HCP should receive a dose of Tdap, regardless of age and regardless of when the last dose of Td was received. Persons ≥65 years of age may be vaccinated (use of Adacel for persons ≥65 years of age is off-label).[65] The dose of Tdap "resets the clock" for subsequent 10-year Td boosters.

■ VAR

Nosocomial transmission of varicella can occur from cases of chickenpox as well as shingles, and the consequences can be devastating to certain patients. The virus is so contagious that it can literally float down the hallway.[66] Providers with unrecognized varicella can expose many patients and other HCP, resulting in time-consuming and costly responses.[67]

All HCP should be immune to varicella (see **Table 26.2** for criteria for evidence of immunity). HCP who are not immune should receive 2 doses of VAR separated by 4 to 8 weeks. Even though VAR is a live vaccine, vaccinated HCP can return to work immediately. However, if a vaccine-related rash develops, they should avoid contact with persons who are not immune and are at risk for severe or complicated disease, at least until the lesions are crusted over (if there are only macules and papules, they should wait until there are no new lesions within a 24-hour period). Vaccinated HCP who are exposed to chickenpox or shingles should be observed carefully during days 8 to 21 postexposure; symptoms suggestive of varicella should prompt a medical leave, and if varicella develops, the worker should remain on leave until all the lesions are crusted or faded and there are no new lesions within a 24-hour period. HCP who have had only one dose of VAR and are exposed to chickenpox or shingles should receive a second dose within 5 days of exposure (as long as it has been at least 4 weeks since the first dose) and should be observed carefully as above. Those who do not receive a second dose, or who receive a second dose >5 days after exposure, should be furloughed during days 8 to 21 postexposure. Exposed HCP with no evidence of immunity should be vaccinated and furloughed as above; those who cannot be vaccinated (eg, pregnant or immunocompromised) and are at risk for complicated disease should receive varicella-zoster immune globulin.

Travel

Travelers going to Canada, Western Europe, Australia, and New Zealand are probably at no higher risk for illness than those traveling within the United States, although the United Kingdom is now considered a measles-endemic region. For other destinations, however, consideration may need to be given to specialized vaccines or to accelerated schedules for routine vaccines, depending to some extent on what circumstances the traveler will encounter.[68] Travel to certain areas may require other measures, including malaria chemoprophylaxis, insect avoidance, food hygiene, and the availability of emergency medical services. Moreover, certain persons may be at higher risk than others for particular diseases. In an international study of nearly 40,000 returned travelers from 1997 to 2007, the most common vaccine-preventable diseases were enteric fever, acute viral hepatitis, and influenza.[69] Risk factors for infection with *S typhi* were traveling to visit friends and relatives and travel to South Central Asia; business travel was a risk factor for influenza and prolonged travel for hepatitis A.

Travel medicine clinics, which may be available at local health departments, academic medical centers, or in private practice settings, maintain up-to-date information and provide vaccination services for travelers. Primary care physicians who choose to provide travel vaccines to their patients should be aware of the following:

- *Planning*—Consultation should take place *at least* 4 to 6 weeks before departure in order to allow for the development of protective immunity after vaccination. More time may be required if certain vaccines will need to be ordered.
- *Itinerary*—It is not enough to know where the person will be traveling. The duration of stay and the particular activities in which the person will be engaged can help determine risk. For example, a 2-day stay in a sophisticated urban hotel carries different risks than extended field work in rural areas.
- *Routine vaccines*—All travelers should be up-to-date on routinely recommended vaccines. Some special considerations are listed below:
  - *Childhood vaccination schedule*: The routine childhood schedules (**Tables 8.1** and **8.3**) provide some flexibility in the timing of doses. For example, Dose 3 of HepB and IPV can be given as early as 6 months of age and Dose 4 of Hib

and PCV13 as early as 12 months of age. Dose 4 of DTaP can be given as early as 12 months of age provided that at least 6 months have elapsed since Dose 3. VAR and HepA can be given as early as 12 months of age. MMR should be given to all infants 6 to 12 months of age who will be traveling outside the United States (reimmunization with 2 doses after the first birthday is necessary); children ≥1 year of age should have 2 doses of MMR before traveling (the minimum interval between doses is 28 days). Two doses of VAR at ≥1 year of age are also recommended (VAR should not be given before 1 year of age); the minimum interval from 1 to 12 years of age is 3 months and at ≥13 years of age is 4 to 8 weeks. Physicians should be aware of flexibility in the schedule and administer all eligible vaccines before the anticipated date of travel.

- *HepA*: For most travelers to endemic areas, vaccination is now preferred over administration of immune globulin and should be initiated as soon as travel is considered.[70] One dose of HepA at any time before departure is likely to provide protection for most healthy people (only monovalent HepA should be used for this purpose). For older adults, immunocompromised persons, and persons with chronic liver disease or other chronic medical conditions, IGIM (0.02 mL/kg) should be given (at a separate site) in addition to vaccine *if* there are <2 weeks before departure. Immune globulin alone should be given to infants <12 months of age and to persons who cannot be or do not want to be vaccinated.
- *HepB*: For those travelers who might have missed universal immunization, HepB should be given if the person might be exposed to blood, have sexual contact with the local population, stay >6 months, or be exposed through medical treatment.
- *Influenza*: Yearly influenza vaccine is now recommended for everyone. High priority should be given to persons traveling to areas with influenza activity. This includes the southern hemisphere during April through September and the tropics at any time of year. Travel with organized tourist groups that include persons from the tropics or southern hemisphere is also a risk factor. People who were vaccinated during the preceding fall or winter *do not* need to be revaccinated before summer travel; however, those who are vaccinated only before summer travel *do* need to be revaccinated the next fall. Vaccine should be given at least 2 weeks before travel, but can be given up to the day of travel if this is not possible. Priority should also be given to persons at risk for complicated influenza. Patients should understand that the vaccine strains used in the northern hemisphere during the

fall may not optimally match the strains circulating in the southern hemisphere during April through September.[71]

- *Polio*: Previously immunized adults traveling to endemic areas should receive one dose of IPV (this does not need to be given again for subsequent travel). If travel of an infant to an endemic area is imminent, 3 doses of IPV can be given at 4-week intervals.
- *PPSV23*: All adults ≥65 years of age and adult smokers and asthmatics should be immunized.
- *Td*: Although boosters are recommended only every 10 years in adults, consideration should be given to a dose if >5 years have elapsed and the person will be working in situations where dirty wounds might be incurred or traveling to regions where diphtheria outbreaks have occurred. If the person has not yet received a dose of Tdap, this should be substituted for Td.

• *Mandatory vaccines*—The only vaccine covered by international health regulations at the present time is YFV, for which travelers to certain countries must have a valid International Certificate of Vaccination or Prophylaxis. However, some countries have their own regulations. For example, Saudi Arabia requires meningococcal vaccine for pilgrims visiting Mecca for the Hajj, and some countries may require the vaccine for persons returning from the Hajj.

• *Recommended vaccines*—**Table 6.6** gives some general guidelines regarding vaccines for travel to certain parts of the world. Specific information about the vaccines is contained in the referenced sections of this book. Since disease outbreaks are always occurring and guidelines frequently change, the best advice is to check updated resources before traveling. The following web sites are useful for this purpose (Accessed November 21, 2011):

- *Centers for Disease Control and Prevention: Travelers' Health*: http://wwwn.cdc.gov/travel/default.aspx
- *World Health Organization: International Travel and Health*: http://www.who.int/ith/en
- *International Society of Travel Medicine*: http://www.istm.org

Other Special Circumstances

Table 6.7 covers other situations and groups that deserve special attention for certain vaccines.

REFERENCES

1. Kroger AT, et al. *MMWR*. 2011;60(RR-2):1-61.
2. American Academy of Pediatrics. *Pediatrics*. 1999;103:1057-1060.
3. Watson JC, et al. *MMWR*. 1998;47(RR-8):1-57.
4. Centers for Disease Control and Prevention. *Epidemiology and Prevention of Vaccine-Preventable Diseases*. 12th ed. Atkinson W, et al, eds. Washington, DC: Public Health Foundation, 2011.
5. Buckley RH. *N Engl J Med*. 2000;343:1313-1324.
6. Lekstrom-Himes JA, et al. *N Engl J Med*. 2000;343:1703-1714.
7. Tedesco F. *Vaccine*. 2008;26S:13-18.
8. Di Sabatino A, et al. *Lancet*. 2011;378:86-97.
9. Mofenson LM, et al. *MMWR*. 2009;58(RR-11):1-166.
10. Kaplan JE, et al. *MMWR*. 2009;58(RR-4):1-207.
11. Panel on Antiretroviral Therapy and Medical Management of HIV-infected Children: Guidelines for the use of antiretroviral agents in pediatric HIV infection. http://aidsinfo.nih.gov/ContentFiles/PediatricGuidelines.pdf. Accessed November 26, 2011.
12. Jones CE, et al. *JAMA*. 2011;305:576-584.
13. Sutcliffe CG, et al. *Lancet Infect Dis*. 2010;10:630-642.
14. Cortese MM, et al. *MMWR*. 2009;58(RR-2):1-25.
15. Marin M, et al. *MMWR*. 2007;56(RR-4):1-40.
16. Chow J, et al. *Clin Infect Dis*. 2009;49:1550-1556.
17. Rahier J-F, et al. *Rheumatology*. 2010;49:1815-1827.
18. CDC. *MMWR*. 2000;49(RR-10):1-125.
19. Tomblyn M, et al. *Biol Blood Marrow Transplant*. 2009;15:1143-1238.
20. Nilsson A, et al. *Pediatrics*. 2002;109:e91.
21. Patel SR, et al. *Clin Infect Dis*. 2007;44:635-642.
22. Esposito S, et al. *Vaccine*. 2010;28:3278-3284.
23. Sawyer MH, et al. *MMWR*. 2011;60:1709-1711.
24. Fiore AE, et al. *MMWR*. 2006;55(RR-7):1-23.
25. Mast EE, et al. *MMWR*. 2006;55(RR-16):1-33.
26. Nuorti JP, et al. *MMWR*. 2010;59(RR-11):1-19.
27. Nuorti JP, et al. *MMWR*. 2010;59:1102-1106.
28. Guidelines for vaccinating pregnant women. Centers for Disease Control and Prevention Web site. http://www.cdc.gov/vaccines/pubs/downloads/b_preg_guide.pdf. Accessed November 26, 2011.
29. Gall SA. *Contemp OB/GYN*. 2011;56:36-48.
30. Fiore AE, et al. *MMWR*. 2010;59(RR-8):1-62.
31. Munoz FM, et al. *Am J Obstet Gynecol*. 2005;192:1098-1106.
32. Beigi RH, et al. *Clin Infect Dis*. 2009;49:1784-1792.
33. Benowitz I, et al. *Clin Infect Dis*. 2010;51:1355-1361.
34. CDC. *MMWR*. 2011;60:1424-1426.

TABLE 6.6 —Vaccine-Preventable Diseases by Region, 2011[a]

Region	Hepatitis A[b]	Japanese Encephalitis[c]	Meningococcus[d]	Polio[e]	Typhoid[f]	Yellow Fever[g]
Caribbean	√				√	√[h]
Central Africa	√		√	√	√	√
East Africa	√		√	√	√	√
East Asia	√[i]	√		√[j]	√	
Eastern Europe and Northern Asia	√	√[k]		√	√	
Indian Ocean Islands	√				√	
Mexico and Central America	√				√	√[l]
Middle East	√		√[m]		√	
North Africa	√				√	
North America						
South Asia	√	√		√	√	
Southeast Asia	√	√			√	
Southern Africa	√				√	
Southern and Western Pacific	√[n]	√[o]			√	

South America					
Temperate	√			√	√[p]
Tropical	√			√	√
West Africa	√	√	√	√	√
Western Europe	√[q]				

[a] Check marks indicate a risk of acquiring the disease in at least one country in the region. Country-specific recommendations can be found at Travelers' Health: Regions. Centers for Disease Control and Prevention Web site. http://wwwnc.cdc.gov/travel/regions/list.htm. Accessed November 14, 2011. Two diseases are not listed but deserve comment:

Hepatitis B: HepB is recommended for all unvaccinated persons traveling to or working in countries with intermediate to high levels of endemic transmission, which includes much of the world. Since exposure to blood or body fluids (through, for example, sexual contact or emergency medical treatment) may not be predictable, all travelers should be immunized.

Rabies: RAB should be considered in most parts of the world if exposure to animals is expected. At particular risk are travelers spending a lot of time outdoors, especially in rural areas, or who are involved in activities such as bicycling, camping, hiking, or outdoor work. Children are considered at higher risk because they tend to play with animals and may not report bites. Spelunkers are also at risk because of potential exposure to bats.

[b] Risk increases with duration of travel and is highest for those who live in or visit rural settings, trek in back-country areas, or frequently eat or drink in areas with poor sanitation.

[c] The risk for short-term travelers and those staying in urban centers is very low. Risk increases with prolonged visits to rural settings, and with extensive outdoor, evening, and nighttime exposures such as bicycling, camping, working outdoors, or sleeping in unscreened structures without bed nets.

[d] Risk is increased for travelers to sub-Saharan Africa (the "meningitis belt") during the dry season, especially if there is prolonged contact with local populations.

Continued

TABLE 6.6 — *Continued*

[e] Adult travelers to endemic or epidemic areas who have had a primary immunization series in the past should receive a dose of IPV before departure.

[f] Risk is higher for those visiting relatives or friends and those who will not have access to cooked foods and safe beverages.

[g] If there is no YF in the country, vaccination may still be required of travelers coming from endemic areas, even if they are just in transit (for example, there is no risk of acquiring YF in Haiti, but the country requires some travelers from endemic areas to have been vaccinated so that YF is not introduced into the country). Vaccination must occur at a certified center and vaccinees must receive an *International Certificate of Vaccination or Prophylaxis* that carries a Uniform Stamp. Some countries with endemic YF may waive the requirements for travelers coming from noninfected areas and staying <2 weeks. Vaccination is also recommended for travel to countries that lie in YF-endemic zones but do not officially report the disease.

[h] Trinidad only.

[i] Except Japan.

[j] China only.

[k] Far eastern Russia only.

[l] Panama only.

[m] Saudi Arabia only. Proof of vaccination with a 4-valent meningococcal vaccine is required of pilgrims traveling to Saudi Arabia for the Hajj.

[n] Except Australia and New Zealand.

[o] Torres Strait, far northern Australia, and Papua New Guinea only.

[p] Northern and northeastern forested areas of Argentina only.

[q] Greenland only.

35. Advisory Committee on Immunization Practices Workgroup on the Use of Vaccines During Pregnancy and Breastfeeding. Guiding principles for development of ACIP recommendations for vaccination during pregnancy and breastfeeding. Centers for Disease Control and Prevention Web site. http://www.cdc.gov/vaccines/recs/acip/downloads/preg-principles05-01-08.pdf. Accessed November 26, 2011.
36. Sanchez-Schmitz G, et al. *Sci Transl Med.* 2011;3:1-8.
37. Yusuf HR, et al. *JAMA*. 2000;284:978-983.
38. Halasa NB, et al. *J Pediatr*. 2008;153:327-332.
39. Kurikka S, et al. *Pediatrics*. 1995;95:815-822.
40. Denizot S, et al. *Vaccine*. 2011;29:382-386.
41. Pourcyrous M, et al. *J Pediatr*. 2007;151:167-172.
42. Centers for Disease Control and Prevention Web site. Notice of revised vaccination criteria for U.S. immigration. http://www.cdc.gov/immigrantrefugeehealth/laws-regs/vaccination-immigration/revised-vaccination-criteria-immigration.html. Accessed November 26, 2011.
43. Verla-Tebit E, et al. *Arch Pediatr Adolesc Med.* 2009;163:473-479.
44. Greenaway C, et al. *Ann Intern Med.* 2007;146:20-24.
45. Cilleruelo MJ, et al. *Vaccine*. 2008;26:5784-5790.
46. CDC. *MMWR*. 2009;58:1006-1007.
47. Cohen AL, et al. *Pediatrics*. 2006;117:1650-1655.
48. McElhaney JE. *Expert Rev Vaccines*. 2009;8:593-606.
49. Thompson MG, et al. *MMWR*. 2010;59:1057-1062.
50. Falsey AR, et al. *J Infect Dis*. 2009;200:172-180.
51. Huang SS, et al. *Vaccine*. 2011;29:3398-3412.
52. Hung IFN, et al. *Clin Infect Dis*. 2010;51:1007-1016.
53. Prevalence and trends data. Centers for Disease Control Web site. http://apps.nccd.cdc.gov/BRFSS/page.asp?cat=IM&yr=2010&state=UB#IM. Accessed November 21, 2011.
54. CDC. *MMWR*. 1997;46(RR-18):1-42.
55. Shefer A, et al. *MMWR*. 2011;60(RR-7):1-45.
56. Lu P-J, et al. *Vaccine*. 2011;29:7049-7057.
57. Cunney RJ, et al. *Infect Control Hosp Epidemiol*. 2000;21:449-454.
58. Harris KM, et al. *MMWR*. 2011;60:1073-1077.
59. Steingart KR, et al. *Infect Control Hosp Epidemiol*. 1999;20:115-119.
60. Chen SY, et al. *J Infect Dis*. 2011;203:1517-1525.
61. Bonebrake AL, et al. *Emerg Infect Dis*. 2010;16:426-432.
62. Polk BF, et al. *N Engl J Med*. 1980;303:541-545.
63. Calugar A, et al. *Clin Infect Dis*. 2006;42:981-988.
64. Deville JG, et al. *Clin Infect Dis*. 1995;21:639-642.

TABLE 6.7 — Vaccine-Preventable Diseases in Other Special Circumstances[a]

Condition or Circumstance	Possible Increased Risks
Animal workers and veterinarians	Anthrax and rabies
Bleeding diathesis	Bleeding (use IM vaccines with caution); hepatitis A in patients receiving clotting factor concentrates[b]
Children and adolescents taking aspirin	Reye syndrome with influenza or varicella[c]
College students living in dormitories	Influenza and invasive *N meningitidis*
Foreign field personnel	Travel-related vaccine-preventable diseases (see **Table 6.6**)
Food handlers	Transmission of hepatitis A[d]
Foresters	Rabies
Injecting illegal drug users	Hepatitis A and hepatitis B
Laboratory workers	Infection with laboratory pathogens for which vaccines are available
Men who have sex with men	Hepatitis A, hepatitis B, and human papillomavirus
Military personnel	Adenovirus, anthrax, influenza, invasive *N meningitidis*, smallpox, and travel-related vaccine-preventable diseases (see **Table 6.6**)
Morticians	Hepatitis B
Native Americans and Alaskans	Invasive *H influenzae* type b and invasive *S pneumoniae*[e]
Patients with cochlear implants or CSF leaks	Invasive *S pneumoniae*
Providers of essential community services	Influenza
Public safety workers	Hepatitis B
Residents of long-term care facilities	Influenza

Sewage workers	*Not* at increased risk for typhoid or hepatitis A in the United States
Spelunkers	Rabies
Staff of correctional facilities	Hepatitis B and influenza
Staff of day care centers	Influenza
Staff of institutions for developmentally disabled	Hepatitis B and influenza

[a] Risks that are particular to the conditions or circumstances are shown.

[b] Transmission of hepatitis A virus, which is resistant to solvent/detergent-treatment, was documented with older preparations of factor concentrates. Newer virus inactivation procedures, high vaccine coverage, and improved donor screening have dramatically reduced the risk of transmission.

[c] Patients should receive IIV. VAR and LAIV are contraindicated.

[d] HepA is not routinely recommended, but could be considered on a local basis.

[e] Routine immunization of otherwise healthy Native Americans and Alaska Natives with PPSV23 is not recommended, unless called for by public health authorities in specific communities where risk is increased.

65. ACIP provisional recommendations for health care personnel on use of tetanus toxoid, reduced diphtheria toxoid and acellular pertussis vaccine (Tdap) and use of postexposure antimicrobial prophylaxis. Centers for Disease Control Web site. http://www.cdc.gov/vaccines/recs/provisional/downloads/use-of-Tdap-in-hcp.pdf. Accessed November 21, 2011.
66. Gustafson TL, et al. *Pediatrics*. 1982;70:550-556.
67. Weber DJ, et al. *Am J Public Health*. 1988;78:19-23.
68. Travelers' Health—Yellow Book Homepage. Centers for Disease Control and Prevention Web site. http://wwwnc.cdc.gov/travel/page/yellowbook-2012-home.htm. Accessed November 21, 2011.
69. Boggild AK, et al. *Vaccine*. 2010;28:7389-7395.
70. Novak R, et al. *MMWR*. 2007;56:1080-1084.
71. CDC. *MMWR*. 2009;58:312.

7 Addressing Concerns About Vaccines

7

Vaccines have saved more lives than virtually any other public health intervention, and they are safer now than ever before. Despite this, providers face the daily challenge of convincing parents and patients that vaccines are safe, effective, and necessary. Good things have come from public concern about vaccines—the replacement, for example, of DTwP with the less reactogenic DTaP. However, the sensational claims made by antivaccination activists, celebrities, wealthy financiers, and rogue researchers have not held up to scientific scrutiny. Despite this, these claims receive airtime and make their way to the Internet. As a result, some well-meaning parents are either refusing to have their children vaccinated or asking for alternative schedules, and adults who should be vaccinated are opting out, translating directly into personal and public harm. This section provides tips on communicating the true risks and benefits of vaccination and gives some background on specific concerns that people have.

Communicating Risks and Benefits

■ The Meaning of Safety

What do we mean when we say that vaccines are *safe*? One definition of the word safe is *harmless*. This definition would imply that any negative consequence of vaccines would make them *unsafe*. But we know that all vaccines have side effects. For example, shots can cause pain, redness, swelling, and tenderness. Some may cause more concerning side effects—MMRV, for example, doubles the risk of febrile seizures when given as the first dose. While febrile seizures do not result in permanent damage, they can be frightening. There are historical examples of more serious side effects—for example, OPV caused paralytic polio, but only one case for every 2.3 million doses distributed. The change to IPV in the year 2000 was based on the occurrence of this extremely rare side effect, which had by then become more of a risk than natural polio itself in the United States.

Few things in life are harmless. Even everyday activities contain hidden dangers. For example, each year in the United States, 350 people are killed in bath- or shower-related accidents and 200 people are killed when food lodges in their windpipe. Just being outdoors can be dangerous—100 people are killed each year by lightning. By the harmless criterion, even routine daily activities could be considered unsafe.

Another definition of the word safe is *having been preserved from a real danger*. Using this definition, the danger (*the disease*) must be significantly greater than the means of protecting against the danger (*the vaccine*). To put it another way, a vaccine's benefits must clearly outweigh its risks. This is the case for all routinely recommended vaccines.

■ How We Think About Vaccination

At the societal level, the perceived value of vaccines paradoxically decreases as their effectiveness increases; when disease is eliminated, the public perceives no benefit from vaccines. The truth is, when vaccines work, *nothing* (as opposed to *disease*) happens. This fact, combined with widespread attention given to rare adverse events, leads to the perception that vaccines do more harm than good.

Scientists, public health officials, and providers think about these things in terms of probability and expected utility. The health value of getting a vaccine, and presumably the basis for decision making, can simplistically be seen as the difference between two things: 1) the probability of avoiding the disease multiplied by the *utility*, or value, of avoiding the disease; and 2) the probability of a vaccine side effect multiplied by the *disutility* of that side effect. For example, the probability of avoiding measles through vaccination is nearly 100%, and the utility of avoiding measles for any given individual is very high (because 1 in 100 patients develop pneumonia and 1 in 1000 die). On the other hand, the probability of getting fever and rash from MMR is low, say 5%, and the disutility of fever and rash is low, since these side effects are self-limited. Thus, the disutility of an uncommon side effect does not detract appreciably from the utility of preventing disease, and the overall mental model overwhelmingly favors vaccination. This is an example of *probabilistic thinking*.

Life is too complicated, however, to create a formula for every decision we need to make. Therefore, many people tend to think *heuristically*—that is, they employ (subconsciously or consciously) shortcut ways of thinking, rules of thumb if you will, to simplify complex decision-making.[1] One example of heuristic thinking is *do no harm*—here, a bad outcome is more tolerable if it occurs from *inaction* rather than *action*. In other words, hospitalization with influenza (something that just *happens*) is more tolerable than side effects of the vaccine (something that a person *causes* by choice). Another example is *avoidance of ambiguity*—here, a *known* risk is more acceptable than an *unknown* risk. In other words, the complications of chickenpox (a disease with which people are familiar) seem more acceptable than the potential risks of the vaccine (with which people are not familiar). One more example: *availability and representativeness*—here, the ease with which a person remembers something, and the degree to

which the circumstances are similar to one's own, correlates with the perceived probability that it will occur. Thus a graphic news story about a child who has an anaphylactic reaction to a vaccine might make someone think that anaphylaxis is more common than it really is (in truth, the risk of anaphylaxis after vaccination is less than 1 in a million[2]). Sometimes we identify so strongly with people in similar circumstances that we feel we actually *know* them. For example, in a 2009 survey,[3] 40% of parents said they personally knew of someone who experienced a harmful adverse event from MMR, something that would be impossible given the established rarity of serious adverse events.[4] It should be men- 7
tioned that not all heuristic thinking leads to vaccine hesitancy. For example, *bandwagoning*, the tendency for people to choose the decision of the majority as what might be wise for themselves, and *altruism*, a willingness to take on personal risks if it is for the benefit of others, might favor vaccination.

Vaccine hesitancy is driven by other thought processes as well. For example, there is *confirmation bias*, our tendency to seek out confirmatory evidence for what we already believe and to ignore contradictory evidence (we begin with the *belief* that vaccines must be harmful, then seek *validation* for this belief). And there is *folk numeracy*, our intuitive sense of numbers that upholds small, anecdotal experiences and makes it difficult for us to see the big picture.[5] So, for example, we intuitively "get" 3 kids with diabetes in the same school but we have difficulty conceptualizing a prospective cohort study with 4.7 million person-years of follow-up. Likewise, we have trouble coming to terms with background rates of adverse events. According to one study, if 10 million women were given a shot today, 86 would develop optic neuritis within 6 weeks, and if all 10 million women were pregnant, 16,684 would have a spontaneous abortion.[6] All of this would happen—*if the shot were a placebo*!

Human beings also have a tendency to find meaningful patterns in meaningless noise, something referred to as *patternicity* ("Almost all children with autism have received the MMR, so there *must* be a connection"). We also intrinsically believe that if one event closely follows another, it must have been *caused* by it (articulated in the Latin phrase, *post hoc ergo propter hoc*, or *after this, therefore because of this*). And there is *agenticity*, our belief that something or someone must be behind things ("There *must* be a conspiracy to cover up the dangers of vaccines, otherwise we would know about them").[7] Each of these is part of our evolved psychology, and understanding this is a starting place for shepherding parents and patients from ill-founded beliefs to rock-solid science. The task is all the more difficult in an age of consumerism, pop culture, and celebrity, where likeable actors and sports figures are entrusted as anti-establishment heros and truth-seekers.[8]

■ Communication Strategies

People will not undertake a risk-control measure such as vaccination unless they believe they can effectively control the risk. In other words, they need to understand that the vaccine really *does* prevent the disease. In addition, the risk should be personally relevant and serious. Nothing substitutes for a straightforward discussion about risks and benefits.

There is a disconnect between what physicians do and what patients want. For example, people want personal verbal communication from their physicians that conveys a sense of trust and respect. Time-motion studies, however, show that physicians spend <2 minutes discussing vaccines with their patients.[9] Physicians are sometimes reluctant to mention risks for fear of "opening a can of worms," but patients are interested in relevant, practical information that can be easily understood.[10] Here are some tips on getting to the point of what parents want to know about routine childhood vaccinations[11]:

- Describe which vaccines the child will receive today.
- Give the pertinent Vaccine Information Statements (VISs) to the parent (see *Chapter 3: Standards, Principles, and Regulations—Vaccine Information Statements [VISs]*).
- Explain why these vaccines are important.
- Review contraindications to each vaccine.
- Give a detailed account of the common, mild side effects and how to manage them.
- Give a brief account of any severe risks.
- Place today's vaccinations in the context of the overall schedule.

In addition, here are some suggestions regarding communication in the office setting:

- *Begin the discussion early*—One of the advantages of the birth dose of HepB is that it opens the door to discussing vaccines immediately after parenthood has begun. Similarly, doses of Tdap and/or IIV for mom (and dad!) during pregnancy are a good way to emphasize the importance of adult immunization, especially as this relates to protecting kids. In the initial discussions before hospital discharge, vaccines should be portrayed as part routine child care. Parents who express doubt or concern should be targeted for further discussion and should receive printed materials and other resources well before the 2-month visit.
- *Use a team approach*—Communication should be a coordinated effort between doctors, nurses, and other office personnel. Even the receptionist can provide an introduction to the vaccination visit, give VISs, and direct the parent or guardian to informational materials in the waiting room. Office nurses are accessible, highly invested in immunization, and can have a great impact on parents. Each member of the team should be

empowered and should know his or her function during the vaccination visit.

- *Be consistent*—Try to reach consensus on how the practice will handle specific issues. Communication is that much more difficult when some providers in the practice endorse "alternative schedules" while others do not.
- *Organize the visit effectively*—Face-to-face time with the doctor can be increased by building efficiencies into the visit, beginning with a preparatory phone call to remind the parent or guardian to bring the child's shot record and perhaps introducing the vaccines that are scheduled for the visit. Use of a screening questionnaire for contraindications (**Table 4.6**) can be helpful. Development of simple, direct messages and easy-to-understand printed materials can eliminate some questions and help focus the discussion. Ultimately, the use of high-valency combination vaccines may increase office efficiency and allow more time for communication. DVDs, books, and other printed materials that can be taken home may solidify concepts that were initiated during the visit. Consider scheduling vaccination visits at off-peak hours.
- *Understand individual backgrounds*—Many factors affect risk perception, including educational, emotional, religious, psychological, spiritual, philosophical, and intuitive foundations. Families differ in their orientation toward the medical establishment—some are traditional and trusting, others are cautious, challenging, and oriented toward alternative practices. Vaccine messages should be delivered with these differences in mind.
- *Layer information appropriately*—Information should be presented with sensitivity to individual intellectual needs. Providers should be aware of the patient's cognitive foundation and begin with information appropriate to that level. Parents who want to know more will ask.
- *Put risks into perspective*—Help parents and patients understand that there is often a difference between what we are afraid of and what the real risks are. For example, we are afraid of shark attacks, but we are 160,000 times more likely to be bitten by dogs.[12] We may be afraid of vaccines, but the diseases represent a much greater risk.
- *Engage patients in a decision-making partnership*—Research shows that parents depend on their health care providers for accurate, honest information (**Figure 7.1**). Building on this trust, the approach should be nonjudgmental, empathetic, and mutually respectful. That said, a physician's direct, personal advocacy ("I get a flu shot every year") carries the most weight.
- *Be aware of pitfalls*—Avoid the tendency to extrapolate from limited data and to fit equivocal data into preconceived notions. Consciously avoid being paternalistic and belittling.

FIGURE 7.1 — Sources of Information About Vaccinations

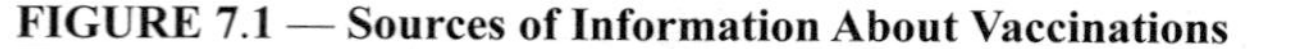

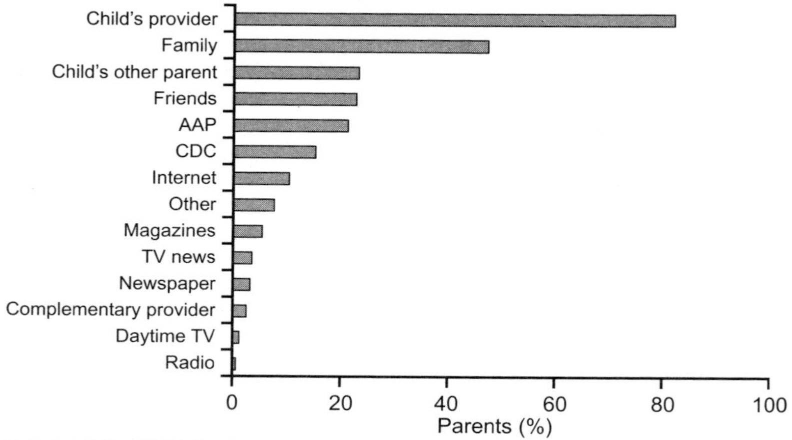

The graph shows the weighted proportion of parents (N=475) responding to the 2009 HealthStyles survey who indicated that these were important sources of information in deciding about vaccinating their youngest child.

Adapted from Kennedy A, et al. *Pediatrics*. 2011;127:S92-S99.

Understand how words and phrases can be misconstrued (**Table 7.1**).

- *Check for understanding*—Make sure parents and patients understand what you have told them and ask if they have any questions.

Vaccine Refusal

7

Many parents are requesting alternative schedules, agreeing to only selected formulations and antigens, or refusing to have their children vaccinated altogether—despite the best efforts of providers and public health agencies to address their concerns. Surveys show that the majority of pediatricians and family practitioners have had at least one family in their practice that has refused vaccination.[13,14] In 2004, it was estimated that slightly more than 1% of the birth cohort in the United States was underimmunized due to parental concerns about safety.[15] Ironically, *unvaccinated* children are more likely to come from well-off backgrounds with ready access to health care, in contrast to *undervaccinated* children—those from less well-off backgrounds who might be vaccinated if they had better access.[16] In a study published in 2008, about 28% of a national sample of parents had significant concerns about vaccinating their children.[17] In a national survey conducted in 2009, 11.5% of parents reported refusing at least one vaccination for their children.[3] The good news is that 90% believed that vaccines are a good way to protect their children and that a majority trust their doctors' recommendations. The disturbing news is that over half were concerned about serious adverse effects, and 25% believed that vaccines cause autism.

How should vaccine refusal be handled? First, listen to what the parent is saying. Providers may mistake the need for information or reassurance for flat-out refusal. Some parents may be refusing a single vaccine; others may be refusing all the vaccines that are due at a single visit. Few parents refuse all vaccines at all visits. Second, it must be recognized that whereas the decision not to vaccinate goes against the best medical advice, it rarely puts a child directly in harm's way. Ironically, this is due to the success of vaccination programs. The truth is that indigenous polio has been eliminated from the Western Hemisphere; therefore, any given unvaccinated child in the United States is, on the whole, unlikely to get polio. In this context, refusing to allow a child to receive the polio vaccine can hardly be interpreted as actionable medical neglect. On the other hand, there are some situations where vaccine refusal could bring immediate harm to a child—during an epidemic, for example, or after a tetanus-prone injury. In such situations, it would be appropriate to involve governmental agencies or the courts to force action in the child's best interest. While states may be reluctant to act unless there is immediate

TABLE 7.1 — Language and Meaning

Expression or Word	Technical Meaning	Common Interpretation
Biased	Having a systematic error that could lead to the wrong conclusion	Not having an open mind
Favor rejection of hypothesis	The data suggest that the hypothesis should be rejected	They do not know
Not statistically significant	The findings are likely to be due to chance alone	The findings are not important
Plausible	Theoretically possible	Factual or worthy of belief
Positive	Value greater than zero	Good
Relative risk	The ratio of two rates of risks	A relationship between risks
Statistically significant	The findings are not likely to be due to chance alone	The observed differences are important
Vaccine adverse event	Something temporally associated with vaccination	Side effect of vaccination

Adapted from Myers MG, Pineda D. Misinformation about vaccines. In: Barrett ADT, Stanberry LR. *Vaccines for Biodefense and Emerging and Neglected Diseases*. Maryland Heights, MO: Elsevier, Inc; 2009.

and substantial danger, it is notable that the courts have repeatedly upheld compulsory immunization laws as a reasonable exercise of the state's power, even in the absence of an epidemic (see *Chapter 3: Standards, Principles, and Regulations—Mandates*).

Third, parents need to understand that the decision not to immunize their children places other children at risk. Outbreaks are spread by unvaccinated persons, and even vaccinated children whose parents have diligently tried to protect them can still get the disease—this is due to the real phenomena of primary vaccine failure and waning immunity. In addition, some children cannot be immunized for medical reasons and can therefore only be protected by herd immunity. Thus, immunization can be construed as a *civic duty*, and failure to immunize can be seen as indirectly bringing the possibility of harm to others. Interestingly, some religious traditions may see immunizations as an imperative—Judiasm, for example, where immunizations may be seen to fulfill the obligation to guard one's own health and to prevent others from becoming sick.[18] If parents understood the scientific facts about the safety of vaccines—and that is a big "if"—it is hard to imagine that most parents would not agree to have their children immunized on the basis of altruism alone. Many parents, however, fear things that have not been, and may not ever be, studied—side effects that could appear decades down the road, for example.

Yet there are still parents who will not agree to vaccination. For these situations, the American Academy of Pediatrics[19] and the Immunization Action Coalition[20] developed refusal to vaccinate forms that can be signed by the parent. It is not clear what legal protection these forms would afford the practitioner in the case of a bad outcome from a vaccine-preventable disease (nevertheless, the signed form should be placed in the permanent medical record). The idea here is to encourage parents to rethink the issue and to document the provider's efforts to communicate the true risks and benefits of immunization. By signing a form, the parent acknowledges that he or she understands the purpose of the vaccine, why it is recommended, what the risks of vaccination are, and what the consequences of infection may be, including disease, death, permanent impairment, transmission to others, and exclusion from school during outbreaks. Some providers place an expiration date on the form in order to encourage readdressing the issue in the future.

Some parents want a modified schedule for their children, one that spreads the shots out over time. Whereas the end of negotiation in this case—namely that the child receives all recommended vaccines—might justify the means, it also places a burden on the provider to prioritize the immunizations. If the parent will only allow two shots on a given day, which ones should be given and which ones deferred? The decision should be made based on the epidemiology and potential consequences of infection. So, for example, given the above discussion about polio, it might make sense to defer IPV in favor of DTaP, since pertussis is still prevalent. Deferral prolongs the period of vulnerability to disease, which in the case of polio may not be consequential; however, it also increases the likelihood that the vaccine series will not be completed.

In a 2005 clinical report (reaffirmed in 2009), the AAP took the position that negotiation is in the best interest of the child, and that physicians should avoid discharging patients from their practices because of vaccine refusal.[21] However, there is no law that says a provider must acquiesce to a parent's wishes. Some providers are not willing to accept the potential exposure to liability that is inherent in negotiating a modified schedule, and they worry about unimmunized kids in their waiting rooms. Others feel that negotiation is a slippery slope—what if the next request is for half doses, or worse yet homeopathic ones? Still other providers feel that drawing a hard line behind the recommended schedule is the best way to send the message that vaccinations—at the proper time, in the proper doses, and according to the proper schedule—are a critical component of preventive medicine; this alone might be enough to change some parents' minds.

Ultimately, failure to come to terms about immunization may predict a poor therapeutic relationship in general, which could affect the care of the child. In this situation, the AAP suggests that families may be encouraged to find another physician or practice. It should be noted that the American Medical Association Code of Ethics, Section E-8.115, states that physicians have the option of withdrawing from a case, so long as notice is given far enough in advance as to permit another medical provider to be secured.[22] Bear in mind that despite the risks, retention allows continued opportunities to break down barriers and protects the child from seeking care from chiropractors and alternative medicine practitioners.

Many studies suggest that the most trusted person in this whole debate is you—the provider.[23] Personally advocating for vaccination, tempered by compassionate engagement and recognition of a shared, firm commitment to the child's well-being, underpinned by scientific data, is the most important thing you can do to ensure the protection of children. Parents should be part of the decision-making process, but many parents will want to know what you have done or would do with your own children.

Antivaccinationism

A simple Internet search using terms such as vaccines or immunization yields a multitude of web sites that contain non–peer-reviewed data, frightening anecdotes, and pseudoscientific arguments intermingled with legitimate concerns for adverse events such as fever, redness, and swelling. Parents may have trouble separating the *information* from the *misinformation*. In fact, in a study published in 2010, 71% of Google "hits" using the term "vaccination" were opposed to vaccination.[24] Many of these web sites are sponsored by organizations that claim authority, credibility, and scientific rigor, which, along with some lay people, vocal celebrities, and fringe researchers, collectively constitute a modern antivaccination movement.[25,26] In truth, antivaccinationism is as old as vaccination itself.[27] It is rooted in a host of underlying sentiments, from libertarianism to distrust of government and science to naturopathy and even religious fundamentalism; it is fueled by sensationalistic and irresponsible journalism, easy access to unfiltered analyses, and a pervasive cultural lack of critical thinking and understanding of science. Superb books on antivaccinationism and its consequences have been published.[28-30]

Antivaccinationists offer strong emotive or political appeals, make explicit claims about vaccines that are unsupported or even contradicted by published data, and they call people to action in opposing vaccine policy. Examples of explicit claims include the following: vaccines cause idiopathic diseases; adverse reactions are underreported; vaccines erode immunity; vaccine policy is motivated by profit; vaccines are ineffective; diseases declined without vaccines; and vaccination is a violation of civil liberties.[24,31,32] **Table 7.2** summarizes some of the rhetorical appeals that are used.

Table 7.3 lists some web sites (and their sponsoring organizations) that have an antivaccination orientation. Providers should remain informed about the content of these sites in order to be better prepared to address issues that patients may raise. Some of the claims made on these sites are patently false, if not ridiculous—claims, for example, that smallpox is harmless and not very infectious; that diseases are caused by imbalanced bodily conditions and lifestyle choices rather than microorganisms; that polio is caused by sugary foods; and that rabies might be psychosomatic.[24]

Individuals and organizations that oppose immunization or argue for "alternative" approaches share common sentiments. **Table 7.4** lists some of those ideas and the reasons why they represent flawed thinking.

The Costs of Public Concern

It is one thing to understand that unvaccinated persons are at increased risk of disease. This makes common sense and has been repeatedly demonstrated, even in the era when most people are vaccinated and many vaccine-preventable diseases are less common. The risk of measles, for example, is 35-fold higher in exemptors, even in communities where >90% of children are

TABLE 7.2 — Rhetorical Appeals Made by Vaccine-Protest Organizations on the Internet

Authoritative and Scientific
• Present their organization as a legitimate, official body with scientific credibility
• Reference self-published works and alternative medicine literature
• Use indiscriminate citations (eg, letters to newspapers, television interviews)
• Draw alternative conclusions from peer-reviewed studies
• Claim to present "both sides"
• Provide links to provaccine sites
Emotive Appeals
• Paint an "us" (the organization, concerned parents) vs "them" (the medical establishment, government, pharmaceutical industry) picture
• Describe physicians as willing conspirators or manipulated pawns
• Pit parents' love and compassion against cold, analytical science
• Feature anecdotal accounts of purported vaccine injury
• Suggest that responsible parenting means refusing vaccination
• Urge parents to resist coercion
• Warn the public about conspiracy
• Characterize vaccines as "unnatural" and suggest that a natural lifestyle will prevent disease
Search for Truth
• Depict their struggle as a search for truth against a backdrop of cover-up
• Highlight excavated "facts" that were hitherto neglected
• Portray rank-breaking doctors as enlightened heroes

Adapted from Davies P, et al. *Arch Dis Child.* 2002;87:22-25.

immunized.[33] The risk of pertussis is also high,[34] and a study from Michigan demonstrated that the highest risk of pertussis was in areas with the highest rates of nonmedical exemption.[35]

It is another thing to connect public fear of vaccination to public harm. The best example is what happened in the United Kingdom in the late 1970s. Anecdotal reports claiming that the whole-cell pertussis vaccine caused encephalopathy, popularized in the lay press, led to widespread fear of the vaccine and to a dramatic decline in immunization rates. The result was a tragic increase in pertussis cases and many infant deaths. Not surprisingly, the same scenario played out in other countries where antivaccination movements gained traction, but not in countries

TABLE 7.3 — Web Sites With a Vaccine-Protest Orientation

URL	Sponsor or Name of Web Site
http://www.ageofautism.com/	Age of Autism
http://canaryparty.org/	The Canary Party
http://www.cryshame.co.uk/	Cryshame!
http://generationrescue.org/	Generation Rescue
http://www.gval.com	Global Vaccine Awareness League
http://www.jabs.org.uk/	Justice Awareness and Basic Support (JABS)
http://www.know-vaccines.org	Kids Need Options With Vaccines (KNOW Vaccines)
http://mvvic.org	International Medical Council on Vaccination
http://www.nvic.org/	National Vaccine Information Center
http://vaccineinfo.net	Parents Requesting Open Vaccine Education (PROVE)
http://www.vaccineeducation.org/	People Advocating Vaccine Education (PAVE)
http://safeminds.org/	Safe Minds
http://thinktwice.com/	Thinktwice Global Vaccine Institute
http://www.vaccination.co.uk/	Vaccination
http://vran.org/	Vaccination Risk Awareness Network (VRAN)
http://www.nccn.net/~wwithin/vaccine.htm	Vaccination Information & Choice Network
http://www.vaclib.org	Vaccination Liberation
http://www.vaccinetruth.org/	Vaccine Information

Accessed September 28, 2011.

TABLE 7.4 — Flawed Thinking About Vaccines

Claim	Why This is Incorrect or Misleading
Doctors do not read the primary data and do not fully understand vaccines.	Committees of experts review the primary data. Their record has been spot-on.
There is a conspiracy to misrepresent the data.	There is no evidence of a conspiracy.
Vaccine-preventable diseases are rarely seen in practice.	This is evidence that vaccines work. Some diseases are not rare. Surveillance data trump antecdotal experiences.
Natural immunity is better than vaccine-induced immunity.	The cost of natural immunity is the risk of serious disease.
Vaccines are not adequately tested for safety.	Vaccines are among the most thoroughly tested pharmaceuticals.
Vaccines protect the public but not individuals.	Individuals benefit by becoming immune and, *as long as others are immunized*, by having less chance of exposure.
Reports in VAERS and language in the package insert constitute accurate profiles of vaccine side effects.	VAERS reports do not establish causality. Package inserts list events that may not be causally related to vaccination.
There is a middle ground between causality and coincidence.	Either vaccine *do* or *do not* cause certain adverse events.
Science fails because it cannot prove there is no connection between vaccines and certain adverse events.	Science works by rejecting or failing to reject the null hypothesis.

Adapted from Offit PA, Moser CA. *Pediatrics* 2009;123:e164-e169.

that had sustained vaccine use. Similarly, claims in the late 1990s that MMR vaccine causes autism led to dramatic declines in MMR uptake in the United Kingdom—and subsequent outbreaks of measles. More examples of the connection between fear of vaccines and harm are given in **Table 7.5**.

To understand the impact of vaccine refusal, one need go no further than Indiana, where in 2005 an unvaccinated teenager returned from a mission trip to Romania, unknowingly incubating measles.[36] The next day she attended a gathering of approximately 500 church members, and the result was 33 cases of measles among church members and 1 case in a hospital phlebotomist (who was not a church member). Three people were hospitalized and one spent 6 days on a ventilator. The vast majority of cases occurred in unvaccinated persons. Several important things can be gleaned from this outbreak. First, fear of adverse events was the main reason people refused vaccination. In testament to the prevalence of misinformation, some families feared MMR because of the preservative thimerosal, which has *never* been part of the vaccine. Second, the church was largely white, middle class, and well educated, reflecting the demographics of vaccine refusal. Third, the church itself had no official position on immunization—vaccine refusal was a subcultural phenomenon (20 of the 28 affected children were home-schooled, suggesting that there are other sociodemographic correlates of vaccine refusal). Fourth, even though the attack rate was much higher in unvaccinated persons, some vaccinated people still got measles. This illustrates the real issue of primary vaccine failure and the fact that unvaccinated people place vaccinated people at risk. Fifth, the outbreak was almost entirely confined to church members—coverage rates in the surrounding community were high enough to prevent spread. Finally, the case could not be made more clearly that diseases such as measles are literally a plane flight away, and that all it takes to ignite an outbreak is for the virus to land in a community with enough susceptible individuals.

Specific Concerns

Here are some specific questions about vaccines that are on the minds of parents and patients. The information provided should serve as a foundation for effective communication of the true risks and benefits.

■ Are Vaccines Still Necessary?

Everyone agrees that vaccine-preventable diseases are less prevalent now than they were before vaccines were introduced (**Table 1.5**). However, the myth still circulates that the diseases were disappearing before we had the vaccines. Nothing could be farther from the truth, to which anyone whose medical career has

TABLE 7.5 — Fear of Vaccines Leads to Public Harm

Vaccine[a]	Event or Finding	Evidence that Event Resulted From Willful Refusal to Vaccinate
DTwP	Outbreaks of pertussis in the United Kingdom, associated with hundreds of deaths,[b] late 1970s	Intense media coverage of anecdotal reports of neurological reactions resulted a drop in vaccination rates from 81% to 31%. Outbreaks were not seen in countries without antivaccine movements.[c]
DTaP	Higher risk of pertussis in certain states	Risk correlates with availability of personal belief exemptions and the ease with which such exemptions are granted.[d]
	Pertussis cases and controls in Colorado	Odds of vaccine refusal 23-times higher among cases. Virtually all cases among refusers, and 11% of cases in the whole population, were due to refusal itself.[e]
MMR	Measles eliminated from the United Kingdom in 1994 but endemic again in 2008[f]	Immunization rates fell dramatically after Wakefield's 1998 article that suggested a causal link with autism.[g]
	33 cases of measles among members of a church in Indiana, 2005	31 cases occurred among members who refused vaccination because they feared adverse reactions.[h]
	Measles outbreaks in the United States, 2008 and 2011	The majority of cases were unvaccinated or vaccination status unknown. Of eligible persons, many were not vaccinated because of religious or personal beliefs.[i,j]
Hib	*H influenzae* disease in Minnesota in 2008—highest number of cases since 1992	3 of the 5 cases were intentionally not immunized, including one who died.[k]
VAR	Varicella cases and controls in Colorado	Odds of vaccine refusal 9-times higher among cases. Virtually all cases among refusers, and 5% of cases in the whole population, were due to refusal itself.[l]

[a] In some cases, the concern may have been about all vaccines, or multiple vaccines, rather than the one cited.
[b] Cherry JD. *Curr Prob Pediatr*. 1984;14:1-78.
[c] Gangarosa EJ, et al. *Lancet.* 1998;351:356-361.
[d] Omer SB, et al. *JAMA.* 2006;296:1757-1763.
[e] Glanz JM, et al. *Pediatrics*. 2009;123:1446-1451.
[f] Measles once again endemic in the United Kingdom. Eurosurveillance Web site. http://www.eurosurveillance.org/viewarticle.aspx?articleid=18919. Accessed September 28, 2011.
[g] Leask J. *Nature*. 2011;473:443-445.
[h] Parker AA, et al. *N Engl J Med.* 2006;355:447-455.
[i] CDC. *MMWR*. 2008;57:893-896.
[j] CDC. *MMWR*. 2011;60:666-668.
[k] CDC. *MMWR*. 2009;58(3):58-60.
[l] Glanz JM, et al. *Arch Pediatr Adolesc Med*. 2010;164(1):66-70.

7

spanned the demise of *H influenzae* type b can testify. In the early 1980s, 1 in 200 children developed invasive *H influenzae* disease. Call nights in the hospital were replete with cases of bacteremia, meningitis, periorbital cellulitis, and the like. Today's pediatric residents have never seen a case—and the change occurred in the early 1990s, after the institution of universal infant Hib immunization. There is an undeniable association between the introduction of new vaccines and the beginning of the end of the respective diseases, as has been seen in the last 2 decades with varicella, hepatitis A, *S pneumoniae*, and rotavirus.

Now that many of these diseases are rare, it is hard for parents and patients to understand why vaccines are still important. Here are a few reasons.

- *Some diseases are still prevalent*—Despite our successes, many vaccine-preventable diseases are still around. The choice not to vaccinate against pertussis, for example, is a choice to take a significant risk of getting the disease. The same is true for *S pneumoniae*. Influenza kills 36,000 people and human papillomavirus infects millions every year in the United States.
- *Diseases could easily re-emerge*—Some diseases continue to circulate at very low levels. If immunization rates decrease, outbreaks are likely to occur. This is exactly what happened between 1989 and 1991 in the United States, when 55,622 cases of measles and 123 deaths from the disease were reported.[37] The single most important contributing factor was low vaccine coverage, especially among preschoolers in inner cities. By 2003, after renewed efforts to achieve universal vaccination and the implementation of a 2-dose schedule, measles was no longer endemic in the United States. This means that there was enough population immunity to prevent sustained transmission, but the situation could change dramatically if coverage rates fall. Outbreaks of mumps in 2006,[38] measles in 2008[39] and 2011[40], and pertussis in 2010[41] are further evidence that diseases can re-emerge.
- *Infections can easily be imported from other parts of the world*—Diseases such as polio and diphtheria still occur in other countries. Tourism, immigration, and international business travel contribute to the ease with which these diseases can be imported into the United States. The outbreaks of measles mentioned above were due to importation.
- *Some diseases cannot be eradicated or extinguished*—Tetanus, which is acquired from the environment as opposed to person-to-person transmission, is a good example.

■ Is Natural Infection Better at Inducing Immunity?

Natural infection may induce stronger and longer-lasting immunity than vaccines. Whereas immunity from disease often follows a single natural infection, immunity from vaccines usually occurs only after several doses and, in some cases, wanes with time. A notable example of waning immunity occurs with the pertussis vaccine—by the time children are teenagers, they have lost the protective immunity imparted by the childhood DTaP series (even natural pertussis immunity wanes with time). As a result, teenagers account for a large proportion of reported cases and serve as a reservoir for transmission in the community. Fortunately, there are now vaccines that can boost immunity in adolescents and adults.

There are some diseases for which vaccines are actually *better* at inducing immunity than natural infection. Infants who are infected with *H influenzae* do not develop effective antibody responses due to an inherent maturational defect in recognizing polysaccharide antigens (see *Chapter 1: Introduction to Vaccinology—Active Immunization*). Hib vaccines, on the other hand, are very effective in young infants because, in coupling the polysaccharide to protein, they are capable of enlisting T-cell help in driving antibody production by B-cells.

The difference between vaccination and natural infection is the price paid for immunity. For chickenpox, the price paid for natural immunity might be pneumonitis, respiratory failure, encephalitis, or necrotizing fasciitis. For *S pneumoniae*, it might be mental retardation from meningitis—and that would only buy you immunity to the one serotype that caused the infection. Likewise, for human papillomavirus, the price might be cervical dysplasia—and if you are lucky enough to resolve the dysplasia without progression to cancer, you are left with immunity to only one human papillomavirus type (the vaccines are only labeled for protection against two of the many cancer-causing serotypes). The price of immunity to shingles is a case of shingles, and, in some cases, postherpetic neuralgia. The cost of vaccine-induced protection against shingles is the cost of the vaccine, plus minor reactogenicity.

■ Can Multiple Vaccines Overload the Immune System?

One hundred years ago, children were routinely vaccinated against one disease—smallpox. Forty years ago, it was five diseases—diphtheria, pertussis, tetanus, polio, and smallpox, necessitating as many as eight shots by 2 years of age. The routine childhood immunization schedule in 2012 calls for over 50 separate vaccine doses by 18 years of age. The good news is that through all of this, 16 different diseases are prevented; the bad news is that some people wonder if it is just too much.

The possibility of immune overload must be put into perspective. Every day, people are bombarded by antigens to which their immune systems must respond. This includes viruses and bacteria from the external environment as well as organisms from within, particularly those in the mouth, nasopharynx, and gut. Most people are not sick most of the time—this speaks to the robustness of the immune system's ability to meet these challenges. Even the most vulnerable people—neonates—seem to do just fine. Within a matter of hours of birth, the initially sterile gastrointestinal tract becomes heavily colonized with a wide variety of bacteria, some of which are potentially harmful. Yet the specific secretory IgA responses that are stimulated by colonization are, by and large, adequate to prevent invasion.

Even though children receive more vaccines today than they did 40 years ago, the number of separate immunologic challenges (ie, proteins or polysaccharides) represented by the routine childhood schedule has drastically decreased (**Table 7.6**). The main reason for this is the elimination of smallpox vaccine, which contained about 200 antigens, and the whole-cell pertussis vaccine, which contained about 3000 antigens. In this sense, the vaccine schedule is "purer" than it used to be.

People fear that vaccines might weaken the immune system and thereby increase susceptibility to infectious agents not contained in the vaccines (so-called *heterologous infections*). Vaccines may cause temporary suppression of delayed-type hypersensitivity skin reactions or transiently alter certain lymphocyte function tests. MMR may decrease the immune response to VAR if the latter is administered within 30 days (and not given on the same day). However, the short-lived immunosuppression caused by certain vaccines does not result in an increased risk of heterologous infections. In fact, just the opposite has been seen. For example, a study from California showed a *decrease* in invasive heterologous infections in the few months following immunization.[42] Similarly, a study from Germany found that children who received the diphtheria, pertussis, tetanus, Hib, and polio vaccines in the first 3 months of life actually had *fewer* infections with vaccine-related as well as vaccine-unrelated pathogens.[43] A study in Denmark that included 2,900,463 person-years of follow-up found no causal association between any of the childhood vaccines and hospitalization for any of seven different infectious diseases unrelated to the vaccine-preventable diseases themselves.[44] Other studies also refute the notion that vaccines increase susceptibility to infection.[45,46]

Bacterial and viral infections, on the other hand, often *do* predispose children and adults to severe infections with other pathogens. For example, influenza infection predisposes patients to pneumococcal and staphylococcal pneumonia. Similarly, varicella infection increases susceptibility to invasive group A beta-hemolytic streptococcal infections. Thus, if susceptibility to heterologous infection is the concern, vaccination makes more sense than no vaccination.

■ Are Adjuvants Dangerous?

Adjuvants are substances that enhance the immune response to vaccine antigens (see *Chapter 1: Introduction to Vaccinology—*

TABLE 7.6 — Maximum Number of Separate Antigens Represented by Vaccines Routinely Recommended for Children and Adolescents

Vaccine	1960	1980	2000	2012
Smallpox[a]	200			
Diphtheria	1	1	1	1
Tetanus	1	1	1	1
Pertussis	3000[b]	3000[b]	5[c]	5[c]
IPV	15	15	15	15
MMR[a]		24	24	24
Hib			2	2
VAR[a]			69	69
PCV			8	14[d]
HepB			1	1
HepA				4
HPV				4[e]
RV[a]				20[f]
MCV4				5
IIV[g]				12[h]
Total	~3217	~3041	126	177

[a] These are live vaccines. Estimates are given of the number of different proteins expressed during infection. Not all of these proteins necessarily represent an antigenic challenge to the host.

[b] Estimate of the number of proteins contained in DTwP.

[c] DTaP contains anywhere from 2 to 5 separate pertussis antigens.

[d] In 2010, PCV13 replaced PCV7.

[e] HPV2 contains 2 separate antigens and HPV4 contains 4.

[f] Rotavirus codes for 12 proteins, 6 structural and 6 nonstructural. RV1 therefore expresses 12 separate antigens and RV5, because it contains a mixture of reassortants, expresses a total of 20 separate antigens (some proteins expressed by each reassortant are the same).

[g] Contains 3 different strains of influenza virus.

[h] The influenza virion contains 8 structural proteins, 3 of which (hemagglutinin, neuraminidase, and M2) are embedded in the lipid envelope and one of which, M1, is closely associated with the envelope. Vaccines are made from the solubilized lipid envelope and therefore are estimated to contain as many as 4 antigens from each strain. However, only the hemagglutinin and neuraminidase are immunologically relevant.

Adapted from Offit PA, et al. *Pediatrics.* 2002;109:124-129.

Basic Vaccine Immunology). Aluminum salts have been used as adjuvants for over 80 years, and hundreds of millions of people have received vaccines containing them.[47] Whereas local reactions such as erythema, nodules, hypersensitivity, and granuloma formation have been reported, serious or persistent adverse events have not. A meta-analysis published in 2004 included studies that compared alum-adjuvanted DTP vaccines to their nonadjuvanted counterparts.[48] In children ≤18 months of age, vaccines containing aluminum hydroxide caused nearly twice as much erythema and induration but there was no increase in collapse, convulsions, or persistent screaming or crying. In older children, aluminum-containing vaccines caused more localized, persistent pain, but not erythema, induration or fever. In a sense, the pain is part of the gain—the irritation or inflammation (and hence pain) caused by the adjuvant also drives the immune response.

Large quantities of aluminum can cause neurologic disease.[49] However, the burden of aluminum exposure through vaccines is far less than the guidelines for safe exposure established by the Agency for Toxic Substances Disease Registry. In fact, infants are exposed to much more aluminum through their diets than through vaccines. Whereas the total aluminum exposure from vaccines in the first 6 months of life is <5 mg, breast-fed infants ingest 7 mg and formula-fed infants as much as 38 to 117 mg over the same period of time, depending on the type of formula.[50]

The newest adjuvant to be used in the United States, AS04 (used in HPV2), contains a derivative of lipopolysaccharide, a major component of bacterial cell walls. Patients may cite this when they say that vaccines "contain toxins." However, they need to understand that exposures to toxins like lipopolysaccharide occur continuously given our symbiotic relationship with bacteria.[51] The truth is that anything (even water!) can be dangerous if taken in large amounts. The amount of lipopolysaccharide in AS04-adjuvanted vaccines is just enough to stimulate a robust antibody response but not nearly enough to cause major problems. This is borne out by many studies demonstrating excellent tolerability and no association with serious adverse events. Even more insidious events have been carefully studied; for example, in an integrated analysis of randomized controlled trials involving nearly 70,000 vaccinees, autoimmune events occurred in the same proportion (about 0.5%) of both AS04-exposed and nonexposed individuals after a mean follow-up period of 21 months.[52]

■ Are the Additives in Vaccines Harmful?

We think of vaccines as antigens, but in truth, vaccines contain additional ingredients that have functions ranging from stabilizing the antigens to preventing them from sticking to the vial. The nature of these substances varies widely and includes the following: proteins; sodium and potassium salts; buffers; sugars; antibiotics; preservatives; amino acids; inactivating agents; and detergents. Some of these are added purposefully in small quantities—gelatin or sucrose, for example, used as stabilizers. Others "leak through" from the manufacturing process and are present in only trace amounts—formaldehyde and sodium deoxycholate, for example, used to inactivate and disrupt viruses. All of the "extra" substances contained in each vaccine are listed in the tables in *Section B: Diseases and Vaccines* under "Excipients and contaminants" (technically, an excipient is an inert substance used as a diluent or vehicle for a drug, but here it has a broader meaning, something along the lines of "everything except the antigen and adjuvant").

Some vaccine ingredients can trigger allergic reactions in sensitized individuals. A classic example is the residual egg protein in influenza vaccines, which can trigger anaphylaxis in those who are severely egg-allergic. Other examples include the gelatin and neomycin in MMR. To some extent, these reactions can be avoided through proper screening (see *Chapter 4: Vaccine Practice—Screening*). 7

None of the other ingredients in vaccines have been demonstrated to be harmful in the quantities used. For example, influenza vaccines may contain at most 100 mcg of residual formaldehyde; for a 10-kg child, that would amount to 10 mcg/kg of exposure *on one day*. The (oral) reference dose for formaldehyde, which is an estimate of *daily* exposure that is likely to be without appreciable risk of deleterious effects *during a person's lifetime*, is 200 mcg/kg.[53] Moreover, a 10-kg child would be expected to have more than 2000 mcg of formaldehyde circulating in the blood at any given time, the result of normal biosynthetic processes.[47]

■ Are "Alternative Schedules" a Good Idea?

Many parents are leery of a "one size fits all" vaccine schedule and are interested in "alternative" schedules that "spread the vaccines out" over time.[54] One of their main concerns, addressed above, is that too many vaccines in one visit could overwhelm the immune system. They also worry about the potential for serious reactions and the cumulative effects of chemical additives (also addressed above) and "toxins" derived from pathogens. Sympathetic voices are easily found.[55] Alternative schedules are seductive—they reduce the cognitive dissonance between wanting to remain in favor of protection but fearing that vaccines are harmful. The problem is that alternative schedules do not provide optimal protection. Moreover, there is no scientific basis for their implementation; in fact, the "basis" for alternative schedules, like so many other antivaccination positions, is anecdotal experience, conjecture, false assumptions, misinterpretation of published data, and a failure to understand the workings of science.[56]

Here are some take-home points:

- *Tailor-made schedules violate an implicit social contract.* This is perhaps the most egregious aspect of schedules that delay vaccinations. Any given individual has the personal luxury of delaying certain vaccines because the diseases are uncommon. But *the diseases are uncommon because the other children are immunized on time*. To put it another way, the other children and their families have taken on the personal risk of immunization (eg, sore arms and low-grade fevers) in part so that all children are protected; in this context, delaying vaccinations in one's own child exploits the goodwill of others. If everyone chose delay, the diseases would come back in full force.

- *Alternative schedules necessitate prioritizing some vaccines over others*. None of the vaccines in the routine childhood schedule have priority over the others. This is because the occurrence, by importation or otherwise, of any of these diseases is completely unpredictable.
- *Spreading out vaccines requires more visits*. With the routine childhood schedule, series completion occurs in 4 or 5 visits by 15 or 18 months of age. Some alternative schedules require as many as 15 visits, delaying series completion until 42 months of age. At a time when health care costs are under scrutiny, it seems wrong to spend money on unnecessary visits. In addition, the more scheduled visits there are, the more visits that will be missed, leading to further delays and costs.
- *Delaying vaccines creates risk*. Here is an example. Some advocate delaying the birth dose of HepB until the third year of life. As we learned in 1999, when hospitals deferred the birth dose because of the thimerosal scare, this practice will inevitably result in some infants who should have been protected by vaccination but were not (the issue is that the mother's HBsAg status at delivery may be unknown or inaccurate).[57] Here is another example: intentionally delaying vaccinations markedly increases the risk that children will not be fully covered by the second year of life.[58] Clearly, the only accomplishment of delayed vaccination is increased susceptibility to disease.
- *On-time vaccination is not harmful*. Even though the total number of vaccines given to infants (and consequently the number given per visit) has increased, the risk of adverse events, such as medically attended visits for fever, has not.[59] Moreover, a study published in 2010 showed that on-time immunization had no adverse effect on neuropsychological outcomes 7 to 10 years later.[60]

■ Do Vaccines Cause Allergies and Autoimmune Disease?

The Hygiene Hypothesis

There has been an increase in the incidence of allergic diseases in developed countries. The *hygiene hypothesis* holds that "clean living" brought on by economic development and the move from an agrarian to an urban lifestyle is responsible for this increase. The idea is that less exposure to micribiota early in life, while the immune system is maturing, results in more Th2-cells and fewer T regulator cells (see *Chapter 1: Introduction to Vaccinology—The*

Germinal Center Reaction), immunological biases that promote allergy and autoimmunity.[61] In fact, a study published in 2011 showed that children who lived on farms had a lower prevalence of asthma and atopy than a reference group, and the risk of these conditions was inversely related to the intensity and diversity of microbial exposures.[62] The question is, are vaccinations part of "clean living" and do they, by preventing childhood infections, contribute to the same immunological biases? Several large epidemiologic studies suggest the answer is "no."[63] Furthermore, for live vaccines at least, there is an inherent inconsistency in the idea, because in this case, vaccination *is* infection!

Asthma

A well-controlled study in the United States identified 18,407 children with asthma who were born between 1991 and 1997 and compared them with a control group without asthma.[64] Exposure to DTwP, OPV, MMR, Hib, or HepB was no more common among cases than controls. Another population-based cohort study was performed in Leicestershire, United Kingdom.[65] A total of 6811 children were enrolled between 1993 and 1997 and questioned about respiratory symptoms repeatedly until 2003. Data on pertussis vaccinations were independently acquired, and the study included 23,201 person-years of follow-up. No association between vaccination and wheezing or asthma was seen. In a subsequent analysis, it was shown that delaying the first immunization beyond the first 2 months of life did not protect against wheezing at 5 to 10 years of age.[66] Other studies also refute an association between vaccinations and the development of asthma.[67]

Other Forms of Atopy

A well-controlled study of over 600 children prospectively evaluated the risk of allergies following receipt of the pertussis vaccine.[68,69] Infants were randomized beginning at 2 months of age to receive a 2-component DTaP vaccine, a 5-component DTaP, DTwP, or DT and were followed up at 7 years of age. No difference in the incidence of allergic diseases was observed between children who did or did not receive pertussis vaccine. Of interest, children who acquired natural pertussis infection were more likely to have allergic diseases than children who were not infected with pertussis.

A cohort study from Tasmania published in 2007 showed small and inconsistent associations between receipt of diphtheria toxoid and asthma, eczema, and food allergies.[70] The authors, however, acknowledged the problems with this and other similar studies: the possibility of recall bias (parents of children with allergies may falsely recall immunizations that were not actually given), difficulty ascertaining the timing of vaccination and types of vaccines that were given, inaccurate reporting of allergies by parents, and health care–seeking behavior on the part of parents (certain parents may seek both immunizations and diagnoses of allergy). Many of these factors could have led to an increased association between immunizations and atopic conditions.

One of the strongest studies to date was the PARSIFAL (Prevention of Allergy-Risk Factors for Sensitization in Children Related to Farming and Anthroposophic Lifestyle) study, conducted in five European countries and involving over 12,000 children born between 1987 and 1996.[71] No association between measles vaccination and allergy was seen (interestingly, measles *infection* was associated with a *reduced* risk of allergy). One strength of this study was the inclusion of allergen-specific serum IgE levels as a marker of allergic sensitization in a subset of children.

Diabetes

The purported link between vaccines and type 1 diabetes is vaccine-induced enhancement of preexisting (subclinical) islet cell autoimmunity. The data, however, do not support an association. One study from the Vaccine Safety Datalink (VSD) compared 252 cases of type 1 diabetes with 768 matched controls without diabetes.[72] No association was found between diabetes and any routinely administered vaccine; for HepB, there was also no association with the timing of doses (birth vs ≥2 months of age). In another study, 21,421 children who received Hib between 1988 and 1990 in the United States were followed for 10 years; the risk of type 1 diabetes was 0.78 when compared with a group of 22,557 children who did not receive the vaccine.[73] Several other well-controlled retrospective studies also found that immunizations are not associated with an increased risk of diabetes.[74-76]

A total of 739,694 children were included in the Danish cohort study of childhood vaccination and type 1 diabetes, and there were 4,720,517 person-years of follow-up.[77] Not surprisingly, the risk of diabetes was much higher in children who had at least one sibling with diabetes. None of the childhood vaccines, however, in any number of doses, was associated with diabetes.

■ Are Vaccines Made From Fetal Tissue?

Some vaccines—rubella, adenovirus, HepA, RAB-HDC, VAR, ZOS, and one form of IPV (the Poliovax contained in Pentacel)—are grown in cultured human embryo fibroblast cell lines (WI-38 or MRC-5) because these are the only cells that replicate the viruses in high enough titer for mass production. Each of these cell lines was first obtained from an aborted fetus in the early 1960s (the rubella vaccine strain itself was originally isolated from an aborted fetus with intrauterine infection). These very same embryonic cells have been passaged in tissue culture in the laboratory since then, and no new fetal material has ever been involved. Receiving vaccines grown in these cells represents a moral dilemma for some people.[78,79] In helping patients work through this, it may be worth emphasizing that the original abortions were done for therapeutic reasons, not for purposes of making vaccines, or even cell lines for that matter—cells were cultured from fetuses that were already dead in order to study immortalization and oncogenesis. Modern day vaccine producers never intended for fetuses to be aborted, and arguably the moral imperative to save lives through vaccination might outweigh the objection to a singular, distant moral transgression. Some religious organizations, including the United States Conference of Catholic Bishops, have used these arguments to justify vaccination despite their opposition to abortion.[80]

■ Does MMR Cause Autism?

In 1998, Wakefield and colleagues described 12 children with chronic enterocolitis and regressive developmental disorder.[81] Ten of these children had autism, and in eight, the onset of regression was linked to receipt of MMR. The authors suggested that replication of the three vaccine viruses in gut tissues caused a unique form of intestinal inflammation. They speculated that this led to the absorption of toxins that affected the brain, resulting in regressive autism.

Since a control group that was never exposed to the vaccine was not included in the study, a causal relationship between MMR and autism could not be established. Moreover, some of the patients in the study may have made their way to Wakefield *because* of his interest in this—in other words, the study population might have been biased toward patients who already thought their symptoms were caused by the vaccine. By 2004, these and other concerns prompted 10 of the 13 original authors to retract their previous interpretation of the study.[82] In 2010, the United Kingdom's General Medical Council found evidence of serious professional misconduct by Wakefield and two of his colleagues,[83] and in February 2010, *The Lancet* formally retracted the original paper.[84] By 2011, it had become clear that the 1998 study was fraudulent.[85]

Unfortunately, the damage had already been done. The notion that MMR causes autism fed directly into the public's natural tendency to assume causality when two events are temporally associated—children get MMR at 1 year of age and the signs of autism become apparent right around the same time. A new wave of antivaccinationism had begun.

MMR does not cause autism. Here is a summary of the evidence:

- *Biological studies*—A 1998 study of 30 patients with IBD, all of whom had had either natural measles infection or MMR vaccination, found no measles genomic sequences in bowel biopsies or blood lymphocytes using a sensitive nested PCR technique.[86] A 2006 study found no differences in antimeasles antibody titers between 54 autistic children (51 had received MMR) and 34 controls (31 had received

MMR), and no study subjects had detectable measles virus gene sequences in their peripheral blood mononuclear cells.[87] Finally, in 2008 investigators studied 25 children with autism and gastrointestinal disturbances and 13 children with gastrointestinal disturbances without autism.[88] Ileal and cecal tissues were obtained and probed for measles virus sequences using molecular amplification techniques in three blinded laboratories, including the one wherein the original association between persistent measles virus and autism was reported. Only one case and one control had positive results, directly refuting Wakefield's hypothesis.

- *Epidemiological studies*—Most studies show that autism cases among children are increasing, but epidemiologists believe this is a reflection of expanded case definitions, diagnostic substitution for other neurodevelopmental conditions, and more public awareness rather than a true increase in incidence.[89] This notion is supported by the finding of nearly identical rates of autism spectrum disorder among adults as among children.[90] In any event, studies done in very different settings—the United Kingdom,[91] California,[92] and Montréal,[93] to name a few—consistently show that the incidence of autism over time does not parallel the uptake of MMR, as it would if MMR caused autism. Another study from the United Kingdom showed no increase in cases of autism after introduction of MMR, which occurred in 1988.[94] In addition, there was no clustering of cases of autism after receipt of MMR vaccine, even when the observation period was extended to many years.[95] Finally, no new form of gastrointestinal disease or autism arises when MMR is introduced into populations.[96,97]
- *Case-control studies*—One study done through the VSD showed no more risk of exposure to MMR among 142 cases with IBD compared with 432 controls without IBD.[98] Another study in the United Kingdom found that 78.1% of 1010 cases had received MMR before being diagnosed with autism, compared with 82.1% of 3671 controls without autism, for an adjusted odds ratio of 0.86 (95% CI 0.68, 1.09).[99] This means that the odds of being diagnosed with autism among persons who had received MMR were essentially the same as those who had not received MMR. Another study from Atlanta showed there was no difference in the proportion of children vaccinated with MMR before 18 or before 24 months of age among 624 case children and 1824 matched controls.[100] Finally, a study from Poland actually showed that the risk of autism was lower among MMR-vaccinated children than among unvaccinated ones.[101]
- *Cohort studies*—Cohort studies are among the most rigorous epidemiologic investigations. The methodology is simple—a

group of subjects is assembled, exposure or nonexposure to the risk factor is determined, and the subsequent development of the outcome is ascertained. The rate of the outcome is then compared between exposed and nonexposed persons; the ratio of the two is called the relative risk (RR), and an RR of 1 means there is no association between the exposure and the outcome. The beauty of retrospective cohort studies, wherein the cohort is identified in the past and followed to the present, is that the exposure and outcomes have already taken place, so that measurement of the exposure (in this case, receipt of MMR) cannot be biased by knowledge of the outcome (autism), allowing for robust inferences. **Figure 7.2** shows the results of the Danish cohort study, which involved 537,303 children.[102] The outcomes of autism or autistic-spectrum disorder were no more common in 1,647,504 person-years of exposure to MMR than they were in 482,360 person-years of nonexposure. The study further showed no association with age at vaccination, interval since vaccination, or the date of vaccination.

There is no scientific rationale for giving the monovalent components of MMR in lieu of the combination, and, in fact, as of 2008 the separate components were no longer available in the United States. The IOM favors rejection of the MMR-causes-autism hypothesis (**Table 2.3**) and the US Court of Federal Claims has rejected claims based on this theory *(see discussion of thimerosal below)*.

■ Did the Thimerosal Used as a Preservative in Vaccines Cause Autism?

High levels of mercury can damage the nervous system and kidneys, and fetuses can be harmed when pregnant women ingest large quantities of mercury. For these reasons, the FDA Modernization Act of 1997 required the FDA to compile a list of drugs and foods that contain mercury. At that time (and really since the beginning of the modern vaccine era), thimerosal, an *ethylmercury* (as opposed to *methylmercury*, which is much more toxic) compound, was added to some vaccines in order to prevent microbial contamination of multidose vials. The cumulative level of mercury represented by the routine vaccine schedule for infants was slightly above the level considered to be safe by the Environmental Protection Agency (EPA). Because of this, the Public Health Service and the AAP issued a joint statement on July 9, 1999, calling for manufacturers to eliminate thimerosal from vaccines as a precautionary measure, stating the following: "The current levels of thimerosal will not hurt children, but reducing those levels will make safe vaccines even safer."[103]

One might wonder how safe vaccines can be made safer, particularly by removing a component that had not been shown

FIGURE 7.2 — Danish Cohort Study of MMR and Autism

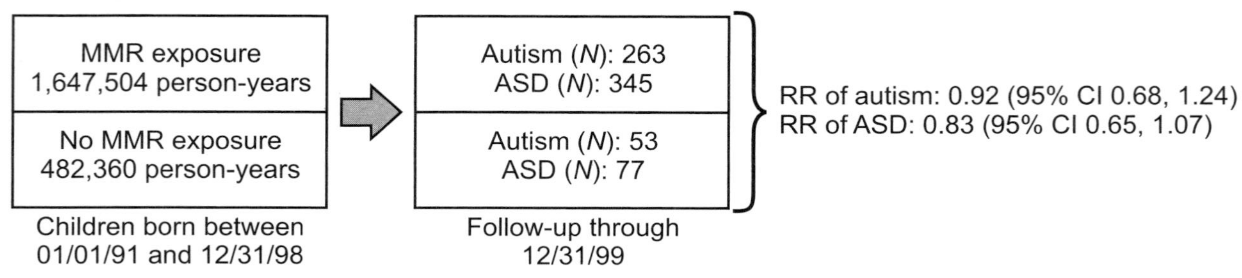

A cohort of children was retrospectively assembled and exposure or nonexposure to MMR was ascertained. The occurrence of autism or autistic-spectrum disorder (ASD) among cohort children was determined, and the rates of the outcome in the exposed and nonexposed groups were compared.

Adapted from Madsen KM, et al. *N Engl J Med*. 2002;347:1477-1482.

to be harmful in the first place. The consequences of this statement included confusion on the part of providers, dismantling of the machinery that had been put in place to deliver the birth dose of HepB, failure to give HepB to some high-risk infants, an onslaught of litigation, and a loss of public confidence.[57,104,105] The effects are still evident today, as celebrities claim that thimerosal is responsible for the "epidemic" of autism and nearly 5000 thimerosal injury claims are pending under the National Vaccine Injury Compensation Program (VICP; see *Chapter 3: Standards, Principles, and Regulations—National Vaccine Injury Compensation Program [VICP]*). The issue reached a penultimate climax in early 2008, when the special federal court for the VICP ruled that multiple vaccinations received in a single day had aggravated the underlying mitochondrial disorder in a child, ultimately manifesting as regressive encephalopathy with features of autistic-spectrum disorder.[106] This reignited the controversy, even though the ruling was strictly applicable only to this case of a child with a previously undiagnosed and rare metabolic defect.

The climax itself occurred in early 2009. Because of the overwhelming burden of petitions before the VICP claiming that vaccines cause autism, the vaccine court asked the petitioners to put forward three test cases for each of three theories, in what became known as the Omnibus Autism Proceedings.[107] The theories were that 1) MMR and thimerosal-containing vaccines combine to cause autism; 2) thimerosal-containing vaccines alone cause autism; and 3) MMR alone causes autism (this theory was subsequently dropped because the evidence was presented as part of the first theory). The petitioners only had to prove their case by a "preponderance of the evidence." On February 12, 2009, the court handed down its decision in the test cases for the first theory.[108] Compensation was denied, and the judges stated unequivocally in each case that the theory was incorrect and that the evidence presented was marginal, paling in comparison to the validated, reproducible, rigorous scientific evidence that had been generated over the years. Appeals in two of the test cases were denied.

On March 12, 2010, the decisions for the test cases of the second theory were handed down.[109] Once again, the court unequivocally rejected the claim that thimerosal caused autism in these children. And, once again, the judges were unequivocal. Special Master Vowell, for example, wrote in the Dwyer case, "The witnesses setting forth this improbable sequence of cause and effect were outclassed in every respect by the impressive assembly of true experts in their respective fields who testified on behalf of respondent."

Thimerosal in vaccines did not cause autism or any other neurodevelopmental problem. Here is a summary of the evidence:

- *Biological studies*—In a pilot study published in 2002, 40 full-term infants ≤6 months of age were given vaccines containing thimerosal and 21 were given thimerosal-free vaccines.[110] No infants had blood mercury concentrations exceeding 29 parts per billion, the level thought to be safe in cord blood. Stool concentrations were high, suggesting elimination through the gastrointestinal tract. A follow-up study looking at 216 infants was published in 2008.[111] The half-life of mercury in blood after administration of thimerosal-containing vaccines was 3.7 days. The highest levels of mercury were seen in the first 24 hours after vaccination, and all were ≤8 ng/mL (some infants received as much as 57.5 mcg of mercury at one time through the vaccinations). Inorganic mercury was detected in stools within days. The results suggest rapid elimination of ethylmercury from the body after vaccination with thimerosal-containing vaccines.
- *Epidemiological studies*—Whether one looks in Denmark[112] and Sweden,[113] where thimerosal was removed from vaccines in 1992, or Canada,[93] where no vaccines contained thimerosal after 1996, the data are remarkably consistent—continued increases in reported cases of autism. A study from California showed no decrease in autism prevalence by age or birth cohort several years after the last lots of thimerosal-containing vaccines would have expired.[114] As discussed earlier, epidemiologists do not uniformly agree that there is a *true* increase in the incidence of autism. However, there *are* many cases being diagnosed, and while the causes remain elusive, the ecologic data argue strongly against thimerosal being one of them.
- *Case-control studies*—The strongest study to date involved 256 children with autism spectrum disorder (ASD) and 752 matched controls from three managed care organizations participating in the VSD.[115] No relationship was found between ethylmercury exposure from vaccines or immunoglobulin preparations and ASD, nor with the subcategories of autistic disorder or ASD with regression. Several periods of exposure were examined, including prenatal, birth to 1 month, birth to 7 months, and birth to 20 months of age. Other strengths included careful individual assessments, good documentation of exposures, and surveillance for undiagnosed autism. **Table 7.7** shows some of the data from this study, which document that cases and controls had similar exposures to ethylmercury at the end of various time periods.
- *Cohort studies*—A retrospective cohort study involving 109,863 children in the United Kingdom born between 1988 and 1997 found no convincing association between thimerosal exposure and developmental disorders.[116] **Figure 7.3** shows the results of the Danish cohort study, which involved

TABLE 7.7 — Cumulative Exposure to Ethylmercury (mcg) From Thimerosal-Containing Vaccines and Immunoglobulins

Exposure Period	Cases (*N*=256)	Controls (*N*=752)
Prenatal	2.70	2.35
Birth to 1 month	9.01	8.99
Birth to 7 months	101.13	103.54
Birth to 20 months	133.58	137.00

Adapted from Price CS, et al. *Pediatrics* 2010;126:656-664.

467,450 children.[117] The outcomes of autism or autistic-spectrum disorder were no more common in 1,220,006 person-years of exposure to thimerosal than they were in 1,660,159 person-years of nonexposure. The study further showed no evidence of a dose-response relationship between cumulative amounts of ethylmercury exposure and autism. A prospective cohort study in the United Kingdom involving over 14,000 children showed that poor prosocial behavior at 47 months of age was correlated with ethylmercury exposure by 3 months of age.[118] However, the same study showed that ethylmercury exposure was associated with *better* outcomes in eight other areas, including conduct, fine motor development, reported tics, and the need for special education. A 2-phase retrospective cohort study in the United States involving over 100,000 children also found no consistent associations with neurodevelopmental outcomes.[119] Finally, in a 2007 study, 1047 children were given a 3-hour assessment involving 42 different neuropsychologic tests; no consistent associations were seen between earlier exposure to thimerosal-containing vaccines and the test results.[120]

Authoritative bodies are virtually unanimous in rejecting the purported link between thimerosal and autism. As of 2012, the only routine childhood vaccines that still contain thimerosal as a preservative are some brands of IIV, although preservative-free formulations for children are available. Activists argue, however, that vaccines labeled *preservative-free* are still not safe because they contain trace amounts of thimerosal (a product cannot be labeled *thimerosal-free* if thimerosal is used in the manufacturing process).

Some autism advocacy groups have urged that we turn our attention away from vaccines and towards more promising lines of research.[121] In fact, there is a growing body of evidence that genetic abnormalities play a role in the development of autism.[122,123]

FIGURE 7.3 — Danish Cohort Study of Thimerosal and Autism

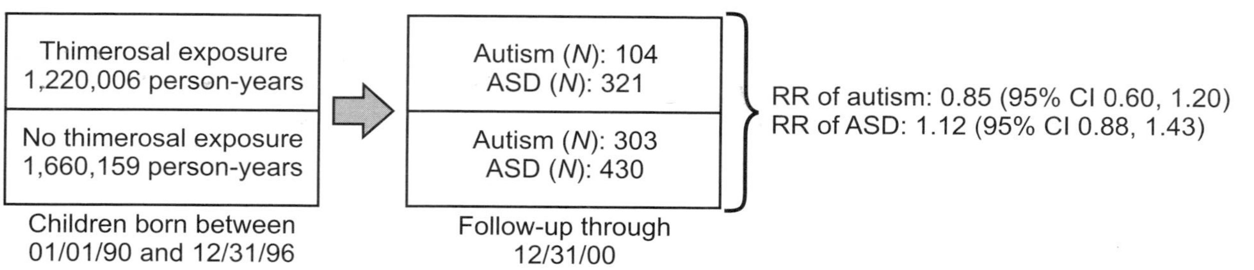

A cohort of children was retrospectively assembled and exposure or nonexposure to thimerosal in vaccines was ascertained. The occurrence of autism or autism spectrum disorder (ASD) among cohort children was determined, and the rates of the outcome in the exposed and nonexposed groups were compared.

Adapted from Hviid A, et al. *JAMA*. 2003;290:1763-1766.

■ Does Pertussis Vaccine Cause Brain Damage?

In 1974, an uncontrolled case series was published describing children who allegedly developed mental retardation and epilepsy following receipt of the whole-cell pertussis vaccine.[124] Over the next several years, fear of the pertussis vaccine generated by media coverage of this report caused a decrease in pertussis immunization rates in British children from 81% to 31%; the decrease in vaccine use resulted in >100,000 cases and over 600 deaths from pertussis.[125] Decreased immunization rates and increased pertussis deaths also were seen in Japan, Sweden, and Wales.[126]

The National Childhood Encephalopathy Study (NCES), conducted in the United Kingdom from 1976 to 1979, suggested the possibility of a relationship between the vaccine and encephalopathy, although methodological problems with this study were quickly highlighted.[127,128] The Institute of Medicine (IOM) independently analyzed NCES data in 1991 and concluded that there was a rare but causal relationship with encephalopathy in the immediate postvaccination period, even though there was no evidence that permanent brain damage occurred.[129] A reanalysis by the IOM in 1994 concluded that the whole-cell pertussis vaccine did not cause encephalopathy.[130]

Other studies also refuted the initial findings of the NCES. For example, a UK study compared over 130,000 children who had received DTwP with a similar number who had received only DT and found no association with encephalopathy.[131] In Denmark, a shift to administration of pertussis vaccine earlier in life was not followed by a shift in diagnosis of neurological disorders.[132] A study in Tennessee found 2 cases of encephalitis among 38,171 children who had received 107,154 DTwP shots; in both cases, the onset of symptoms was >2 weeks following immunization.[133] Finally, in a case-control study conducted in Washington and Oregon involving 218,000 children, 424 cases with neurological illness were each matched with 2 controls.[134] No association was seen with DTwP administration, even when the analysis was restricted to encephalopathy or complicated seizures and adjusted for factors that might have affected vaccine administration.

In a study published in 2006, the records of four large US health maintenance organizations were used to address this issue once again.[135] A total of 452 children with encephalopathy diagnosed between 1981 and 1995 were compared with matched controls without encephalopathy. Exposure to pertussis vaccine in any postvaccination time period was no more common among cases than controls. The maximum possible all-cause incidence of encephalopathy after pertussis immunization was 1 in 370,000, which is no different from the background rate of encephalopathy in young children.

The availability of new tools has shed light on the issue of pertussis vaccine and brain damage. In a landmark 2006 study, de novo mutations in the gene encoding a neuronal sodium channel protein were found in 11 of 14 patients who allegedly had suffered vaccine encephalopathy[136]; since then additional cases have been reported.[137] These individuals are born with a molecular defect that would cause seizures and regression, *vaccines or no vaccines*. Despite this finding, and despite the fact that acellular pertussis vaccines have replaced whole-cell vaccines, encephalopathy remains an injury that can be compensated through the Vaccine Injury Table under the VICP (see *Chapter 3: Standards, Principles, and Regulations—National Childhood Vaccine Injury Act*).

■ Do Vaccines Cause Guillain-Barré Syndrome?

GBS is an acute, immune-mediated, demyelinating peripheral neuropathy characterized by progressive symmetric weakness. Cases usually occur after an infectious event, most notably *Campylobacter jejuni* enteritis. In 1976, there was an outbreak of a new H1N1 influenza strain among soldiers at Fort Dix, New Jersey.[138] The virus, dubbed A/New Jersey/76 (Hsw1N1) and known to be closely related to the deadly 1918 pandemic strain, had circulated in pigs for years and had apparently jumped to humans. Fearing the start of a new pandemic, the US government instituted a mass immunization campaign. In retrospect, the outbreak may have been an anomaly—an animal virus introduced into a stressed, crowded, closed population, with little potential to spread in normal communities (in fact, the virus never spread beyond the military installation). Unfortunately, the mass immunization campaign was not benign. Over 45 million people were immunized over a 3-month period, resulting in more than 500 cases of GBS; the attributable risk of GBS to swine flu vaccination was estimated to be 1 in 100,000.[139] The mechanism may have involved some form of molecular mimicry, supported by the observation that mice receiving the vaccine develop anti-ganglioside antibodies.[140]

While some studies have suggested a possible causal relationship between seasonal influenza vaccine and GBS,[141] most have not. One, for example, looked at two influenza seasons in the United States in the early 1990s and found a RR of 1.7 (95% CI 1.0, 2.8), corresponding to approximately one additional case of GBS per million people vaccinated.[142] It is important to keep a perspective here: in any given 6-week period of time, somewhere between 1 in 220,000 and 1 in 1.4 million people will develop GBS—*vaccine or no vaccine*.[143] Another study in the United Kingdom spanning the years 1992 to 2000 found 228 incident cases of GBS; seven cases occurred within 42 days of any immunization (three were after influenza immunization) and 221 were not associated with immunization, for a RR of 1.03 (95% CI 0.48, 2.18).[144] A study from Canada published in 2006 demonstrated no seasonality of GBS and no increase in hospital admissions for GBS after the introduction of a universal influenza immunization program.[145] Preliminary analysis of data from the Emerging Infections Program showed a small, statistically significant association between receipt of 2009 H1N1 vaccine and GBS, of the order of 0.8 excess cases per 1 million vaccinations.[146] This was much smaller than the association seen with the 1976 vaccine, and, importantly, no clustering of cases occurred in the second week after vaccination, as was seen with the former vaccine. Similar results were seen in Europe.[147]

By September 2006, 17 cases of GBS associated with MCV4-D administration had been reported to VAERS (the vaccine was licensed in January 2005).[148] Most of the cases occurred within 2 weeks of vaccination, a timeframe that would fit with a causal relationship. The rate of GBS among immunized teenagers, calculated based on doses distributed, was estimated to be about 0.20 per 100,000 person-months. This rate was similar to the background rate of GBS calculated from the VSD database, but it was slightly higher than that seen in the Healthcare Cost and Utilization Project, a multistate hospital discharge database. It was estimated that if GBS was truly caused by MCV4-D, there would be 1 extra case for every 800,000 teenagers vaccinated. However, combined data from two very large studies showed no incident cases of GBS within 6 weeks of 2.3 million vaccinations, for an estimated upper 95% confidence limit of the attributable risk of 1 case per million doses, which is not above background rates.[149] In June 2010, the ACIP removed history of GBS as a precaution for receipt of MCV4, which had been in place since the initial VAERS data came to light.

■ Do Vaccines Cause Multiple Sclerosis (MS)?

The hypothesis that vaccines might cause MS was fueled by anecdotal reports of MS following HepB administration and two case-control studies showing an increase in the incidence of MS in vaccinated persons that was not statistically significant. However, two large case-control studies evaluated whether HepB causes MS or whether HepB, tetanus, or influenza vaccines exacerbate symptoms of MS. The first study in a cohort of nurses identified 192 women with MS and 645 matched controls.[150] There was no association between MS and any exposure to HepB, exposure within the 2 years before diagnosis, or the number of doses of HepB received. The second study included 643 patients in Europe with MS relapse occurring between 1993 and 1997.[151] No association was found between relapse and exposure to any vaccine, or specifically HepB, tetanus, or influenza vaccines, in the 2-month period before relapse, compared with the four previous 2-month periods. In a case-control study in France, 143 cases of MS in children <16 years of age were matched to 1122 controls; 32% of cases and 32% of controls had received HepB in the 3 years before the index date.[152] A subsequent study by the same group looked at first-ever episodes of acute inflammatory demyelination in children, irrespective of the subsequent course of the disease.[153] The rates of HepB vaccination in the 3 years before the index date were 24.4% for 349 cases and 27.3% for 2941 matched controls, for an adjusted odds ratio of 0.74 (95% CI 0.54, 1.02), although a possible trend was seen for one vaccine type.

Other well-controlled studies also found that influenza vaccine did not exacerbate symptoms of MS. In a retrospective study of 180 patients with relapsing MS, *infection* with influenza virus was more likely than *immunization* with influenza vaccine to cause an exacerbation of symptoms, suggesting that influenza vaccine may actually *prevent* exacerbations of MS.[154] In a multicenter, prospective, randomized, double-blind trial of influenza vaccine among 104 patients with MS, immunization was not associated with exacerbation of symptoms or change in disease course.[155]

■ Can Vaccines Transmit Mad Cow Disease (MCD)?

By July 2000, more than 176,000 cows in the United Kingdom had developed bovine spongiform encephalopathy, more commonly referred to as MCD, a progressive deterioration of the nervous system. At the same time, >70 people in the United Kingdom had developed a progressive neurologic condition termed *variant Creutzfeldt-Jakob disease* (vCJD) that likely resulted from eating meat prepared from cows with MCD. Both MCD and vCJD are caused by prions, which are proteinaceous, self-replicating infectious particles. Because bovine-derived materials such as serum, albumin and gelatin have been used in vaccine manufacture, there was theoretical concern that prions could be transmitted through vaccination. The FDA recommended that vaccines use bovine materials originating from countries without endogenous MCD.[156] Mathematical models suggest that the agent of MCD first entered cattle feed in the United Kingdom around 1980; since the vast majority of initial cases of vCJD were born well before then, childhood vaccines were not likely to be the cause.[157]

There is no evidence that any case of vCJD was acquired from vaccination.[158] In fact, there are many reasons for reassurance. Prions are found in neuronal tissues of infected cows, tissues that are not used in vaccine manufacture. Fetal bovine serum, used to support cell growth in culture and ultimately removed from the final product, and gelatin, used as a stabilizer in vaccine preparations and derived from connective tissues of cows and pigs, are not known to contain prions or transmit vCJD.

■ Did SV40 Contamination of Vaccines Cause Cancer?

The polio vaccine used in the late 1950s and early 1960s was contaminated with a monkey virus called simian virus 40

(SV40), present in the monkey kidney cells used to grow the vaccine.[159] Investigators found SV40 DNA in biopsy specimens obtained from patients with mesothelioma, osteosarcoma, and non-Hodgkin's lymphoma. Interestingly, SV40 DNA was present in the cancers of people who had received the polio vaccine that was contaminated with SV40, but it was also present in those who had not. SV40 DNA was even found in the cancers of people born after 1963, a time when the vaccine no longer contained SV40. A study published in 2004 shed some light on this.[160] Some of the primers that were being employed in the PCR reactions used to amplify DNA sequences of SV40 were directed at a region of the T antigen. As it turns out, these sequences are also present in common laboratory plasmids. How did they get there? They were engineered into the plasmids during the first attempts to create expression vectors for eukaryotic cells, but this happened so long ago that their presence was not well known. When alternative T-antigen primers were used, only a few cancers were positive. Moreover, this study found no evidence of T-antigen RNA transcript production and no T-antigen protein expression in the tumors. Finally, epidemiologic studies do not show an increased risk of cancers in those who received polio vaccine between 1955 and 1963.

■ Did the Polio Vaccine Cause the AIDS Pandemic?

In his 1999 book entitled *The River: A Journey to the Source of HIV and AIDS*, Edward Hooper claimed that the origin of AIDS could be traced back to oral poliovirus vaccines that were administered in the Belgian Congo between 1957 and 1960. This assertion was based on the following assumptions: 1) all poliovirus vaccines were grown in monkey kidney cells; 2) those cells were contaminated with simian immunodeficiency virus (SIV), which is closely related to HIV; and 3) people were inadvertently infected with SIV that then mutated to HIV and caused the AIDS epidemic. The following facts, however, exonerate polio vaccines as a cause of AIDS:

- SIV is found in chimpanzees, not monkeys, and chimpanzee cells were never used to grow polio vaccine.[161,162]
- SIV and HIV are not very close genetically and mutation from SIV to HIV would have required centuries, not years.[163,164]
- Both SIV and HIV are enveloped viruses that are easily disrupted by extremes of pH; if given by mouth (as was OPV), both of these viruses would likely be destroyed in the acid environment of the stomach.
- Original lots of the polio vaccine (including those used in Africa for the polio vaccine trials) did not contain HIV, SIV, or chimpanzee genetic sequences when analyzed by molecular amplification techniques.[165,166]

Unfortunately, fears of polio vaccine based on this unfounded theory adversely affected vaccine use where it is need most—in the developing world where the last vestiges of wild-type poliovirus reside.[167]

■ Can Vaccines Cause SIDS?

In the early 1990s there were 5000 annual SIDS deaths in the United States. In 1991, routine vaccination of infants with HepB was recommended—theoretically, every one of the 4 million babies born each year would receive 3 doses of HepB during the first 6 months of life. Under this scenario, there will inevitably be infants who die from SIDS the very day they receive the vaccine—and there were, sparking concerns that HepB caused SIDS.

By 2001, HepB uptake in infants had increased to about 90% and the incidence of SIDS had *decreased* dramatically to about 1600 cases per year. What happened? Reports from Europe and Australia suggested that prone sleeping position was a risk factor for SIDS, and in 1994 the "Back to Sleep" campaign, in which parents were encouraged to place their infants on their backs or sides when going to sleep, was initiated. VAERS data published in 1999 showed very few neonatal deaths following HepB after approximately 86 million doses were given.[168] Several studies actually show *lower* SIDS rates among infants who receive vaccines when compared with those who do not.[169,170] While this may reflect biases wherein healthier or better-cared-for infants are the ones who are immunized, the data clearly do not implicate vaccines as a risk factor for SIDS.

A study published in 2004 looked at a cohort of 361,696 infants born between 1993 and 1998.[171] A total of 1363 infants in the cohort died in the first 29 days of life; only 5% of them had been vaccinated with HepB, whereas 66% of those who survived the first month of life had been immunized. Moreover, there was no difference in the proportion of vaccinated and unvaccinated infants who died of unexpected causes, and the SIDS death rate was the same (3.3 per 100,000) for vaccinated and unvaccinated infants.

More recent data suggest that infants who die from SIDS have abnormalities of the medullary serotonin system, which controls autonomic function and breathing.[172]

■ Do Vaccines Trigger Kawasaki Disease (KD)?

KD is an acute, inflammatory, small-to-medium sized vessel vasculitis manifest by prolonged high fever and some combination of rash, conjunctival suffusion, changes in the oral mucosa or peripheral extremities, and cervical lymphadenopathy; desquamation occurs in the convalescent phase, and ectasia or aneurysms can develop in the coronary arteries. An infectious etiology is suspected based on clustering of cases, but a genetic predisposition is likely based on widely varying incidence in different racial and ethnic groups.

In phase 3 clinical trials of RV5, KD was reported in 5 of 36,150 vaccinees and 1 of 35,536 placebees within 42 days of vaccination, for an unadjusted RR of 4.9 (95% CI 0.6, 239.1); even with such wide confidence intervals, this finding raised some concern. Early reassurance came from the VSD, where there had been only one unconfirmed case of KD within 30 days of 65,000 RV5 doses.[173] A study published in 2009 provided further reassurance that RV5 does not cause KD.[174] VAERS reports from 1990 through mid-2007 were analyzed, yielding only 97 cases. No clustering of cases was seen after vaccination. The reporting rates for KD in the 30 days following vaccination were 0.65 per 100,000 person-years before the RV5 label was changed to include KD as a reported adverse event, and 2.78 per 100,000 person-years after the change; both rates were lower than the expected background incidence of 9 to 19 per 100,000 person-years.

A subsequent study from the VSD looked at 207,621 doses of RV5 given from 2006 to 2008.[175] The age-adjusted odds ratio for KD in RV5 recipients was 0.28 (95% CI 0.07-1.09). Finally, in a postmarketing study (presented at the October 2009 ACIP meeting) that looked at approximately 85,000 infants who received at least one dose of RV5, there was no evidence of an association with KD during any follow-up period after any dose.[176]

■ Do Vaccines Contain Adventitious Agents?

Live vaccines are often attenuated by serial passage in animal cell culture. Some, such as RV5, are actually derived from animal viruses (the genetic backbone of RV5 is a bovine strain of rotavirus). Animal products, such as bovine fetal serum, may be used in the propagation of vaccine virus strains or may be added to the final product as stabilizers, as in the case of gelatin. For these reasons, contamination with animal agents is possible. Moreover, vaccines grown in human cell lines could potentially pick up unwanted infectious agents or genetic material. Despite rigorous screening procedures designed to detect contaminants before licensure, as time goes by and as our magnifying glass gets bigger, we are likely to find more of these contaminants, or *adventitious* agents. Then the question will be whether or not these agents represent a health threat.

The case of polio vaccine contaminated with SV40 is discussed above. There are many other examples of known contamination with adventitious agents. For example, measles vaccine, mumps vaccine, and YFV harbor endogenous avian retrovirus particles.[177,178] These viruses are intrinsic to the chick embryo fibroblasts in which the vaccines are propagated and they arise even though the chick embryo cells are derived from pathogen-free flocks. These viruses are not infectious for humans; they do not replicate in human cells nor are they capable of integrating their genetic material into human host chromosomes—they therefore represent no safety issue for vaccinees. In some cases, the DNA of adventitial agents can be detected in vaccines, without live particles.[179] This is the case, for example, with the detection of simian retrovirus proviral DNA in RV5 preparations—these sequences are present in the Vero (African green monkey kidney) cells in which the vaccine is grown. Vaccines grown in human cell lines, including rubella vaccine and VAR, may also harbor genetic sequences of human endogenous retroviruses—these sequences are present in our own genomes.[179]

In March 2010, it was discovered that RV1 (Rotarix) was contaminated with porcine circovirus 1 (PCV1) DNA.[179] Subsequent studies showed that the vaccine contained full length PCV1 DNA in intact viral particles; one study suggested that these were not infectious[180] while another suggested that they were.[181] RV5 (RotaTeq) was also found to harbor PCV DNA sequences, albeit in fragments rather than intact particles (initial studies suggested that both PCV1 and PCV2 DNA was present,[181] but later studies demonstrated only PCV2).[182] In the case of RV1, the porcine virus was probably replicating in the Vero cells used to make the vaccine; in the case of RV5, the DNA fragments were introduced by the trypsin used in the manufacturing process.

PCV1 and PCV2 are not pathogenic for humans. In fact, these viruses are ubiquitous in pork products and can be found in human feces.[183] PCV1 has been in RV1 since the early stages of development, and tens of millions of doses have been given with no discernible related adverse events. For RV1, steps are being taken to remove PCV, and for RV5 to ensure that the trypsin supply is PCV-free. In the meantime, the contamination with PCV represents no threat to vaccinees.

■ Can Vaccines Cause Febrile Seizures?

The first dose of MMRV causes fever more often than MMR and VAR given separately on the same day.[184] Since some young children are predisposed to seizures when they get fever (2% to 5% of all children experience at least one febrile seizure in their lifetime[185]), it is not surprising that some children will have a seizure after they receive MMRV. In fact, a postlicensure study conducted at Kaiser Permanente Southern California showed that the rate of febrile seizures after the first dose of MMRV was approximately twice as high (about 7 per 10,000) as after the separate vaccines in the 5 to 12 days following vaccination.[186] Similarly, a study from the Vaccine Safety Datalink showed an elevated risk of febrile seizures from days 7 to 10 postvaccination.[187] These studies suggest that one febrile seizure attributable to the vaccine will occur for every 2300 to 2600 children vaccinated.

Febrile seizures also may occur when PCV13 and IIV are given on the same day. The risk here, as derived from preliminary analysis of VSD data, is about one in every 2200 children 12 to 23 months of age.[188]

While considered benign by medical professionals, these events can be frightening for children and their parents. Ironically, each of these vaccines can *prevent* febrile seizures by preventing the respective diseases. Since febrile seizures occur early when the temperature is rapidly rising, management of fever with antipyretics is not likely to prevent them, and prophylaxis with antipyretics is not warranted since fever from MMRV can occur anywhere from 5 to 12 days after vaccination. The finding that febrile seizures can occur after vaccination has not altered any immunization recommendations, other than the removal of a preference for MMRV over MMR plus VAR for the first dose.

■ Do Rotavirus Vaccines Cause Intussusception?

The first rotavirus vaccine, rhesus-human reassortant rotavirus vaccine-tetravalent (RRV-TV; RotaShield), was licensed in the United States in August 1998. Licensure was based on demonstrated safety and efficacy in clinical trials wherein nearly 11,000 children received the vaccine in its final formulation. With universal use, RRV-TV was expected to prevent 55,000 hospitalizations and 25 deaths each year. A few cases of intussusception (IS, a form of bowel obstruction) occurred in the clinical trials, but there was no evidence of a statistically significant association with vaccination. Nevertheless, the package insert listed IS as a possible adverse reaction and postlicensure surveillance was mandated. By July 1999, there were 15 reports of IS in the VAERS database, and several population-based investigations suggested a causal relationship. The CDC recommended suspension of vaccination, and by October 1999, the product was withdrawn from the market.[189] The highest incidence of vaccine-associated IS was in the first 2 weeks after Dose 1, a time when viral replication peaks.

It is estimated that IS attributable to RRV-TV occurred once for every 10,000 children vaccinated, although some argue that the risk was actually much less (for reference, the natural risk of IS in about 1 in 2000). The risk was so small that it could not have been detected in the prelicensure trials, given the number of children enrolled. As a result of this experience, the new-generation rotavirus vaccines, RV5 (RotaTeq) and RV1 (Rotarix), were each tested in approximately 70,000 children before licensure, and no evidence of an association with IS was found.[190,191] Even these massive trials, however, cannot detect extremely small associations. Therefore, rigorous postmarketing studies have been conducted.

By August 2007, over 9 million doses of RV5 had been distributed in the United States and there were 160 reports of IS in VAERS.[192] Assuming 75% reporting and 75% administration of distributed vaccine, the number of VAERS reports was about half that expected in the first 21 days after vaccination, providing reassurance that RV5 does not cause IS. In a VSD study involving 207,621 doses (42% were Dose 1) of RV5 given from 2006 to 2008, there were only 2 confirmed cases of IS; neither of these was after Dose 1 and both occurred >14 days after vaccination.[175] Finally, a large postmarketing study (presented at the October 2009 ACIP meeting) looked at over 50,000 infants who received 3 doses of RV5 and compared them to concurrent controls (who received DTaP but not RV5) and historical controls—there was no increase in IS during any time period within 30 days of any dose.[176]

Postmarketing studies of RV1 in the United States are difficult to do because the vaccine was licensed 2 years after RV5. However, active surveillance in Mexico and Brazil, where RV1 is used exclusively, demonstrated an increased risk of IS after Dose 1 in Mexico and after Dose 2 (but not Dose 1) in Brazil.[193] The respective attributable risks of IS to vaccination were 1 in 51,000 infants in Mexico and 1 in 68,000 infants in Brazil. In Australia, where both vaccines are used about equally, there appeared to be an association with IS after Dose 1—in the first 7 days after Dose 1 of RV5, the RR was 5.3 (95% CI 1.1, 15.4), and for RV1 it was 3.5 (95% CI 0.7, 10.1). This suggests that live rotavirus vaccines as a class may slightly increase the risk of IS.

In the Australian study, there was no increased risk of IS when all exposure windows were aggregated after each dose through 9 months of age. This suggests that an increase in IS after Dose 1 was offset by fewer cases later in infancy. Similar observations were made during the RRV-TV era.[194] Thus, it is possible that, for whatever reason, some infants are predisposed to developing IS, and that administration of live oral rotavirus vaccines "brings out" the IS that would have occurred eventually.[195] Either way, the risk, if confirmed, is very small, and the benefits of vaccination far outweigh those risks. However, in October 2011, because of these data and the risk of recurrent IS, the ACIP added personal history of intussusception to the list of contraindications for RV.

REFERENCES

1. Evans G, Bostrom A, Johnston RB, Fisher BL, Stoto MA. *Risk Communication and Vaccination: Summary of a Workshop*. Washington, DC: National Academy Press; 1997.
2. Bohlke K, et al. *Pediatrics*. 2003;112:815-820.
3. Freed GL, et al. *Pediatrics*. 2010;125:654-659.
4. Patja A, et al. *Pediatr Infect Dis J*. 2000;19:1127-1134.
5. Shermer M. *Sci Amer*. 2008;September:40.
6. Black S, et al. *Lancet*. 2009;374:2115-2122.
7. Shermer M. *Sci Amer*. 2009;June:36.
8. Opel DJ, et al. *Arch Pediatr Adolesc Med*. 2009;163:432-437.
9. LeBaron CW, et al. *Arch Pediatr Adolesc Med*. 1999;153:1154-1159.
10. Davis TC, et al. *Pediatrics*. 2001;107:e17.
11. Fredrickson DD, et al. *Pediatr Ann*. 2001;30:400-406.
12. Kalb C, et al. *Newsweek*. 2010;155(22).
13. Flanagan-Klygis EA, et al. *Arch Pediatr Adolesc Med*. 2005;159: 929-934.
14. Freed GL, et al. *Am J Prev Med*. 2004;26:11-14.
15. Gust DA, et al. *Pediatrics*. 2004;114:e16-e22.
16. Smith PJ, et al. *Pediatrics*. 2004;114:187-195.
17. Gust DA, et al. *Pediatrics*. 2008;122:718-725.
18. Eisenberg D. The ethics of smallpox immunization. Aish.com Web site. http://www.aish.com/ci/sam/48943486.html. Accessed February 15, 2010.
19. Refusal to vaccinate. American Academy of Pediatrics Web site. http://www.aap.org/immunization/pediatricians/pdf/RefusaltoVaccinate.pdf. Accessed September 30, 2011.
20. Refusal of vaccination for my child. Immunization Action Coalition Web site. http://www.immunize.org/catg.d/p4059.pdf. Accessed October 30, 2011.
21. Diekema DS, et al. *Pediatrics*. 2005;115:1428-1431.
22. AMA Code of Medical Ethics. American Medical Association Web site. http://www.ama-assn.org/ama/pub/category/2498.html. Accessed January 22, 2010.
23. Freed GL, et al. *Pediatrics*. 2011;127:S107-S112.
24. Kata A. *Vaccine*. 2010;28:1709-1716.
25. Poland GA, et al. *Vaccine*. 2001;19:2440-2445.
26. Blume S. *Soc Sci Med*. 2006;62:628-642.
27. Poland GA, et al. *N Engl J Med*. 2011;364:97-99.
28. Colgrove J. *State of Immunity: The Politics of Vaccination in Twentieth-Century America*. Berkeley, CA: University of California Press; 2006.
29. Offit PA. *Autism's False Prophets: Bad Science, Risky Medicine, and the Search for a Cure*. New York, NY: Columbia University Press; 2008.

30. Offit PA. *Deadly Choices: How the Anti-Vaccine Movement Threatens Our Children*. New York, NY: Basic Books; 2011.
31. Wolfe RM, et al. *JAMA*. 2002;287:3245-3248.
32. Bean SJ. *Vaccine.* 2011;29:1874-1880.
33. Salmon DA, et al. *JAMA*. 1999;282:47-53.
34. Feikin DR, et al. *JAMA*. 2000;284:3145-3150.
35. Omer SB, et al. *Am J Epidemiol*. 2008;168:1389-1396.
36. Parker AA, et al. *N Engl J Med* 2006;355:447-455.
37. The National Vaccine Advisory Committee. *JAMA*. 1991;266:1547-1552.
38. Dayan GH, et al. *N Engl J Med.* 2008;358:1580-1589.
39. CDC. *MMWR*. 2008;57:893-896.
40. CDC. *MMWR*. 2011;60:666-668.
41. California Department of Public Health. http://www.cdph.ca.gov/programs/immunize/Documents/PertussisReport20119.pdf. Accessed October 1, 2011.
42. Black SB, et al. *Am J Dis Child.* 1991;145:746-749.
43. Otto S, et al. *J Infect.* 2000;41:172-175.
44. Hviid A, et al. *JAMA.* 2005;294:699-705.
45. Storsaeter J, et al. *Pediatr Infect Dis J.* 1988;7:637-645.
46. Davidson M, et al. *Am J Dis Child.* 1991;145:750-754.
47. Offit PA, et al. *Pediatrics*. 2003;112:1394-1397.
48. Jefferson T, et al. *Lancet Infect Dis*. 2004;4:84-90.
49. Keith LS, et al. *Vaccine*. 2002;20:S13-S17.
50. Hot topics: aluminum. The Children's Hospital Vaccine Education Center Web site. http://www.chop.edu/service/vaccine-education-center/hot-topics/aluminum.html. Accessed October 4, 2011.
51. Beutler B, et al. *Nat Rev Immunol*. 2003;3:169-176.
52. Verstraeten T, et al. *Vaccine*. 2008;26:6630-6638.
53. Integrated Risk Information System. Formaldehyde (CASRN 50-00-0). U.S. Environmental Protection Agency Web site. http://www.epa.gov/ncea/iris/subst/0419.htm#reforal. Accessed October 4, 2011.
54. Dempsey AF, et al. *Pediatrics*. 2011;128:1:doi:10.1542/peds.2011-0400.
55. Sears R. *The Vaccine Book: Making the Right Decision for Your Child*. New York, NY: Little, Brown and Co; 2007.
56. Offit PA, et al. *Pediatrics*. 2009;123:e164-e169.
57. Hurie MB, et al. *Pediatrics*. 2001;107:755-758.
58. Smith PJ, et al. *Pub Health Rep*. 2010;125:534-541.
59. Lin ND, et al. *Vaccine*. 2010;28:4169-4174.
60. Smith MJ, et al. *Pediatrics*. 2010;125:1134-1141.
61. Schaub B, et al. *J Allergy Clin Immunol.* 2006;117:969-977.
62. Ege MJ, et al. *N Engl J Med.* 2011;364:701-709.
63. Offit PA, et al. *Pediatrics.* 2003;111:653-659.
64. DeStefano F, et al. *Pediatr Infect Dis J.* 2002;21:498-504.

65. Spycher BD, et al. *Pediatrics*. 2009;123:944-950.
66. Spycher BD, et al. *J Allerg Clin Immunol*. 2008;37:656.
67. Anderson HR, et al. *Am J Public Health.* 2001;91:1126-1129.
68. Nilsson L, et al. *Arch Pediatr Adolesc Med.* 1998;152:734-738.
69. Nilsson L, et al. *Arch Pediatr Adolesc Med*. 2003;157:1184-1189.
70. Nakajima K, et al. *Thorax*. 2007;62:270-275.
71. Rosenlund H, et al. *Pediatrics*. 2009;123:771-778.
72. DeStefano F, et al. *Pediatrics*. 2001;108:e112.
73. Black SB, et al. *Pediatr Infect Dis J.* 2002;21:568-569.
74. Heijbel H, et al. *Diabetes Care.* 1997;20:173-175.
75. Graves PM, et al. *Diabetes Care.* 1999;22:1694-1697.
76. Hummel M, et al. *Diabetes Care.* 2000;23:969-974.
77. Hviid A, et al. *N Engl J Med*. 2004;350:1398-1404.
78. Grabenstein JD. *Catholic Pharmacist.* 1996;29:2-4.
79. Zimmerman RK. *Vaccine.* 2004;22:4238-4244.
80. United States Conference of Catholic Bishops. Fact Sheet: Embryonic stem cell research and vaccines using fetal tissue. USCCB Web site. http://old.usccb.org/prolife/issues/bioethic/vaccfac2.shtml. Accessed October 1, 2011.
81. Wakefield AJ, et al. *Lancet.* 1998;351:637-641.
82. Murch SH, et al. *Lancet*. 2004;363:750.
83. Dr. Andrew Jeremy Wakefield: Determination on serious professional misconduct (SPM) and sanction: 24 May 2010. General Medical Council Web site. http://www.gmc-uk.org/Wakefield_SPM_and_SANCTION.pdf_32595267.pdf. Accessed October 4, 2011.
84. Editors. *Lancet*. 2010;375:445.
85. Godlee F, et al. *BMJ*. 2011;342:64-66.
86. Afzal MA, et al. *Lancet.* 1998;351:646-647.
87. D'Souza Y, et al. *Pediatrics.* 2006;118:1664-1675.
88. Hornig M, et al. *PLoS ONE*. 2008;9:e3140(1-8).
89. Shattuck PT. *Pediatrics.* 2006;117:1028-1037.
90. Brugha TS, et al. *Arch Gen Psychiatry*. 2011;68:459-466.
91. Kaye JA, et al. *BMJ.* 2001;322:460-463.
92. Dales L, et al. *JAMA*. 2001;285:1183-1185.
93. Fombonne E, et al. *Pediatrics*. 2006;118:139-150.
94. Taylor B, et al. *Lancet*. 1999;353:2026-2029.
95. Farrington CP, et al. *Vaccine.* 2001;19:3632-3635.
96. Taylor B, et al. *BMJ.* 2002;324:393-396.
97. Fombonne E, et al. *Pediatrics.* 2001;108:e58.
98. Davis RL, et al. *Arch Pediatr Adolesc Med*. 2001;155:354-359.
99. Smeeth L, et al. *Lancet.* 2004;364:963-969.
100. DeStefano F, et al. *Pediatrics*. 2004;113:259-266.
101. Mrożek-Budzyn D, et al. *Pediatr Infect Dis J*. 2010;29:397-400.
102. Madsen KM, et al. *N Engl J Med*. 2002;347:1477-1482.

103. CDC. *MMWR.* 1999;48:563-565.
104. Freed GL, et al. *Pediatrics.* 2002;109:1153-1159.
105. Luman ET, et al. *JAMA.* 2004;291:2351-2358.
106. Offit PA. *N Engl J Med.* 2008;358:2089-2091.
107. U.S. Court of Federal Claims. Autism decisions and background information. Available at: http://www.uscfc.uscourts.gov/node/5026. Accessed October 4, 2011.
108. Cedillo vs Secretary of Health and Human Services, No. 98-916V; Hazlehurst vs Secretary of Health and Human Services, No. 03-654V; Snyder vs Secretary of Health and Human Services, No. 01-162V.
109. Dwyer vs Secretary of Health and Human Services, No. 03-1202V; King vs Secretary of Health and Human Services, No. 03-584V; Mead vs Secretary of Health and Human Services, No. 03-215V.
110. Pichichero ME, et al. *Lancet.* 2002;360:1737-1741.
111. Pichichero ME, et al. *Pediatrics.* 2008;121:e208-e214.
112. Madsen KM, et al. *Pediatrics.* 2003;112:604-606.
113. Stehr-Green P, et al. *Am J Prev Med.* 2003;25:101-106.
114. Schechter R, et al. *Arch Gen Psychiatry*. 2008;65:19-24.
115. Price CS, et al. *Pediatrics*. 2010;126:656-664.
116. Andrews N, et al. *Pediatrics.* 2004;114:584-591.
117. Hviid A, et al. *JAMA*. 2003;290:1763-1766.
118. Heron J, et al. *Pediatrics.* 2004;114:577-583.
119. Verstraeten T, et al. *Pediatrics.* 2003;112:1039-1048.
120. Thompson WW, et al. *N Engl J Med.* 2007;357:1281-1292.
121. Autism Science Foundation Web site. http://www.autismscience foundation.org. Accessed October 4, 2011.
122. Eichler EE, et al. *N Engl J Med*. 2008;358:737-739.
123. Weiss LA, et al. *Nature*. 2009;461:802-808.
124. Kulenkampff M, et al. *Arch Dis Child.* 1974;49:46-49.
125. Cherry JD. *Curr Prob Pediatr*. 1984;14:1-78.
126. Gangarosa EJ, et al. *Lancet.* 1998;351:356-361.
127. Miller DL, et al. *BMJ*. 1981;282:1595-1599.
128. Miller D, et al. *BMJ.* 1993;307:1171-1176.
129. Howson CP, Howe CJ, Fineberg HV, eds. *Adverse Effects of Vaccines: A Report of the Committee to Review the Adverse Consequences of Pertussis and Rubella Vaccines.* Washington, DC: National Academy Press; 1991.
130. Stratton KR, Howe CJ, Johnston RB, eds. *DPT Vaccine and Chronic Nervous System Dysfunction: A New Analysis.* Washington, DC: National Academy Press; 1994.
131. Pollock TM, et al. *Lancet.* 1983;1:753-757.
132. Shields WD, et al. *J Pediatr.* 1988;113:801-805.
133. Griffin MR, et al. *JAMA.* 1990;263:1641-1645.
134. Gale JL, et al. *JAMA.* 1994;271:37-41.

135. Ray P, et al. *Pediatr Infect Dis J.* 2006;25:768-773.
136. Berkovic SF, et al. *Lancet Neurol.* 2006;5:488-492.
137. Reyes IS, et al. *Pediatrics.* 2011;128:e699-e702.
138. Gaydos JC, et al. *Emerg Infect Dis.* 2006;12:23-28.
139. Haber P, et al. *Drug Safety.* 2009;32:309-323.
140. Nachamkin I, et al. *J Infect Dis.* 2008;198:226-233.
141. Haber P, et al. *JAMA.* 2004;292:2478-2481.
142. Lasky T, et al. *N Engl J Med.* 1998;339:1797-1802.
143. Evans D, et al. *J Infect Dis.* 2009;200:321-328.
144. Hughes RA, et al. *Arch Intern Med.* 2006;166:1301-1304.
145. Juurlink DN, et al. *Arch Intern Med.* 2006;166:2217-2221.
146. Prothro C, et al. *MMWR.* 2010;59:657-661.
147. Dieleman J, et al. *BMJ.* 2011;343:d3908.
148. CDC. *MMWR.* 2006;55:1120-1124.
149. ACIP Summary Report, June 23-24, 2010. Centers for Disease Control and Prevention Web site. http://www.cdc.gov/vaccines/recs/acip/downloads/min-jun10.pdf. Accessed October 1, 2011.
150. Ascherio A, et al. *N Engl J Med.* 2001;344:327-332.
151. Confavreux C, et al. *N Engl J Med.* 2001;344:319-326.
152. Mikaeloff Y, et al. *Arch Pediatr Adolesc Med.* 2007;161:1176-1182.
153. Mikaeloff Y, et al. *Neurology.* 2009;72:873-880.
154. De Keyser J, et al. *J Neurol Sci.* 1998;159:51-53.
155. Miller AE, et al. *Neurology.* 1997;48:312-314.
156. CDC. *MMWR.* 2000;49:1137-1138.
157. Minor PD, et al. *Vaccine.* 2000;19:409-410.
158. Recommendations for the use of vaccines manufactured with bovine-derived materials. U.S. Food and Drug Administration Web site. http://www.fda.gov/BiologicsBloodVaccines/SafetyAvailability/ucm111476.htm. Accessed October 2, 2011.
159. Ferber D. *Science.* 2002;296:1012-1015.
160. López-Ríos F, et al. *Lancet.* 2004;364:1157-1166.
161. Plotkin SA. *Clin Infect Dis.* 2001;32:1068-1084.
162. Plotkin SA. *Vaccine.* 2004;22:1829-1830.
163. Korber B, et al. *Science.* 2000;288:1789-1796.
164. Worobey M, et al. *Nature.* 2004;428:820.
165. Berry N, et al. *Nature.* 2001;410:1046-1047.
166. Poinar H, et al. *Science.* 2001;292:743-744.
167. Butler D. *Nature.* 2004;428:109.
168. Niu MT, et al. *Arch Pediatr Adolesc Med.* 1999;153:1279-1282.
169. Griffin MR, et al. *N Engl J Med.* 1988;319:618-623.
170. Fleming PJ, et al. *BMJ.* 2001;322:822.
171. Eriksen EM, et al. *Pediatr Infect Dis J.* 2004;23:656-662.
172. Duncan JR, et al. *JAMA.* 2010;303:430-437.

173. Kawasaki syndrome and RotaTeq vaccine. Centers for Disease Control and Prevention Web site. http://www.cdc.gov/vaccinesafety/Vaccines/Rotavirus.html. Accessed October 2, 2011.

174. Hua W, et al. *Pediatr Infect Dis J*. 2009;28:943-947.

175. Belongia EA, et al. *Pediatr Infect Dis J*. 2010;29:1-5.

176. ACIP Summary Report, October 21-22, 2009. Centers for Disease Control and Prevention Web site. http://www.cdc.gov/vaccines/recs/acip/downloads/min-oct09.pdf. Accessed October 2, 2011.

177. Tsang SX, et al. *J Virol*. 1999;73:5843-5851.

178. Hussain AI, et al. *J Virol*. 2003;77:1105-1111.

179. Victoria JG, et al. *J Virol*. 2010;84:6033-6040.

180. Baylis SA, et al. *Vaccine*. 2011;29:690-697.

181. McClenahan SD, et al. *Vaccine*. 2011;29:4745-4753.

182. Ranucci CS, et al. *J Pharm Sci Technol*. 2001;65:589-598.

183. Li L, et al. *J Virol*. 2010;84:1674-82.

184. Kuter BJ, et al. *Hum Vaccine*. 2006;2:205-214.

185. AAP. *Pediatrics*. 2011;127:389-394.

186. Jacobsen SJ, et al. *Vaccine*. 2009;27:4656-4661.

187. Klein NP, et al. *Pediatrics*. 2010;126:e1-e8.

188. Update on febrile seizures in children following vaccination with influenza vaccines and pneumococcal vaccines. Centers for Disease Control and Prevention Web site. http://www.cdc.gov/vaccinesafety/Concerns/FebrileSeizures.html. Accessed October 4, 2011.

189. Peter G, et al. *Pediatrics*. 2002;110:e67.

190. Vesikari T, et al. *N Engl J Med*. 2006;354:23-33.

191. Cheuvart B, et al. *Pediatr Infect Dis J*. 2009;28:225-232.

192. Haber P, et al. *Pediatrics*. 2008;121:1206-1212.

193. Patel MM, et al. *N Engl J Med*. 2011;364:2283-2292.

194. Simonsen L, et al. *Lancet*. 2001;358:1224-1229.

195. Greenberg HB. *N Engl J Med*. 2011;364:2354-2355.

8 Schedules

As discussed in *Chapter 2: Vaccine Infrastructure in the United States—Policy and Recommendations*, the Advisory Committee on Immunization Practices (ACIP) has permanent working groups that make recommendations for changes to the routine childhood/adolescent and adult vaccination schedules.

Since 1995, the childhood schedule has been "harmonized" in its current graphic layout with the recommendations of the American Academy of Pediatrics (AAP) and the American Academy of Family Physicians (AAFP). The new schedule is released at the beginning of each year. Since 2007, the schedule has been split into two—one giving the routinely recommended vaccines for children 0 to 6 years of age (**Figures 8.1** and **8.2**) and the other giving the recommendations for children and adolescents 7 to 18 years of age (**Figure 8.3**). Two additional charts—the catch-up schedules (**Figures 8.4** and **8.5**)—are used to bring unimmunized and underimmunized children up-to-date as soon as possible. Catch-up can be accomplished by giving all vaccines for which a person is eligible at each visit, keeping in mind the minimum intervals between doses (**Table 5.1**). Remember, routine vaccine series do not need to be restarted, regardless of the time that has elapsed between doses.

The adult schedule, first published in its current form in 2002, is also updated at the beginning of each year. The recommendations are developed in conjunction with the AAFP, the American College of Obstetricians and Gynecologists, and the American College of Physicians. The schedule is given in two different formats—by age group (**Figure 8.6**) and by underlying medical condition (**Figure 8.7**).

In this chapter, the routine schedules for 2012[1,2] are given in simplified format. Details, which include information from the footnotes of the published schedules as well as certain flexibilities in the schedules, are contained in the individual vaccine chapters in *Section B*. Vaccination of high-risk groups and other special populations is discussed in more detail in *Chapter 6: Vaccination in Special Circumstances*.

REFERENCES

1. CDC. *MMWR.* 2012;61(5):1-4.
2. CDC. *MMWR.* 2012;61(4):1-7.

FIGURE 8.1 — Routine Schedule for Children 0 to 6 Years of Age, 2012

<table>
<tr><th rowspan="2">Vaccine</th><th rowspan="2">Birth</th><th colspan="9">Months</th><th colspan="2">Years</th></tr>
<tr><th>1</th><th>2</th><th>4</th><th>6</th><th>9</th><th>12</th><th>15</th><th>18</th><th>19-23</th><th>2-3</th><th>4-6</th></tr>
<tr><td>HepB</td><td>Dose 1</td><td colspan="2">Dose 2</td><td></td><td colspan="4">Dose 3</td><td></td><td></td><td></td><td></td></tr>
<tr><td>RV</td><td></td><td></td><td>Dose 1</td><td>Dose 2</td><td>(Dose 3)</td><td></td><td></td><td></td><td></td><td></td><td></td><td></td></tr>
<tr><td>DTaP</td><td></td><td></td><td>Dose 1</td><td>Dose 2</td><td>Dose 3</td><td></td><td></td><td colspan="2">Dose 4</td><td></td><td></td><td>Dose 5</td></tr>
<tr><td>Hib</td><td></td><td></td><td>Dose 1</td><td>Dose 2</td><td>(Dose 3)</td><td></td><td colspan="2">Dose 3 or Dose 4</td><td></td><td></td><td></td><td></td></tr>
<tr><td>PCV</td><td></td><td></td><td>Dose 1</td><td>Dose 2</td><td>Dose 3</td><td></td><td colspan="2">Dose 4</td><td></td><td></td><td colspan="2">PPSV for high-risk</td></tr>
<tr><td>IPV</td><td></td><td></td><td>Dose 1</td><td>Dose 2</td><td colspan="4">Dose 3</td><td></td><td></td><td>Dose 4</td></tr>
<tr><td>Influenza</td><td></td><td></td><td></td><td></td><td colspan="8">Annual</td></tr>
<tr><td>MMR</td><td></td><td></td><td></td><td></td><td></td><td></td><td colspan="2">Dose 1</td><td></td><td></td><td></td><td>Dose 2</td></tr>
<tr><td>VAR</td><td></td><td></td><td></td><td></td><td></td><td></td><td colspan="2">Dose 1</td><td></td><td></td><td></td><td>Dose 2</td></tr>
<tr><td>HepA</td><td></td><td></td><td></td><td></td><td></td><td></td><td colspan="3">Dose 1</td><td>Dose 2</td><td colspan="2">High-risk</td></tr>
<tr><td>MCV</td><td></td><td></td><td></td><td></td><td></td><td colspan="7">High-risk</td></tr>
</table>

Doses shown in parentheses may not be necessary, depending on which product is used.

Adapted from CDC. *MMWR*. 2012;61(5):1-4.

FIGURE 8.2 — Use of Combination Vaccines in Children 0 to 6 Years of Age, 2012

<table>
<tr><th rowspan="2">Combination Vaccine</th><th rowspan="2">Birth</th><th colspan="9">Months</th><th colspan="2">Years</th></tr>
<tr><th>1</th><th>2</th><th>4</th><th>6</th><th>9</th><th>12</th><th>15</th><th>18</th><th>19-23</th><th>2-3</th><th>4-6</th></tr>
<tr><td>HepB-Hib</td><td>HepB</td><td></td><td>Dose 1</td><td>Dose 2</td><td colspan="2"></td><td colspan="2">Dose 3</td><td colspan="4"></td></tr>
<tr><td>DTaP-HepB-IPV</td><td>HepB</td><td></td><td>Dose 1</td><td>Dose 2</td><td>Dose 3</td><td colspan="2"></td><td colspan="2">DTaP</td><td colspan="2"></td><td>DTaP
IPV</td></tr>
<tr><td>DTaP-IPV/Hib</td><td colspan="2"></td><td>Dose 1</td><td>Dose 2</td><td>Dose 3</td><td colspan="2"></td><td colspan="2">Dose 4</td><td colspan="2"></td><td>DTaP
IPV</td></tr>
<tr><td rowspan="2">DTaP-IPV</td><td rowspan="2" colspan="2"></td><td rowspan="2">DTaP
IPV</td><td rowspan="2">DTaP
IPV</td><td>DTaP</td><td colspan="2"></td><td colspan="2">DTaP</td><td rowspan="2" colspan="2"></td><td rowspan="2">Dose 1</td></tr>
<tr><td colspan="5">IPV</td></tr>
<tr><td>MMRV</td><td colspan="6"></td><td colspan="2">MMR + VAR
or
Dose 1</td><td colspan="3"></td><td>Dose 1
or
Dose 2</td></tr>
</table>

Only the vaccination series relevant to each combination vaccine are shown. For example, infants receiving DTaP-IPV/Hib at 2, 4, 6, and 15-18 months of age should also receive the birth dose of HepB, but it is not shown here because HepB is not contained in the combination vaccine.

Adapted from CDC. *MMWR*. 2012;61(5):1-4.

8

FIGURE 8.3 — Routine Schedule for Children 7 to 18 Years of Age, 2012

<table>
<tr><th>Vaccine</th><th>7-10 Years</th><th>11-12 Years</th><th colspan="2">13-18 Years</th></tr>
<tr><td>Tdap</td><td>If pertussis series incomplete</td><td>Dose 1</td><td colspan="2">Catch-up</td></tr>
<tr><td>HPV</td><td></td><td>Dose 1, Dose 2, Dose 3
(Females: HPV2 or HPV4)
(Males: HPV4)</td><td colspan="2">Catch-up
(Females: HPV2 or HPV4)
(Males: HPV4)</td></tr>
<tr><td rowspan="2">MCV</td><td rowspan="2">High-risk</td><td rowspan="2">Dose 1</td><td></td><td>Dose 2
(16 years)</td></tr>
<tr><td>Catch-up
(13-15 years)
Dose 1</td><td>Catch-up
(16-18 years)
Dose 1 or
Dose 2</td></tr>
<tr><td>Influenza</td><td colspan="4">Annual</td></tr>
<tr><td>PCV, PPSV</td><td colspan="4">High-risk</td></tr>
<tr><td>HepA</td><td colspan="4">High-risk or catch-up (based on local recommendations)</td></tr>
<tr><td>HepB</td><td colspan="4">Catch-up</td></tr>
<tr><td>IPV</td><td colspan="4">Catch-up</td></tr>
<tr><td>MMR</td><td colspan="4">Catch-up</td></tr>
<tr><td>VAR</td><td colspan="4">Catch-up</td></tr>
</table>

Adapted from CDC. *MMWR*. 2012;61(5):1-4.

8

This page left intentionally blank.

FIGURE 8.4 — Catch-Up Schedule for Children 4 Months to 6 Years of Age, 2012

Vaccine	Minimum Age for Dose 1	Minimum Interval to...			
		Dose 2	Dose 3	Dose 4	Dose 5
HepB	Birth	4 weeks	8 weeks and ≥16 weeks after Dose 1 (minimum age 24 weeks)		
RV	6 weeks	4 weeks	(4 weeks)		
DTaP	6 weeks	4 weeks	4 weeks	6 months	6 months
Hib	6 weeks	Dose 1 at <12 months: 4 weeks Dose 1 at 12-14 months: 8 weeks (final dose) Dose 1 at ≥15 months: no further doses	Age <12 months: 4 weeks Age ≥12 months, Dose 1 at <12 months and Dose 2 at <15 months: 8 weeks (final dose) Any dose at ≥15 months: no further doses	Age 12-59 months and 3 doses at <12 months: 8 weeks (final dose)	

PCV	6 weeks	Dose 1 at <12 months: 4 weeks Dose 1 at ≥12 months: 8 weeks (final dose) Age 24-59 months: 8 weeks (final dose) Dose 1 at ≥24 months: no further doses	Age <12 months: 4 weeks Age ≥12 months: 8 weeks (final dose) Age ≥24 months: no further doses	Age 12-59 months and 3 doses at <12 months: 8 weeks (final dose)	
IPV	6 weeks	4 weeks	4 weeks	6 months (minimum age 4 years)	
MCV	9 months	8 weeks			
MMR	12 months	4 weeks			
VAR	12 months	3 months			
HepA	12 months	6 months			

This schedule should be used for children who start late or who are >1 month behind. Some combinations may be used for catch-up. Doses shown in parentheses may not be necessary, depending on which product is used.

Adapted from CDC. *MMWR*. 2012;61(5):1-4.

FIGURE 8.5 — Catch-Up Schedule for Children 7 to 18 Years of Age, 2012

Vaccine	Minimum Age for Dose 1	Minimum Interval to...			
		Dose 2	Dose 3	Dose 4	Dose 5
Td, Tdap	7 years	4 weeks	Dose 1 at <12 months: 4 weeks Dose 1 at ≥12 months: 6 months	Dose 1 at <12 months: 6 months	
HPV	9 years	4 weeks	12 weeks and ≥24 weeks after Dose 1		
HepA	12 months	6 months			
HepB	Birth	4 weeks	8 weeks and ≥16 weeks after Dose 1		
IPV	6 weeks	4 weeks	4 weeks	6 months	
MCV	9 months	8 weeks			
MMR	12 months	4 weeks			
VAR	12 months	Age <13 years: 3 months Age ≥13 years: 4 weeks			

This schedule should be used for children who start late or who are >1 month behind. Some combinations may be used for catch-up. Doses shown in parentheses may not be necessary, depending on which product is used.

Adapted from CDC. *MMWR*. 2012;61(5):1-4.

8

This page left intentionally blank.

FIGURE 8.6 — Routine Schedule for Adults by Age, 2012

<table>
<tr><th rowspan="2">Vaccine</th><th colspan="6">Age Group (Years)</th></tr>
<tr><th>19-21</th><th>22-26</th><th>27-49</th><th>50-59</th><th>60-64</th><th>≥65</th></tr>
<tr><td>Influenza</td><td colspan="6">Annual</td></tr>
<tr><td>Td, Tdap</td><td colspan="5">Substitute Tdap for Td one time, then Td every 10 years</td><td>Tdap one time if in contact with infants, otherwise Td every 10 years[a]</td></tr>
<tr><td>VAR</td><td colspan="6">2 doses</td></tr>
<tr><td rowspan="2">HPV</td><td colspan="2">Females: 3 doses (HPV2 or HPV4)</td><td colspan="4" rowspan="2"></td></tr>
<tr><td>Males:
3 doses (HPV4)</td><td>High-risk males:
3 doses (HPV4)</td></tr>
<tr><td>ZOS</td><td colspan="4"></td><td colspan="2">1 dose</td></tr>
<tr><td>MMR</td><td colspan="3">1 or 2 doses</td><td colspan="3">1 or 2 doses if high-risk</td></tr>
<tr><td>PPSV</td><td colspan="5">1 or 2 doses if high-risk</td><td>1 dose</td></tr>
<tr><td>MCV, MPSV</td><td colspan="6">≥1 dose if high-risk</td></tr>
<tr><td>HepA</td><td colspan="6">2 doses if high-risk</td></tr>
<tr><td>HepB</td><td colspan="6">3 doses if high-risk</td></tr>
</table>

These recommendations apply if a person was not previously vaccinated and is not otherwise immune (except in the case of influenza, where vaccination should occur every year). Thus, for example, MMR and VAR should be given to adults who have not previously been vaccinated and who do not meet the criteria for immunity. For Tdap, HPV, ZOS, influenza, PPSV, and MCV or MPSV, vaccination should occur even if disease has been previously documented. Thus, for example, HPV is given to women known to have had cervical dysplasia or human papillomavirus infection, since the vaccine may prevent infection with serotypes that have not yet been encountered.

[a] In February 2012, the ACIP voted to extend this recommendation to all persons ≥65 years of age.

Adapted from CDC. *MMWR*. 2012;61(4):1-7.

FIGURE 8.7 — Routine Schedule for Adults by Medical and Other Indications, 2012

Vaccine	Indication									
	Pregnancy	Immune comprom-ised	HIV		Men who have sex with men	Heart disease, chronic lung disease, alcoholism	Asplenia, persistent comple-ment deficiency	Chronic liver disease	Diabetes, kidney failure, end-stage renal disease, hemodialy-sis	Health care personnel
			<200 CD4 per µL	≥200 CD4 per µL						
Influenza	Annual IIV				Annual IIV or LAIV	Annual IIV				Annual IIV or LAIV
Td, Tdap	Substitute Tdap for Td one time, then Td every 10 years									
VAR	*Contraindicated*			2 doses						
HPV		Females: ≤26 years (HPV2 or HPV4)				Females: ≤26 years (HPV2 or HPV4)				
		Males: ≤26 years (HPV4)				Males: ≤21 years (HPV4)				

ZOS	*Contraindicated*			1 dose ≥60 years					
MMR	*Contraindicated*			1 or 2 doses					
PPSV	*If otherwise indicated*	1 or 2 doses							*If otherwise indicated*
MCV, MPSV	*If otherwise indicated*					≥2 doses	*If otherwise indicated*		
HepA	*If otherwise indicated*			2 doses	*If otherwise indicated*		2 doses	*If otherwise indicated*	
HepB	*If otherwise indicated*		3 doses		*If otherwise indicated*		3 doses		

Adapted from CDC. *MMWR*. 2012;61(4):1-7.

9 Adenovirus

Pathogen

Adenovirus is a nonenveloped, double-stranded DNA virus in the Adenoviridae family. The viral capsid consists of 252 capsomeres, each of which in turn consists of 240 hexons and 12 pentons. The pentons form the vertices of an icosahedron, and each has a projecting fiber, giving the virion a satellite-like appearance with "antennae." The fibers interact with cell surface ligands on epithelial cells, including CD46 (a complement regulatory protein) and CAR (the coxsackie virus and adenovirus receptor) to initiate infection, and antibodies to the fibers and pentons are neutralizing. After acute infection, latency is established (probably in mucosa-associated lymphoid cells) [1]; subsequent reactivation and shedding contribute to endemnicity in populations. Over 50 serotypes of human adenovirus are described, most of which cause respiratory disease but some of which cause gastroenteritis. The virion is very stable and can survive in the environment for long periods of time, facilitating transmission.

Clinical Features

Adenovirus is most commonly associated with respiratory disease.[2] Types 1, 2, 3, 5, and 7 cause *nasopharyngitis*, *pharyngitis*, *tonsillitis*, *acute laryngotracheitis*, and *bronchitis*. Respiratory symptoms, which last 5 to 7 days, may be accompanied by fever, cervical adenopathy, headache, malaise, myalgia, chills, and rash. Rarely, extrapulmonary manifestations including hepatitis, splenomegaly, nephritis, myocarditis, seizures, meningitis, and encephalitis can be seen, as can permanent respiratory sequelae such as *bronchiolitis obliterans*. Types 4 and 7 cause *epidemic acute respiratory disease*, classically seen in military installations and characterized by high attack rates and high rates of hospitalization.[3] Types 3, 4, 7, and 21 rank third behind respiratory syncytial virus and parainfluenza virus as causes of *pneumonia* in young children. Some strains, particularly type 5, can cause a *pertussis-like illness* in infants and young children with paroxysmal cough, whoop, post-tussive emesis, cyanosis, and lymphocytosis.

Other syndromes caused by adenovirus include *pharyngoconjunctival fever* (types 3, 4 and 7), *epidemic keratoconjunctivitis* (types 8 and 37), *hemorrhagic conjunctivitis* (type 11), *hemorrhagic cystitis* (type 11), and *acute gastroenteritis* (types 31,

40, and 41). Mortality rates are high in immunocompromised persons.[4]

Epidemiology and Transmission

Infection rates peak between 6 months and 5 years of age such that by school age, most children have been infected with several serotypes. Epidemic respiratory disease is seen more often in winter and spring, but sporadic disease occurs throughout the year. Epidemics of pharyngoconjunctival fever typically occur during the summer and have been associated with camps and swimming pools. Epidemics that occur during basic training may involve over 90% of military recruits in first 8 weeks.

Transmission occurs by close physical contact with respiratory secretions, small droplet aerosols, and fomites or, in the case of enteric adenoviruses, by the fecal-oral route. Inoculation takes place at mucosal surfaces such as the conjunctiva, nose, and throat. In the military setting, contamination of environmental surfaces and prolonged shedding facilitate outbreaks.[5]

Immunization Program

Despite the significance of adenoviral disease in children, there has never been a concerted effort to develop a vaccine for generalized use in this population. In contrast, the heavy burden of disease among military recruits provided adequate justification for vaccine development. Beginning in 1971, an adenovirus types 4 and 7 vaccine manufactured by Wyeth (acquired by Pfizer in 2009) was routinely administered to recruits at US military training centers. Wyeth stopped producing the vaccine in 1996, and by 1997 outbreaks of adenovirus-associated acute respiratory disease were again rampant at training posts,[6] and studies suggested that reinstating an immunization program would be cost-saving.[7] In 2001, the Department of Defense awarded a contract to Barr Laboratories to develop and remanufacture the vaccine with cooperation from Wyeth, and the vaccine was relicensed in 2011.

Vaccines

Characteristics of the adenovirus vaccine licensed in the United States are given in **Table 9.1**. This is a live vaccine that consists of lyophilized viruses embedded in enteric-coated tablets. The viruses are not attenuated; rather, because they are given enterically rather than in the respiratory tract, they are capable of inducing immunity without causing disease. The enteric coating allows the vaccine to bypass the stomach, where it might be inactivated, and establish infection in the small intestine.

TABLE 9.1 — Adenovirus Vaccine

Trade Name	—
Abbreviation	—
Manufacturer/distributor	Barr Labs/Teva Pharmaceuticals
Type of vaccine	Live
Composition	Non-attenuated, lyophylized adenovirus types 4 and 7 in enteric-coated tablets (white and peach, respectively) Propagated in human diploid lung fibroblast (WI-38) cells At least 32,000 tissue-culture infective doses per tablet
Adjuvant	None
Preservative	None
Excipients and contaminants	Monosodium glutamate Sucrose D-mannose D-fructose Dextrose Human serum albumin Potassium phosphate Plasdone C Anhydrous lactose Microcrystalline cellulose Polacrilin potassium Magnesium stearate Cellulose acetate phthalate Alcohol Acetone Castor oil FD&C Yellow #6 aluminum lake dye
Latex	None
Labeled indications	Prevention of febrile acute respiratory disease in military populations[a]
Labeled ages	17 to 50 years
Dose	2 tablets (swallowed whole)
Route of administration	PO
Labeled schedule	1 dose
Recommended schedule	Same
How supplied (number in package)	100-dose bottles (1 bottle of type 4 and 1 bottle of type 7)
Reference package insert	March 2011

[a] The vaccine is not licensed for use in civilians.

Efficacy and/or Immunogenicity

Field trials of the previously licensed adenovirus vaccine in military settings demonstrated over 90% effectiveness in preventing hospitalization.[8-10] During the years that the vaccine was used, except for a period when vaccine potency was compromised in the 1970s, there was never an outbreak of acute adenovirus type 4 or 7 respiratory disease in any vaccinated group.

The relicensed vaccine was studied in 4041 US military recruits who were randomized to receive vaccine or placebo in a 3:1 ratio. Efficacy against febrile respiratory disease caused by adenovirus type 4 was 99% and seroconversion rates were 95%. The seroconversion rate for type 7 was 94% (there was not enough type 7 disease to allow for an efficacy assessment).

Safety

Approximately 30% of vaccinees shed type 4 in the stool and 60% shed type 7, but this occurs exclusively in the first 28 days. Vaccine virus is not detectable in the throat. Solicited adverse events include headache (30%), nasal congestion (15%), nausea (14%), sore throat (13%), cough (12%), and diarrhea (10%), but these rates are similar to those seen in placebees. Fever is reported in 1% of vaccinees.

- *Contraindications*
  - Severe allergic reaction (eg, anaphylaxis) to previous dose of vaccine or any vaccine component (risk of recurrent allergic reaction)
  - Pregnancy (theoretical risk to the fetus of live-virus vaccine or attribution of birth defects to vaccination). The military recommends that vaccinees avoid pregnancy for 6 weeks.
  - Inability to swallow an entire tablet whole without chewing
- *Precautions*
  - Moderate or severe acute illness (difficulty distinguishing illness from vaccine reaction)
  - Vomiting and/or diarrhea (potential interference with effectiveness or difficulty distinguishing illness from vaccine reaction)
  - Immunodeficiency or immunosuppression (risk of disease caused by live virus)
  - Breast-feeding (risk of disease caused by live virus)

Recommendations

Adenovirus vaccine is routinely given to all enlisted basic trainees 17 to 50 years of age as soon as they arrive at the accession site.[11] There are no booster doses. The vaccine is not used in civilians.

REFERENCES

1. Zhang Y, et al. *J Virol*. 2010;84:8799-8810.
2. Lenaerts L, et al. *Rev Med Virol*. 2008;18:357-374.
3. Dingle JH, et al. *Am Rev Resp Dis*. 1968;97:1-65.
4. Echavarria M. *Clin Microbiol Rev*. 2008;21:704-715.
5. Russell KL, et al. *J Infect Dis*. 2006;194:877-885.
6. Kolavic-Gray SA, et al. *Clin Infect Dis*. 2002;35:808-818.
7. Howell MR, et al. *Am J Prev Med.* 1998;14:168-175.
8. Stallones RA, et al. *JAMA*. 1957;163:9-15.
9. Hilleman MR, et al. *Arch Intern Med*. 1958;102:428-436.
10. Peckinpaugh RO, et al. *JAMA*. 1968;205:75-80.
11. Implementation guidance for administration of adenovirus type 4 and type 7 vaccine live, oral. Milvax Web site. http://www.vaccines.mil/documents/1459ADENO_IMPLEMENTATION_PLAN_army.pdf. Accessed January 16, 2012.

10 Anthrax

Pathogen

Bacillus anthracis is a large, aerobic, spore-forming, toxin-producing gram-positive rod with a "jointed bamboo-rod" appearance and "Medusa's head" colony morphology. Pathogenicity is mediated by two secreted virulence factors: lethal toxin and edema toxin.

Clinical Features

10

Inhalational anthrax is characterized by a flu-like illness, dyspnea, and hemorrhagic thoracic lymphadenitis and mediastinitis.[1] *Cutaneous anthrax* is characterized by a painless ulcer with extensive surrounding edema, eschar formation, and regional adenopathy. Both of these forms of disease would be seen after a bioterrorism attack and either can lead to meningitis. The *gastrointestinal* (bloody diarrhea, hemorrhagic mesenteric adenitis) and *oropharyngeal* (oral or esophageal ulcers and regional adenopathy) forms of anthrax result from ingestion of large numbers of vegetative bacilli (usually in poorly cooked meat) and would therefore be unlikely to result from an attack. After the spores are ingested by phagocytes, they are transported to regional lymph nodes, where they germinate into vegetative cells after variable (and potentially extended) periods of time. Replicating cells then elaborate toxins that lead to massive hemorrhage, edema, necrosis, and cytokine release. Early antibiotic therapy for symptomatic disease is essential, but the effects of local tissue damage and systemic toxinosis may be irreversible.[2]

Epidemiology and Transmission

Anthrax spores are found in soil worldwide and may remain viable for years. Infection occurs in grazing animals that ingest the spores, and natural human infection occurs almost exclusively after contact with infected animals and animal products (a classic example is *woolsorter's disease*, inhalational anthrax linked to the processing of hides and wool in enclosed spaces). Up to 20,000 annual cases of anthrax are estimated to occur worldwide, but disease was rare in the United States until 2001. In September and October of that year, at least five letters containing high-grade Ames strain anthrax spores were mailed through the US postal service from Trenton, NJ, to sites in Florida, New York City, and

Washington, DC.[3] One letter was known to contain 2 g of powder and between 100 billion and 1 trillion spores. A total of 22 anthrax cases occurred in seven eastern states between September 22 and November 16; 11 were inhalational (five deaths), 11 cutaneous (no deaths), and 12 victims were mail handlers. Cross-contamination was evidenced by the isolation of anthrax from over 100 environmental samples along the path of the letters.

Anthrax is an attractive bioterrorism agent because infection can be lethal, natural immunity does not exist, the organism can be engineered into antibiotic resistance, and the infectious dose of spores is very low.[4] It is easily grown in the laboratory, and the spores can be weaponized into a highly concentrated powder with uniform small particle size and low electrostatic charge, features that reduce clumping and facilitate aerosol dispersal. Such aerosols are odorless and invisible, can spread over large areas, and would probably not be detected until cases occurred. The lethality of aerosolized weapons-grade anthrax was demonstrated after the accidental release of anthrax spores (possibly as little as 1 g) on April 2, 1979, from a Soviet bioweapons facility in Sverdlovsk (now called Ekaterinburg, a city of over 1 million people).[5] Nearly 100 cases and over 60 deaths occurred downwind of the release, mostly from inhalational disease. Most cases occurred within 10 days, although some occurred 6 weeks later. While the majority of victims were exposed in a narrow 4-km band extending from the military facility to the southern city limit, cases did occur many miles away and livestock in several towns downwind of the release were affected.

A release of 100 kg of spores over Washington, DC would result in as many as 3 million deaths.[6] Unlike smallpox, all cases occurring after an attack would result from primary exposure, because the infection is not transmitted from person to person. However, secondary aerosolization of particles that settle after a primary release could continue to cause disease for some time.

Immunization Program

The latest recommendations for civilian use of anthrax vaccine prior to the 2001 attacks were published in 2000.[7] Following the attacks, occupational health guidelines for remediation workers[8] and vaccination recommendations in response to bioterrorism were released.[9] Updated recommendations for civilians were published in 2010.[10]

Antibiotic therapy after exposure can prevent inhaled spores from germinating and causing disease. In fact, there were no cases of anthrax among over 10,000 people who took antibiotics (primarily ciprofloxacin or doxycycline) for at least 60 days following the 2001 attacks. In 2002, the Working Group on Civilian Biodefense concluded that antibiotic therapy in conjunction with vaccination would be optimal for exposed persons, and current recommendations incorporate that concept.

Pre-exposure vaccination is based on the risk of exposure and is not recommended for the general public. Although a vaccine has been licensed since 1970, it was in limited use until 1991, when the US military immunized 150,000 service members deployed for the Gulf War. The Anthrax Vaccine Immunization Program was started in 1998 with the routine immunization of personnel deployed to high-risk areas. In 2002, the Department of Defense reintroduced the program (which had slowed because of dwindling vaccine supplies) because of intelligence assessments indicating possible risk of exposure to military personnel; the guidelines were updated in 2009.[11]

Vaccines

Characteristics of the anthrax vaccine licensed in the United States are given in **Table 10.1**. This is an inactivated vaccine composed of proteins released by the bacterium into the medium during growth in culture. It contains no intact bacteria, live or dead.

Efficacy and/or Immunogenicity

From 1955 to 1959, a controlled trial of a vaccine similar to the one that is currently licensed was conducted among 1249 mill workers (379 were immunized); efficacy was 92.5%. Case surveillance data from 1962 to 1974 suggest that anthrax in mill workers or those living near mills occurred exclusively in unvaccinated or incompletely vaccinated persons. In a controlled trial conducted from 2002 to 2008 involving 1564 adults, the intramuscular route of administration was found to be noninferior to the subcutaneous route in terms of immunogenicity, and nearly all vaccinees demonstrated a ≥4-fold increase in antibody titer.

Safety

In an open-label safety study, 15,907 doses of BioThrax were administered subcutaneously to 7000 at-risk persons. Mild local reactions occurred after 8.6% of doses administered, moderate reactions after 0.9%, and severe reactions after 0.15%. There were only four reports of systemic reactions such as fever, chills, nausea, and general body aches.

In the 2002 to 2008 trial, intramuscular administration was found to cause less local reactogenicity than subcutaneous administration. Most local and systemic reactions were mild or moderate in severity. Interestingly, injection site reactions

TABLE 10.1 — Anthrax Vaccine

Trade Name	BioThrax
Abbreviation	—
Manufacturer/distributor	Emergent BioDefense Operations Lansing[a]
Type of vaccine	Inactivated, purified subunits
Composition	Cell-free filtrate of microaerophilic cultures of an avirulent, noncapsulated *Bacillus anthracis* strain Includes 83 kDa protective antigen
Adjuvant	Aluminum hydroxide (0.6 mg aluminum)
Preservative	Benzethonium chloride (12.5 mcg) Formaldehyde (50 mcg)
Excipients and contaminants	Sodium chloride (0.85%)
Latex	Vial stopper contains latex
Labeled indications	Pre-exposure prophylaxis
Labeled ages	18 to 65 years
Dose	0.5 mL
Route of administration	Intramuscular (subcutaneous if patient has coagulopathy)
Labeled schedule	0, 4 weeks, 6, 12, 18 months (intramuscular) Booster doses every year (intramuscular)
Recommended schedule	Pre-exposure: same Postexposure:[b] 0, 2, 4 weeks (subcutaneous)
How supplied (number in package)	10-dose vial (1)
Cost per dose ($US, 2011):	
Public	—
Private	99.00
Reference package insert	December 2008

[a] Formerly manufactured by BioPort.

[b] Use of anthrax vaccine for postexposure prophylaxis is off-label, but it may be given under an Investigational New Drug application held by the CDC or under an Emergency Use authorization. Antimicrobials may also be indicated (see **Table 10.2**).

were more common in women, especially with subcutaneous administration. There were 44 pregnancies during the study; the majority of outcomes were good, although there was a spontaneous abortion and a clubbed foot abnormality among infants born to 15 women vaccinated in the first trimester. In an observational study of infants born to US military service women from 1998 to 2004, birth defects were slightly more common (odds ratio 1.18) among the 3465 infants born to women who were vaccinated during the first trimester when compared with the 33,675 infants whose mothers were vaccinated outside of the first trimester (most of these were vaccinated before pregnancy or after delivery).[12]

In a study involving >4300 service personnel in Korea, 2% of persons reported limitation in work performance after Dose 1 or Dose 2 but <1% lost ≥1 day of work. In 2002, an IOM study concluded that the anthrax vaccine is safe,[13] and epidemiologic studies provide no evidence linking the vaccine to Gulf War Syndrome.[14] Finally, from 1998 to 2007, approximately 6 million doses of anthrax vaccine were administered and slightly over 4700 adverse event reports were received by VAERS.[15] No unexpected risks were seen and there was no distinctive pattern of serious events or death.

- *Contraindications*
  - Severe allergic reaction (eg, anaphylaxis) to previous dose of vaccine or any vaccine component (risk of recurrent allergic reaction)
- *Precautions*
  - Moderate or severe acute illness (difficulty distinguishing illness from vaccine reaction)
  - Pregnancy (Pregnancy Category D—vaccine can cause fetal harm, so use only if the potential benefits outweigh the potential risks)
  - Previous anthrax disease (risk of more severe adverse events)

Recommendations

Recommendations for civilian use of anthrax vaccine are given in **Table 10.2**.

Use of anthrax vaccine in the military is summarized below:

- Vaccination is mandatory for Department of Defense service members, emergency-essential designated civilians, and contractor personnel performing mission-essential services assigned to Central Command area of responsibility for ≥15 consecutive days, Korean Peninsula for ≥15 consecutive days, special units with biowarfare or bioterrorism related missions, and specialty units with approved exception to policy.
- Vaccination occurs up to 120 days prior to deployment or arrival in higher threat areas.

TABLE 10.2 — Recommendations for Civilian Use of Anthrax Vaccine

Group	Pre-exposure[a]	Postexposure Prophylaxis[b]
General public	Not recommended	Recommended
Pregnant women	Not recommended	Recommended
Breastfeeding women	Not recommended	Recommended
Children 0 to 18 years of age	Not recommended	Determine on event-by-event basis[c]
Medical professionals	Not recommended	Recommended
Persons engaged in handling animals or animal products	Not routinely recommended[d]	Recommended
Persons engaged in certain laboratory work[e]	Recommended	Based on pre-event vaccination status
Persons working in postal facilities	Not recommended	Recommended
Persons engaged in environmental investigations or remediation efforts	Recommended	Based on pre-event vaccination status
Emergency and other responders[f]	Not routinely recommended[g]	Recommended

[a] Pre-exposure vaccination is recommended for persons who are occupationally at risk for exposure to aerosolized *B anthracis* spores. See **Table 10.1** for vaccination schedule.

[b] Prophylaxis is recommended following natural, occupational, or intentional exposure to *B anthracis* spores in persons who have not completed pre-exposure vaccination. See **Table 10.1** for vaccination schedule. In addition to vaccination, appropriate antimicrobials are given for 60 days (see Anthrax: exposure management/prophylaxis. Centers for Disease Control and Prevention Web site. http://www.bt.cdc.gov/agent/anthrax/exposure. Accessed January 8, 2012.). Persons who already received 5 doses of the vaccine plus annual boosters before exposure do not need

additional vaccination or antimicrobials unless there was a disruption in their personal protective equipment. Use of anthrax vaccine for postexposure prophylaxis is off-label.

[c] Use of anthrax vaccine in persons <18 years of age is off-label.

[d] Recommended if handling potentially infected animals in a research setting, animals with high incidence of enzootic anthrax, or if standards are insufficient to prevent exposure to spores. Potentially contaminated animal products include imported animal hides, furs, bone meal, wool, animal hair, or bristles.

[e] Includes persons handling high concentrations of spores, pure cultures, environmental samples associated with anthrax investigations, spore-contaminated areas or other settings with aerosol exposure. Does not include workers using standard Biosafety Level 2 practices in routine processing of clinical samples or environmental swabs.

[f] Includes police and fire departments, hazmat units, government responders, and National Guard who may perform site investigations, respond to "white powder incidents," perform evacuations, or other activities critical to the maintenance of infrastructure.

[g] Vaccination may be offered on a voluntary basis under a comprehensive occupational health and safety program.

Adapted from CDC. *MMWR*. 2010;59(RR-6):1-30.

- Vaccination is voluntary for Department of Defense service members and government civilian employees of the Department of Defense who are not in the mandatory groups and have received at least one dose of anthrax vaccine during or after 1998.
- Vaccination is voluntary for Department of Defense civilians and adult family members, as well as contractors and their accompanying United States citizen family members.
- Vaccine manufacturing and research personnel and others, as designated by the Assistant Secretary of Defense for Health Affairs, are vaccinated.

REFERENCES

1. Dixon TC, et al. *N Engl J Med*. 1999;341:815-826.
2. Grabenstein JD. *Clin Infect Dis*. 2008;46:129-136.
3. Inglesby TV, et al. *JAMA*. 2002;287:2236-2252.
4. CDC. *MMWR*. 2000;49(RR-15):1-20.
5. CDC. *MMWR*. 2002;51:786-789.
6. CDC. *MMWR*. 2002;51:1024-1026.
7. CDC. *MMWR*. 2010;59(RR-6):1-30.
8. Military Vaccine Agency, Office of the Army Surgeon General. Anthrax vaccine immunization program (AVIP): questions and answers. Anthrax Vaccine Immunization Program Web site. http://www.anthrax.osd.mil/documents/Anthrax_QA.pdf. Accessed January 8, 2012.
9. Ryan MAK, et al. *Am J Epidemiol*. 2008;168:434-442.
10. Joellenbeck LM, et al, editors. *The Anthrax Vaccine: Is It Safe? Does It Work?* Washington, DC: Institute of Medicine, National Academy Press; 2002.
11. Iowa Persian Gulf Study Group. *JAMA*. 1997;277:238-245.
12. Niu MT, et al. *Vaccine*. 2009;27:290-297.

11 Diphtheria, Tetanus, Pertussis

The Pathogens

Diphtheria

Corynebacterium diphtheriae is an aerobic, nonencapsulated, nonspore-forming, pleomorphic gram-positive bacillus that has a club-like appearance on Gram stain.[1] Infection occurs on mucous membranes of the upper respiratory tract or in the skin, where the organism elaborates a potent exotoxin that works by inactivating tRNA transferase, preventing amino acids from being added to nascent polypeptide chains during protein synthesis. On respiratory surfaces like the throat, necrotic cells, inflammatory exudate, bacteria, and fibrin coalesce into adherent *pseudomembranes*. Local effects of the toxin include paralysis of the palate and hypopharynx; distant effects can be seen in the kidneys, liver, heart, and nervous system.

Tetanus

Clostridium tetani is a nonencapsulated, gram-positive, obligately anaerobic bacillus that has a drumstick or tennis racket appearance on Gram stain because of terminally located spores.[2] Initial infection usually takes place in a deep, penetrating wound, where the organism elaborates *tetanospasmin*, a potent neurotoxin. The toxin spreads via the bloodstream and lymphatics to distant sites, where it is taken up into nerves through the neuromuscular junction and transported to the CNS. There it prevents the release of neurotransmitters at inhibitory synapses, causing unopposed lower motor-neuron activity, with resultant spasms and rigidity.

Pertussis

Bordetella pertussis is a tiny, aerobic, gram-negative coccobacillus that is tropic for ciliated respiratory epithelium.[3] Attachment is mediated by several proteins, including *filamentous hemagglutinin* (FHA), *fimbriae* (FIM), and *pertactin* (PRN). The major virulence factor is *pertussis toxin* (PT), a complex molecule that causes increased intracellular levels of cyclic adenosine monophosphate and disruption of cellular function. PT also facilitates adherence, promotes lymphocytosis, inhibits phagocytosis, increases insulin production (causing hypoglycemia) and increases sensitivity to histamine (causing vascular permeability and hypotension). PT and other toxins, including *tracheal cytotoxin* and *adenylate cyclase toxin*, are involved in the genesis of protracted cough.

Clinical Features

■ Diphtheria

The disease most often presents as *membranous nasopharyngitis* or *obstructive laryngotracheitis* associated with low-grade fever.[1] Less commonly, cutaneous, vaginal, conjunctival, or otic infection can occur. Serious complications include upper airway obstruction caused by extensive membrane formation, myocarditis, and peripheral neuropathy. The case fatality rate is as high as 10%, but is higher in young children and adults >40 years of age. Treatment includes antibiotics as well as equine antitoxin (available through the CDC), which neutralizes circulating toxin and prevents disease progression.

■ Tetanus

Most cases occur within 14 days of injury.[2] Shorter incubation periods have been associated with more heavily contaminated wounds, more severe disease, and worse prognosis. *Generalized tetanus* (lockjaw) initially manifests with trismus, followed within a week by neck stiffness, dysphagia, rigidity of the abdominal muscles, and generalized muscle spasms. Severe spasms, often aggravated by external stimuli, persist for 3 to 4 weeks, and complete recovery may take months. *Neonatal tetanus* results from contamination of the umbilical stump. *Localized tetanus* manifests as muscle spasms in areas contiguous with an infected wound. *Cephalic tetanus* refers to cranial nerve dysfunction associated with infected wounds on the head and neck. Both localized and cephalic tetanus may precede generalized tetanus. Treatment includes tetanus immune globulin (TIG), which neutralizes unbound toxin. The case fatality rate is about 10%.

■ Pertussis

Classic *whooping cough* begins with mild upper respiratory tract symptoms (*catarrhal stage*) that last for 1 to 2 weeks.[3] This progresses to severe paroxysms of cough (*paroxysmal stage*), often followed by a characteristic inspiratory whoop, that last for 4 to 6 weeks. Post-tussive emesis is common and the cough can be forceful enough to cause injury—rib fractures and even carotid artery dissections have been reported. Fever is usually absent and symptoms wane gradually (*convalescent stage*) over 6 to 10 weeks, giving rise to the colloquial term "the hundred-day cough." Complications include seizures, pneumonia, and encephalopathy. Pertussis is most severe during the first year of life. During 2000 to 2004, approximately 2500 cases were reported each year in infants <12 months of age—63% were hospitalized for a median duration of 5 days.[4] Almost all deaths occur in young infants; of the 100 pertussis-related deaths reported from 2000 to 2004, 90 were among infants <4 months of age. Disease in infants <6 months of age may be atypical, with prominent apnea and absent whoop. Older children and adults may also have atypical disease, manifested solely as persistent cough, making recognition and treatment difficult. Infection in immunized children and older persons is often mild.

Epidemiology and Transmission

Diphtheria

Humans are the only known reservoir of *C diphtheriae*. Patients excrete the organism for 2 to 6 weeks in nasal discharge, from the throat, or from eye or skin lesions. Antibiotic treatment shortens the period of communicability. Transmission results from intimate contact, and illness is more common in crowded living situations. Although *infection* can still occur in immunized persons, *disease* generally does not because any elaborated toxin is neutralized by antibody. Respiratory diphtheria is seen in winter and spring; summer epidemics can occur in warm, moist climates where skin infections are prevalent. While there are only two or three cases reported each year in the United States, toxigenic *C diphtheriae* can still be found in some populations. Diphtheria continues to be a significant cause of morbidity and mortality in developing countries.

Tetanus

Tetanus is not transmissible from person to person. Spores of *C tetani* are ubiquitous in the environment, especially where there is soil contaminated with excreta. Wounds, recognized or unrecognized, are where the organism multiplies and elaborates toxin. Contaminated wounds, those that result from deep puncture, and those with devitalized tissue are at greatest risk. Disease occurs worldwide but is more frequent in warmer climates and during warmer months, in part because contaminated wounds are more common. In 2003, the number of reported cases in the United States reached a low of 20. Neonatal tetanus is rare in the United States but common in developing countries, where pregnant women may not be fully immunized and nonsterile umbilical cord-care practices are followed.

Pertussis

Humans are the only known hosts for *B pertussis*. Transmission occurs through respiratory droplets and direct contact with respiratory secretions, and acquisition rates approach 80% in susceptible household contacts. Patients are most contagious during the catarrhal stage, before the onset of paroxysms; communicability then diminishes rapidly but may persist for ≥3 weeks after onset of cough. Antibiotic therapy decreases infectivity and may limit spread. Asymptomatic infection has been demonstrated but may not be a significant factor in transmission.

Pertussis is a common cause of prolonged cough illness. One study showed that 26% of university students with cough for ≥6 days had pertussis.[5] Many cases go unrecognized and untreated, and chemoprophylaxis of contacts does not take place, facilitating persistence and spread through communities. In fact, older people in the environment—parents, older siblings, non-household adults—are the most important source of transmission to young infants.[6] Nearly 26,000 cases of pertussis were reported in the United States in 2004, the highest number since 1959[7]; by 2007, the number of cases had fallen to around 10,000.[8] The actual annual disease burden probably exceeds 1 million[9]; in fact, about 1% of adolescents and young adults per year experience pertussis, although only 1 in 6 is symptomatic.[10] The *incidence* of disease—approximately 100 cases per 100,000—is highest among very young infants,[11] and hospitalization rates approach 240 per 100,000.[12] However, the greatest number of reported cases occurs among adolescents and young adults. School-based outbreaks are common.

A resurgence of pertussis occurred in the United States 2010. In California alone there were 9154 cases, including 809 hospitalizations and 10 deaths.[13] This was the highest number of cases reported since 1947.

Immunization Program

Diphtheria

Introduction of diphtheria toxoid vaccines in the United States in the 1940s led to a dramatic reduction in disease. High levels of vaccination have made diphtheria rare in the United States, and most cases today occur in unvaccinated or inadequately vaccinated persons. However, immunization does not completely eliminate the potential for transmission because it does not prevent carriage of the organism in the nasopharynx or on the skin. The consequences of inadequate population immunity were demonstrated by the massive resurgence of diphtheria in the former Soviet Union during the 1990s.[14]

Tetanus

Following the introduction of tetanus toxoid vaccines in the United States, the incidence of tetanus declined from 0.4 per 100,000 in 1947 to 0.05 per 100,000 since the mid 1970s. Currently, the majority of tetanus cases occur in persons who have not completed a 3-dose primary series or who have uncertain vaccination histories. From 1998 to 2000, only one death is known to have occurred in a person who had completed a primary immunization series; in this case, however, the last dose of tetanus toxoid was 11 years before the onset of illness. In contrast, 19 deaths occurred in persons who had not completed a primary series or who had unknown vaccination histories. Because naturally acquired immunity to tetanus toxin does not occur, universal primary vaccination with appropriately timed boosters is the only way to protect persons in all age groups.

■ Pertussis

After the introduction of universal infant immunization in the 1940s, the number of cases dramatically declined; between 1980 and 2004, however, there was a dramatic *increase* in cases, making pertussis the only disease preventable by a routinely recommended vaccine that was on the rise. During this time, from 1991 to 1996, the whole-cell pertussis vaccine was gradually replaced by acellular vaccines, which were less reactogenic.[15] Some of the resurgence in reported pertussis cases was due to the use of polymerase chain reaction for diagnosis as well as increased case-finding, but *waning immunity* also was important. Protection from childhood immunization (and natural infection, for that matter) is thought to wane after about 5 to 10 years, although data from the 2010 California outbreak suggest that the duration of protection may be even shorter.[16]

With the approval of Tdap vaccines for adolescents and adults in 2005, booster immunization became a possibility and, along with that, the opportunity to reduce disease in that age group as well as to impact a reservoir of pertussis in the community. The experience in Canada validated this approach—adolescent booster immunization was started there in 2000, and overall cases of pertussis steadily declined.[17] In 2006, Tdap was recommended for all adolescents and adults in the United States.[4,18] Recommendations for immunization of postpartum women, part of a "cocooning" strategy (see *Chapter 4: Vaccine Practice—Expanding Access*), were published in 2008.[19] However, subsequent data suggested that postpartum immunization of mothers alone is not enough to protect young infants from pertussis.[20] In 2011, routine vaccination of pregnant women beyond 20 weeks' gestation was recommended,[21] with the hope that transplacental antibodies might protect the youngest infants until they develop their own antibodies from immunization. In 2010, Tdap was recommended for incompletely immunized children 7 to 9 years of age and for persons ≥65 years of age anticipating contact infants[22]; in February 2012, the ACIP voted to extend this recommendation to all persons ≥65 years of age. Updated recommendations for prevention of pertussis among HCP were published in 2011.[23]

Vaccines

Characteristics of the diphtheria, tetanus, and pertussis vaccines licensed in the United States are given in **Tables 11.1** and **11.2**. These vaccines contain diphtheria, tetanus, and pertussis toxins that are chemically treated to render them nontoxic but

TABLE 11.1 — Diphtheria, Tetanus, and Pertussis Vaccines[a]

Trade name	Adacel	Boostrix	Daptacel[b]	Infanrix[c]
Abbreviation	Tdap	Tdap	DTaP	DTaP
Manufacturer/distributor	Sanofi Pasteur	GlaxoSmithKline	Sanofi Pasteur	GlaxoSmithKline
Type of vaccine	Inactivated, purified subunits and toxoids	Inactivated, purified subunits and toxoids	Inactivated, purified subunits and toxoids	Inactivated, purified subunits and toxoids
Composition:				
Diphtheria toxoid	2 Lf units	2.5 Lf units	15 Lf units	25 Lf units
Tetanus toxoid	5 Lf units	5 Lf units	5 Lf units	10 Lf units
Inactivated pertussis toxin	2.5 mcg	8 mcg	10 mcg	25 mcg
Filamentous hemagglutinin	5 mcg	8 mcg	5 mcg	25 mcg
Pertactin	3 mcg	2.5 mcg	3 mcg	8 mcg
Fimbriae types 2 and 3	5 mcg	—	5 mcg	—
Adjuvant	Aluminum phosphate (0.33 mg aluminum)	Aluminum hydroxide (≤0.39 mg aluminum)	Aluminum phosphate (0.33 mg aluminum)	Aluminum hydroxide (≤0.625 mg aluminum)
Preservative	None	None	None	None
Excipients and contaminants:				
Formaldehyde	≤5 mcg	≤100 mcg	≤5 mcg	≤100 mcg
Glutaraldehyde	≤50 ng	—	≤50 ng	—
2-phenoxyethanol	3.3 mg[d]	—	3.3 mg[d]	—
Polysorbate 80	—	≤100 mcg	—	≤100 mcg
Sodium chloride	—	4.5 mg	—	4.5 mg

Latex	Tip cap of prefilled syringe contains latex	Tip cap (and plunger for one presentation) of prefilled syringe contains latex	None	Tip cap (and plunger for one presentation) of prefilled syringe contains latex
Labeled indications	Booster immunization against diphtheria, tetanus, and pertussis	Booster immunization against diphtheria, tetanus, and pertussis	Prevention of diphtheria, tetanus, and pertussis	Prevention of diphtheria, tetanus, and pertussis
Labeled ages	11 to 64 years	≥10 years	6 weeks to 6 years	6 weeks to 6 years
Dose	0.5 mL	0.5 mL	0.5 mL	0.5 mL
Route of administration	Intramuscular	Intramuscular	Intramuscular	Intramuscular
Trade name	Adacel	Boostrix	Daptacel[b]	Infanrix[c]
Abbreviation	Tdap	Tdap	DTaP	DTaP
Labeled schedule	1 dose	1 dose	2, 4, 6, 15 to 20 months, 4 to 6 years of age	2, 4, 6, 15 to 20 months, 4 to 6 years of age
Recommended schedule	11 to 12 years of age Catch-up	11 to 12 years of age Catch-up	2, 4, 6, 15 to 18 months, 4 to 6 years of age	2, 4, 6, 15 to 18 months, 4 to 6 years of age
How supplied (number in package):				
1-dose vial	(5, 10)	(10)	(1, 5, 10)	(10)
Prefilled syringe	(5)	(1, 5, 10)	—	(5, 10)

Continued

TABLE 11.1 — *Continued*

Trade name	Adacel	Boostrix	Daptacel[b]	Infanrix[c]
Abbreviation	Tdap	Tdap	DTaP	DTaP
Cost per dose ($US, 2011):				
Public	29.59	29.59	14.51	14.85
Private	38.83	37.55	24.40	20.96
Reference package insert	February 2012	July 2011	July 2011	August 2010

[a] Tripedia (Sanofi Pasteur), which contains diphtheria and tetanus toxoids, inactivated pertussis toxin, and filamentous hemagglutinin, is no longer available as of early 2012.

[b] A DTaP vaccine similar to Daptacel is also available in combination with Hib and IPV (Pentacel; Sanofi Pasteur); in this case, ActHIB is reconstituted with liquid DTaP-IPV that is packaged with the product. Pentacel is usually given at 2, 4, 6, and 15 to 18 months of age.

[c] Infanrix is available in combination with HepB and IPV (Pediarix; GlaxoSmithKline). Pediarix is usually given at 2, 4, and 6 months of age. Infanrix is also available in combination with IPV (Kinrix; GlaxoSmithKline). Kinrix is indicated for the booster dose at 4 to 6 years of age.

[d] Not present as a preservative.

still immunogenic, as well as other physically purified bacterial subunits, such as PRN, FHA, and FIM, some of which are also chemically modified.

TIG is used for postexposure prophylaxis. One product available in the United States is *HyperTET S/D* (Talecris). It consists of IgG derived from pooled plasma of human donors who have been immunized with tetanus toxoid; TIG is therefore polyclonal (contains a variety of antibodies, including antibodies to other organisms). Procedures used to purify the immune globulin and reduce the potential for transmission of blood-borne pathogens include cold ethanol fractionation, solvent-detergent treatment, and filtration. The product is formulated for IM administration.

Efficacy and/or Immunogenicity

Essentially 100% of persons who receive a series of any of the available diphtheria or tetanus toxoid-containing vaccines achieve protective antibody levels. The acellular pertussis vaccines have not been compared directly in head-to-head clinical trials, but efficacy estimates overlap enough so as to consider the products equivalent in terms of protection. 11

Infanrix was tested in an Italian trial sponsored by the NIH that enrolled 15,601 infants, 4481 of whom received 3 doses. Efficacy against typical pertussis (≥21 days of cough plus culture or serologic confirmation) was 84%, and efficacy against milder disease, defined as >7 days of cough, was 71%. Protection against typical pertussis was sustained to 6 years of age. In a German household contact study involving 22,000 children, Infanrix was 89% effective against typical pertussis and 81% effective against disease with ≥7 days of paroxysmal cough. Daptacel was tested in a Swedish trial involving 9829 infants, 2587 of whom received 3 doses. Efficacy against typical pertussis was 85%, and efficacy against milder disease, defined as ≥1 day of cough, was 78%. Protection was sustained during the 2-year follow-up period.

Both Tdap vaccines were licensed on the basis of immunogenicity rather than efficacy. In each case, the antibody response to pertussis antigens after a single dose was noninferior to the analogous infant DTaP vaccine, for which efficacy had been previously demonstrated. In a randomized, double-blind trial among adolescents and adults, 1391 subjects received an acellular pertussis vaccine containing the same antigens as Boostrix and 1390 received HepA as a control.[9] Efficacy against pertussis was 92%, although there was no difference in the incidence of prolonged cough illness.

TABLE 11.2 — Diphtheria and Tetanus Vaccines[a]

Trade name	Tenivac	Diphtheria and Tetanus Toxoids Adsorbed USP (for Pediatric Use)	Tetanus and Diphtheria Toxoids Adsorbed	Tetanus Toxoid Adsorbed
Abbreviation	Td	DT	Td	TT
Manufacturer/distributor	Sanofi Pasteur	Sanofi Pasteur	MassBiologics[b]/Merck	Sanofi Pasteur
Type of vaccine	Inactivated, toxoids	Inactivated, toxoids	Inactivated, toxoids	Inactivated, toxoids
Composition:				
Diphtheria toxoid	2 Lf units	6.7 Lf units	2 Lf units	—
Tetanus toxoid	5 Lf units	5 Lf units	2 Lf units	5 Lf units
Adjuvant	Aluminum phosphate (0.33 mg aluminum)	Aluminum potassium sulfate (≤0.17 mg aluminum)	Aluminum phosphate (≤0.53 mg aluminum)	Aluminum potassium sulfate (≤0.25 mg aluminum)
Preservative	None	None	None	Multidose vial: thimerosal (25 mcg mercury)
Excipients and contaminants:				
Formaldehyde	≤5 mcg	≤0.02%	≤100 mcg	≤0.02%
Sodium chloride	Amount not specified	Isotonic	—	0.85%
Thimerosal	None	≤0.3 mcg mercury[c]	≤0.3 mcg mercury[c]	Preservative-free formulation: ≤0.3 mcg mercury[c]

Latex	Tip cap of prefilled syringe contains latex	Vial stopper contains latex	None	Multidose vial: vial stopper contains latex
Labeled indications	Prevention of diphtheria and tetanus	Prevention of diphtheria and tetanus	Prevention of diphtheria and tetanus	Prevention of tetanus
Labeled ages	≥7 years	6 weeks to 6 years	≥7 years	≥7 years
Dose	0.5 mL	0.5 mL	0.5 mL	0.5 mL
Route of administration	Intramuscular	Intramuscular	Intramuscular	Intramuscular
Labeled schedule	2 doses 2 months apart; Dose 3 6 to 8 months after Dose 2; booster dose	3 doses 4 to 8 weeks apart; reinforcing dose 6 to 12 months after Dose 3; booster dose	2 doses 4 to 8 weeks apart; Dose 3 6 to 12 months after Dose 2; booster dose	2 doses 4 to 8 weeks apart; Dose 3 6 to 12 months after Dose 2; booster dose
Recommended schedule	Same	Same	Same	Same
How supplied (number in package)	1-dose vial (10) Prefilled syringe (10)	1-dose vial (10)	1-dose vial (10)	1-dose vial (10) 10-dose vial (1)
Cost per dose ($US, 2011):				
Public	16.50	—	15.00	—
Private	21.15	29.81	17.99	30.23
Reference package insert	December 2010	December 2005	February 2011	December 2005

[a] Decavac (Sanofi Pasteur), which contains diphtheria and tetanus toxoids, is no longer available as of early 2012.
[b] Formerly Massachusetts Public Health Biologic Laboratories.
[c] Not present as a preservative.

Safety

Local pain, swelling, and erythema are common after DTaP administration, reported in up to 40% of vaccinees during the primary series. The rate of local reactions is higher with Dose 4 and Dose 5, and swelling of the entire limb, sometimes accompanied by fever, has been reported. Such reactions are self-limited, resolve without sequelae, and are not contraindications to further doses.[24] Clinically significant fever is reported in <5% of DTaP recipients. Tdap appears to be slightly more painful than Td, with local pain and/or tenderness in up to 75% of vaccinees (60% to 70% for Td); swelling and erythema occur in around 20% of recipients of either Tdap or Td. Fever occurs in <5%. In a large Vaccine Safety Datalink study, the risk of medically attended local reactions was 2.6 per 10,000 vaccinations.[25] A postmarketing study of Boostrix involving 13,427 adolescents showed no increases in medically attended neurologic, allergic, or hematologic events, and no increased risk of new onset chronic illness.[26]

- DTaP

  Contraindications

  - Allergic reaction to previous dose of vaccine or any vaccine component (risk of recurrent allergic reaction)
  - Encephalopathy within 7 days of receiving a pertussis-containing vaccine (risk of recurrent encephalopathy [causality not established] and difficulty distinguishing illness from vaccine reaction)

  Precautions

  - Moderate or severe acute illness (difficulty distinguishing illness from vaccine reaction)
  - Progressive neurologic disorder, including infantile spasms, uncontrolled epilepsy, and progressive encephalopathy (risk of neurologic deterioration [causality not established] and difficulty distinguishing illness from vaccine reaction)
  - Any of these conditions after receiving a DTaP vaccine:
    - Otherwise unexplained fever ≥105°F (40.5°C) within 48 hours (risk of recurrent fever)
    - Collapse or shock-like state (hypotonic hyporesponsive episode) within 48 hours (risk of recurrent reaction)
    - Persistent, inconsolable crying lasting ≥3 hours within 48 hours (risk of recurrent reaction)
    - Seizure with or without fever occurring within 3 days (risk of recurrent seizure)
  - Personal history of GBS within 6 weeks of receiving a tetanus toxoid-containing vaccine (risk of recurrent GBS; family history not relevant)
  - Severe local (Arthus-type) reaction to previous dose of tetanus and/or diphtheria toxoid-containing vaccine (this

includes MCV4-D) in the last 10 years (risk of recurrent reaction)

- Tdap

  Contraindications

  – Allergic reaction to previous dose of vaccine or any vaccine component (risk of recurrent allergic reaction)

  – Encephalopathy within 7 days of receiving a pertussis-containing vaccine (risk of recurrent encephalopathy [causality not established] and difficulty distinguishing illness from vaccine reaction)

  Precautions

  – Moderate or severe acute illness (difficulty distinguishing illness from vaccine reaction)

  – Progressive or unstable neurologic disorder, uncontrolled seizures, or progressive encephalopathy (risk of neurologic deterioration [causality not established] and difficulty distinguishing illness from vaccine reaction)

  – Personal history of GBS within 6 weeks of receiving a tetanus toxoid-containing vaccine (risk of recurrent GBS; family history not relevant)

  – Severe local (Arthus-type) reaction to previous dose of tetanus and/or diphtheria toxoid-containing vaccine (this includes MCV4-D) in the last 10 years (risk of recurrent reaction)

- DT, Td, TT

  Contraindications

  – Allergic reaction to previous dose of vaccine or any vaccine component (risk of recurrent allergic reaction)

  Precautions

  – Moderate or severe acute illness (difficulty distinguishing illness from vaccine reaction)

  – GBS within 6 weeks of receiving a tetanus toxoid-containing vaccine (risk of recurrent GBS; family history not relevant)

  – Severe local (Arthus-type) reaction to previous dose of tetanus and/or diphtheria toxoid-containing vaccine (this includes MCV4-D) in the last 10 years (risk of recurrent reaction)

Patients with selective IgA deficiency may be at increased risk for anaphylactic reactions to TIG because it may contain minute amounts of IgA.

Recommendations

All persons should be vaccinated against diphtheria, tetanus, and pertussis, and immunity should be maintained through booster immunization. The primary series of DTaP consists of doses at

2, 4, 6, and 15 to 18 months of age; Dose 4 may be given at 12 to 14 months of age if ≥6 months have elapsed since Dose 3 and the child is unlikely to return at 15 to 18 months of age. A booster dose of DTaP is given at 4 to 6 years of age (this is optional if Dose 4 was given at ≥4 years of age), and while there is a preference to use the same brand of DTaP for all 5 doses, any brand may be used if this is not feasible. An additional booster in the form of Tdap is given at 11 to 12 years of age. If contraindications to pertussis immunization exist, DT may be used for children and Td may be used for adolescents. However, if pertussis vaccination is deferred during the first year of life because of the possibility of an evolving neurologic condition, DT should not be given because the risk of diphtheria or tetanus is very low. By 1 year of age, if the neurologic condition is deemed to be nonprogressive, the DTaP series may be initiated; if the condition *is* progressive, the series should be given as DT.

Children who have had well-documented pertussis (ie, laboratory confirmed, or typical symptoms and epidemiological link to a confirmed case) do not need further pertussis immunization until they reach adolescence and become eligible for the booster dose of Tdap. Patients who have had diphtheria or tetanus should still be immunized because natural infection does not confer immunity (the amount of toxin is too small to induce effective immune responses).

All persons ≥11 years of age who have never had a dose of Tdap should have one (final approval of the recommendation to routinely immunize adults ≥65 years of age was pending as of February 2012; use of Adacel in persons ≥65 years of age is off-label). As a matter of routine, a dose of Tdap should replace the next scheduled 10-year Td booster for adults. If not given at 11 to 12 years of age, Tdap should be given at the next available opportunity. The manufacturers recommend a minimum interval of 5 years between the last dose of a tetanus toxoid-containing vaccine and a dose of Tdap, but the ACIP states that Tdap may be given regardless of when the last tetanus toxoid-containing vaccine was received. Tdap may be given at the same time as MCV4 and HPV (the AAP recommends a minimum interval of 1 month between MCV4-D and Tdap if they are not given on the same day; the ACIP does not recommend a minimum interval).

For unimmunized adolescents and adults, Tdap should be given followed by 2 doses of Td at least 4 weeks apart. Tdap should be given to children 7 to 10 years of age who are not fully immunized against pertussis (5 doses of DTaP or 4 doses if the last dose was given at ≥4 years of age); this recommendation is off-label except for use of Boostrix in children 10 years of age. Tdap should be used in place of Td for wound management for all persons ≥11 years of age if they have not previously had a dose *(see above note regarding routine use of Tdap for all adults ≥65 years of age).*

Pregnant women beyond 20 weeks' gestation should receive a dose of Tdap if they have not had one before. Tdap should also be used for wound management in pregnant women who have never received a dose, regardless of trimester. Postpartum women who have never received Tdap should receive a dose before discharge from the hospital. In these situations, the dose of Tdap "resets the clock" for the next decennial dose of tetanus and diphtheria toxoid vaccines. Pregnant women who need primary immunization against tetanus should receive 3 doses of a tetanus and diphtheria toxoid-containing vaccine on a schedule of 0, 4 weeks, and 6 to 12 months; the first of those doses beyond 20 weeks' gestation should be Tdap.

The use of tetanus toxoid-containing vaccines and TIG for wound management is summarized in **Table 11.3**.

TABLE 11.3 — Tetanus Prophylaxis in Wound Management

			Clean, Minor Wounds		Tetanus-Prone Wounds[a]	
Tetanus Toxoid Vaccine	**Age (Years)**	**Last Dose**	**Tetanus Vaccine**	**TIG[b]**	**Tetanus Vaccine**	**TIG[b]**
Complete[c]	≤6[d]	<5 years	None	No	None	No
		≥5 years	DTaP[e,f]	No	DTaP[f]	No
	7 to 10	<5 years	None[g]	No	None[g]	No
		≥5 years	None[g]	No	Tdap or Td[h]	No
	≥11	<5 years	None[g]	No	None[g]	No
		≥5 years	None[g]	No	Tdap or Td[g]	No
Unimmunized, unknown, or incomplete	≤6[d]	Not relevant	DTaP[e,f]	No	DTaP[f]	Yes
	7 to 10		Tdap or Td[h]	No	Tdap or Td[h]	Yes
	≥11		Tdap or Td[g]	No	Tdap or Td[g]	Yes

[a] Includes puncture, avulsion, crush, necrotic, and burn wounds; frostbite; and wounds contaminated with dirt, feces, soil, or saliva. Wounds should be cleaned, necrotic tissue debrided, and foreign material removed.

[b] The dose of TIG is 250 units given intramuscularly. Immune globulin intravenous can be used if TIG is not available. Equine tetanus antitoxin is not available in the United States. Vaccine and TIG should be given at separate sites.

[c] The primary series is considered complete if the patient has received ≥3 doses of an adsorbed (not fluid) tetanus toxoid. HIV-infected persons should be considered *unimmunized* even if they have received the vaccine series; therefore, they should be vaccinated and receive TIG for tetanus-prone wounds, regardless of immunization history.

[d] For infants <6 months of age who have not received the 3-dose primary series, decisions about the use of TIG should be based on the mother's vaccination history. For example, a 4-month-old infant with a tetanus-prone wound whose mother has had a complete primary series, plus a booster dose in the last year, does not need TIG (although he may be eligible for his routine DTaP).

[e] A booster dose of DTaP is routinely indicated for all children at 4 to 6 years of age, so a dose should be given to children who have not received a routine booster, even for clean, minor wounds (vaccination here is for catch-up, not wound management).

[f] Use DT if pertussis immunization is contraindicated.

[g] In situations where tetanus vaccination is not necessary for wound management, Tdap should be given anyway if otherwise indicated. For example, a child 7 to 10 years of age whose pertussis immunization is incomplete should receive Tdap, even if tetanus immunization is not indicated (this recommendation is off-label at 7 to 10 years of age except for use of Boostrix in children 10 years of age). Another example would be any adolescent or adult who has not yet received a dose of Tdap. If a patient $\geq$11 years of age qualifies for tetanus vaccination for wound management and Tdap has never been given, it should be used instead of Td; if Tdap has previously been given, or if pertussis immunization is contraindicated, Td should be used (TT may be used if Td is not available). Tdap may be used in persons $\geq$65 years of age if no previous doses have been received (off-label recommendation for Adacel).

[h] Tdap should be used at 7 to 10 years of age if pertussis immunization is incomplete (this recommendation is off-label except for use of Boostrix in children 10 years of age). Otherwise, Td is preferred but TT can be used; only adsorbed products are indicated.

REFERENCES

1. Vitek CR. *Curr Top Microbiol Immunol*. 2006;304:71-94.
2. Ataro P, et al. *South Med J*. 2011;104:613-617.
3. Cherry JD. *J Infect Dis*. 1996;174:S259-S263.
4. Broder KR, et al. *MMWR*. 2006;55(RR-3):1-34.
5. Mink CM, et al. *Clin Infect Dis*. 1992;14:464-471.
6. Wendelboe AM, et al. *Pediatr Infect Dis J*. 2007;26:293-299.
7. Jajosky RA, et al. *MMWR*. 2006;53:1-79.
8. Hall-Baker PA, et al. *MMWR*. 2009;56:1-94.
9. Ward JI, et al. *N Engl J Med*. 2005;353:1555-1563.
10. Ward JI, et al. *Clin Infect Dis*. 2006;43:151-157.
11. Tanaka M, et al. *JAMA*. 2003;290:2968-2975.
12. Cortese MM, et al. *Pediatrics*. 2008;121:484-492.
13. Pertussis report—January 6, 2012. California Department of Public Health Web site. http://www.cdph.ca.gov/programs/immunize/Documents/PertussisReport1-6-2012.pdf. Accessed February 12, 2012.
14. Vitek CR, et al. *Emerg Infect Dis*. 1998;4:539-550.
15. CDC. *MMWR*. 1997;46(RR-7):1-25.
16. Witt MA, et al. Marked acellular pertussis vaccine failure in 8-14 year olds in a North American outbreak (abstract B-1679a). 51st Interscience Conference on Antimicrobial Agents and Chemotherapy; Chicago, IL: September 20, 2011.
17. Greenberg DP, et al. *Pediatr Infect Dis J*. 2009;28:521-528.
18. Kretsinger K, et al. *MMWR*. 2006;55(RR-17):1-37.
19. Murphy TV, et al. *MMWR*. 2008;57(RR-4):1-51.
20. Castagnini LA, et al. *Clin Infect Dis*. 2012;54:78-84.
21. CDC. *MMWR*. 2011;60:1424-1426.
22. CDC. *MMWR*. 2011;60:13-15.
23. Shefer A, et al. *MMWR*. 2011;60(RR-7):1-45.
24. Rennels MB, et al. *Pediatr Infect Dis J*. 2008;27:464-465.
25. Jackson LA, et al. *Vaccine*. 2009;27:4912-4916.
26. Klein NP, et al. *Pediatr Infect Dis J*. 2010;29:613-617.

12 *Haemophilus influenzae* Type b

The Pathogen

H influenzae type b is an aerobic gram-negative bacterium that appears as pleomorphic coccobacilli on Gram stain. The organism produces a polysaccharide capsule (polyribosylribitol phosphate [PRP]) that contributes to virulence by inhibiting complement-mediated lysis and phagocytosis by neutrophils (antibodies to PRP are protective). Colonization of the nasopharynx is facilitated by factors that mediate adherence to respiratory epithelium and interfere with ciliary clearance, as well as immune evasion mechanisms such as IgA1 protease. Disease results from bacteremia and spread to distant sites like the meninges.

Clinical Features

The most common forms of invasive *H influenzae* type b disease are *meningitis*, *bacteremia*, *epiglottitis*, *pneumonia*, *arthritis*, *periorbital cellulitis*, and *buccal cellulitis*. Meningitis is the most common clinical manifestation, accounting for 50% to 65% of cases in the prevaccine era. Hallmark presenting features include fever, altered mental status, and stiff neck. The mortality rate is 2% to 5%, even with appropriate antimicrobial therapy, and neurologic sequelae occur in 15% to 30% of survivors. Osteomyelitis and pericarditis are less common. Infection with nontypeable (nonencapsulated) strains of *H influenzae*, commonly associated with otitis media and acute bronchitis, is not preventable by currently available vaccines.

Epidemiology and Transmission

Humans are the only natural hosts and transmission occurs by direct person-to-person contact or via respiratory droplets. The organism does not survive on fomites. Asymptomatic nasopharyngeal colonization was seen in 2% to 5% of children in the prevaccine era, but widespread use of *H influenzae* type b conjugate vaccine (Hib) has resulted in much lower colonization rates. Invasive disease now is rare. *H influenzae* type b disease was more frequent in boys, African-Americans, Alaska Eskimos, Apache and Navajo Indians, child care center attendees, children living in overcrowded conditions, and children who were not breast-fed. Unimmunized children, particularly those <4 years of age who were in prolonged close contact with an infected child, were at high risk. Sickle cell disease, asplenia, HIV infection, certain immunodeficiency syndromes, and malignant neoplasms may predispose to invasive infection.

Immunization Program

Prior to the introduction of routine childhood immunization, *H influenzae* type b was a major cause of invasive bacterial infection in the United States, with an estimated 12,000 cases of meningitis and 8000 other invasive syndromes annually. A striking *one out of every 200 children* in the first 5 years of life developed invasive *H influenzae* type b infection, with peak incidence in infants 6 to 12 months of age. In high-risk populations, disease rates were even higher.

After 1991, when Hib was recommended for all infants,[1] the incidence of invasive disease in infants and young children declined by >99% (**Table 1.5**). This remarkable reduction in disease burden was partly due to the ability of conjugate vaccines to reduce nasopharyngeal carriage, leading to reduced rates of exposure and infection even in those not immunized (this is an example of herd immunity; see *Chapter 1: Introduction to Vaccinology—Herd Immunity*). The standing recommendations for Hib were published in 1993[2]; the only recent changes have been updates on available products[3] and use of the vaccine for high-risk persons >5 years of age. Today, invasive *H influenzae* type b disease is seen primarily in underimmunized children and infants too young to have completed the primary series; in 2008, attention focused on a resurgence of cases in infants and children who were intentionally not immunized because of parental concerns about vaccine safety.[4]

Vaccines

Characteristics of the Hib vaccines licensed in the United States are given in **Table 12.1**. Each of these is a protein-polysaccharide conjugate made much the same way as MCV4 and PCV13. Two are available in combination with other antigens.

Efficacy and/or Immunogenicity

Efficacy of Hib-OMP (PedvaxHIB) was first demonstrated in Navajo infants who had very high rates of invasive infection. After a primary regimen given at 2 and 4 months of age, 91% of infants had anti-PRP antibody levels >0.15 mcg/mL (the so-called *short term* correlate of protection) and 60% had levels >1 mcg/mL (the so-called *long-term* correlate of protection). Efficacy at 15 to 18 months of age was 93%. In infants drawn from the general US population who received the 2-dose primary series, 97% achieved anti-PRP antibody levels >0.15 mcg/mL and 80%, >1 mcg/mL; the proportions after a booster at 12 to 15 months were 99% and 95%, respectively. Hib-OMP is the only vaccine that induces significant antibody levels after a single injection in infants <6 months of age.

Licensure of ActHIB (Hib-T) was based on immunogenicity that was comparable to that of the other licensed products. Overall, about 90% of infants achieve anti-PRP antibody levels of ≥1 mcg/mL after the primary series of 3 doses, and 98% achieve this level after a booster dose.

Hiberix (Hib-T) has been used outside the United States for both primary series and booster dose since 1996. Immunogenicity studies conducted in Germany and Canada involving slightly over 200 subjects led to licensure for the booster dose in the United States in 2009. In these studies, the proportion of subjects with anti-PRP antibody levels ≥0.15 mcg/mL went from 71.4%-77.8% to 100% 1 month after a booster dose, and the proportion with anti-PRP antibody levels ≥1.0 mcg/mL went from 12.7%-35.7% to 97.6%-100%.

Children ≥15 months of age respond well to a single dose of any of the vaccines.

Safety

Local reactions such as redness, swelling, and pain occur in 5% to 30% of recipients, but typically are mild and last <24 hours. Systemic reactions, such as high fever and irritability, are infrequent. Serious adverse events such as anaphylaxis are rare.

- *Contraindications*
  - Severe allergic reaction (eg, anaphylaxis) to previous dose of vaccine or any vaccine component (risk of recurrent allergic reaction)
  - Age <6 weeks (risk of induction of immune tolerance)
- *Precautions*
  - Moderate or severe acute illness (difficulty distinguishing illness from vaccine reaction)

Recommendations

All infants should be vaccinated against *H influenzae*. The primary series for Hib-T consists of doses at 2, 4, and 6 months of age; the primary series for Hib-OMP consists of doses at 2 and 4 months of age. For both of these vaccines, booster doses are given at 12 to 15 months of age. Hiberix may be used for the booster dose at 12 to 15 months of age (off-label recommendation). Previously unimmunized children 15 to 59 months should receive

TABLE 12.1 — *H influenzae* Type b Vaccines[a]

Trade name	ActHIB[b,c]	PedvaxHIB[b,d]	Hiberix[b]
Abbreviation	Hib-T	Hib-OMP	Hib-T
Manufacturer/distributor	Sanofi Pasteur	Merck	GlaxoSmithKline
Type of vaccine	Inactivated, engineered subunit	Inactivated, engineered subunit	Inactivated, engineered subunit
Composition	Polyribosylribitol phosphate (10 mcg) conjugated to tetanus toxoid (24 mcg)	Polyribosylribitol phosphate (7.5 mcg) conjugated to *N meningitidis* serogroup B (strain B11) outer membrane protein (125 mcg)	Polyribosylribitol phosphate (10 mcg) conjugated to tetanus toxoid (25 mcg)
Adjuvant	None	Aluminum hydroxide (0.225 mg aluminum)	None
Preservative	None	None	None
Excipients and contaminants	Sucrose (8.5%)	Sodium chloride (0.9%)	Lactose (12.6 mg) Residual formaldehyde (≤0.5 mcg)
Latex	Diluent vial stopper contains latex	Vial stopper contains latex	Tip cap of prefilled syringe contains latex
Labeled indications	Prevention of invasive *H influenzae* type b disease	Prevention of invasive *H influenzae* type b disease	Booster immunization against invasive *H influenzae* type b disease
Labeled ages	2 to 18 months	2 to 71 months	15 months to 4 years

Dose	0.5 mL	0.5 mL	0.5 mL
Route of administration	Intramuscular	Intramuscular	Intramuscular
Labeled schedule	2, 4, 6, 12 to 15 months of age	2, 4, 12 to 15 months of age[e]	15 months of age
Recommended schedule	Same	Same	12 to 15 months of age
How supplied (number in package)	1-dose vial (5), lyophilized, with diluent	1-dose vial (10)	1-dose vial (10), lyophilized, with diluent in prefilled syringes
Cost per dose ($US, 2011):			
Public	9.00	11.64	8.98
Private	24.29	22.77	22.83
Reference package insert	November 2009	December 2010	December 2010

[a] ProHIBit (Hib-D; Connaught), HibTITER (Hib-CRM; Pfizer [formerly Wyeth]), and TriHIBit (Hib-T/DTaP; Sanofi Pasteur) are no longer available.

[b] Hib-T and Hib-OMP are considered interchangeable in the primary series. However, if either the 2-month or 4-month dose is given as Hib-T, a dose of either product must be given at 6 months. If the first 2 doses are Hib-OMP, the 6-month dose is omitted. Hib-OMP and Hib-T are considered interchangeable for the booster dose.

[c] ActHIB is also available in combination with DTaP and IPV (Pentacel; Sanofi Pasteur); in this case, ActHIB is reconstituted with liquid DTaP-IPV that is packaged with the product. Pentacel is usually given at 2, 4, 6, and 15 to 18 months of age.

[d] Hib-OMP is also available in combination with HepB (Comvax; Merck). Comvax is usually given at 2, 4, and 12 to 15 months of age.

[e] The primary series for Hib-OMP consists of only 2 doses.

12

a single dose of ActHIB or PedvaxHIB (Hiberix should not be given as the only Hib dose in a child with no prior Hib doses). Previously unvaccinated persons with functional or anatomic asplenia (including sickle cell disease and splenectomy), immune deficiency (especially IgG2 subclass deficiency), immunosuppression from cancer chemotherapy, HIV infection, and hematopoietic stem cell transplantation should receive one dose of Hib (use of Hib in older children and adults may be off-label, depending on the product).

REFERENCES

1. CDC. *MMWR*. 1991;40(RR-1):1-7.
2. CDC. *MMWR*. 1993;42(RR-13):1-15.
3. CDC. *MMWR*. 2009;58:1008-1009.
4. CDC. *MMWR*. 2009;58(3):58-60.

13 Hepatitis A

The Pathogen

Hepatitis A virus (HAV) is a small, nonenveloped, single-stranded RNA virus in the Picornaviridae family. There is only one known serotype. Initial infection occurs in the pharynx and lower gastrointestinal tract, with hematogenous spread to the liver, where the virus replicates in hepatocytes and Kupffer cells (resident macrophages). It is believed that most of the injury to the liver is immune mediated rather than the direct result of viral replication. Virus is excreted in the bile and ultimately shed in the stool. Unlike hepatitis B virus, HAV does not establish chronic infection and does not cause chronic liver disease.

Clinical Features

Ninety percent of children <5 years of age with HAV infection are asymptomatic, whereas 90% of adults experience symptoms such as jaundice. The incubation period ranges from 15 to 50 days. Onset is usually abrupt, with low-grade fever, myalgia, poor appetite, nausea, vomiting, malaise, and fatigue, followed by dark-colored urine, scleral icterus, pale stools, jaundice, and weight loss. Diarrhea is more common in children. Hepatomegaly, right upper quadrant tenderness, and occasionally splenomegaly or rash may be present. Symptoms generally subside within 3 to 4 weeks, although 10% to 15% of patients experience prolonged or relapsing disease for up to 6 months. Fulminant hepatitis is rare. Extrahepatic manifestations include arthralgias, pruritus, cutaneous vasculitis, cryoglobulinemia, hemophagocytic syndrome, and GBS.

Epidemiology and Transmission

Humans are the only natural hosts and transmission occurs by the fecal-oral route. Peak infectivity occurs during the 2-week period before the onset of jaundice, and infants and children can shed the virus for several months. Since infants and young children often have clinically silent infection and exposure to their feces may be unavoidable, they are often the source of infection for adults in households or day care centers. Contaminated water and undercooked food (especially shellfish) are also common sources of transmission—often a food handler somewhere up the line is infected.[1] Transient viremia in a donor occasionally leads to transmission through transfusion of blood products.

Hepatitis A is most prevalent in Southeast Asia, Africa, and Latin America. In countries with high endemicity, the infection is usually acquired in childhood, whereas in developed countries many adults have not yet been exposed. Childhood disease often correlates with overcrowding, poor sanitation, limited access to clean water, and inadequate sewage systems. Prior to the institution of a universal immunization program in the United States, the incidence of *disease* was highest among children 5 to 14 years of age, but the incidence of *infection* was highest in those <4 years of age. Infection was more common among American Indians, Alaska Natives, and Hispanics. Disease rates were substantially higher in the western United States; between 1987 and 1997, half of all cases occurred in 11 states west of the Mississippi. The majority of patients in the United States in 2007 (67.7%) had no known risk factor for hepatitis A.[2] The most important *known* risk factor was international travel (17.5% of cases)[3]; other risk factors were sexual or household contact with a case (7.8%), male homosexual activity (5.9%), food- or water-borne outbreaks (6.5%), employment or attendance at a day care center (3.8%), contact with a day care employee or attendee (4.6%), injection drug use (1.2%), and other known contact with a case (9.0%).

Immunization Program

In the prevaccine era, there were 22,000 to 36,000 annual reported cases of hepatitis A and an estimated 271,000 annual HAV infections in the United States. Up to 22% of patients were hospitalized, and the average work lost for these patients was 33 days. Annual direct and indirect costs were as high as $488 million (1997 dollars).

In 1996, HepA was recommended for high-risk groups and children living in communities with the highest rates of infection.[4] In 1999, universal vaccination of all children ≥2 years of age was recommended in states, counties, and communities whose average annual reported incidence of hepatitis A was ≥20 cases per 100,000 population (at least twice the national average between 1987 and 1997).[5] At that time, the states meeting that criterion were Arizona, Alaska, Oregon, New Mexico, Utah, Washington, Oklahoma, South Dakota, Idaho, Nevada, and California. Routine immunization was also considered for children living in areas where the average annual reported incidence was ≥10 but <20 cases per 100,000 population; those states were Missouri, Texas, Colorado, Arkansas, Montana, and Wyoming. For areas with high rates of disease, routine vaccination of children beginning at 2 years of age, catch-up vaccination of preschool children, and vaccination of older children (10 to 15 years of age) was recommended.

After these recommendations were instituted, hepatitis A declined dramatically in the United States, a demonstration of the remarkable ability of childhood immunization to prevent disease in an entire population (see *Chapter 1: Introduction to Vaccinology—Herd Immunity* and **Figure 1.8**). In fact, HepA is a model for the benefits of herd immunity effects in immunization programs, more than doubling the expected cost savings compared with direct effects alone.[6] By 2007, there were only 2979 symptomatic cases reported, for an incidence of 1.0 per 100,000, the lowest ever recorded (the estimated number of infections was 25,000).[7] As might have been expected, the disease burden decreased overall and shifted from the West to other regions of the country. In 2006, new age indications (down to 12 months) for both available vaccines made it easier to consider incorporation of HepA into the routine childhood schedule, and the final step in the incremental national strategy to control hepatitis A was taken—the recommendation to immunize all young children.[8] This was seen as creating the foundation for eventual elimination of indigenous transmission. By 2009, there were only 1987 cases reported, for an incidence of 0.6 per 100,000; the estimated number of infections was down to 21,000.[9]

Recommendations for control of hepatitis A in correctional facilities were issued in 2003,[10] updates on postexposure prophylaxis and international travel in 2007,[11] and vaccination of contacts of international adoptees in 2009.[12] In 2010, the recommendations for HepA were broadened to include vaccination of anyone who desires protection from the disease.

Vaccines

Characteristics of the hepatitis A vaccines licensed in the United States are given in **Table 13.1**. These are inactivated, whole-virus vaccines, made much the same way as the Salk polio vaccine.

Efficacy and/or Immunogenicity

Nearly 100% of persons who receive 2 doses of either vaccine achieve protective levels of antibody. Seroconversion rates within 1 month of the first dose exceed 95%. Based on kinetic models of antibody decay, protective antibody may persist for up to 20 years in children and ≥25 years in adults.

The efficacy of Havrix was evaluated in a study of 40,119 school children in Thailand aged 1 to 16 years. Two doses of vaccine (360 ELISA units each) or placebo were administered 1 month apart, and efficacy was estimated at 94%. In children 2 to 19 years of age, 1 dose (720 ELISA units) resulted in seroconver-

TABLE 13.1 — Hepatitis A Vaccines

Trade name	Havrix[a,b]	Vaqta[b]
Abbreviation	HepA	HepA
Manufacturer/distributor	GlaxoSmithKline	Merck
Type of vaccine	Inactivated, whole agent	Inactivated, whole agent
Composition:[c]		
Virus strain	HM175	CR326F
Propagation	Human diploid (MRC-5) cells	Human diploid (MRC-5) cells
Inactivation	Formalin	Formalin
Antigen content:		
Pediatric/adolescent formulation	720 ELISA units/0.5 mL	25 U/0.5 mL
Adult formulation	1440 ELISA units/mL	50 U/mL
Adjuvant	Aluminum hydroxide (0.25 mg/0.5 mL aluminum)	Aluminum hydroxyphosphate sulfate (0.225 mg/0.5 mL aluminum)
Preservative	None	None
Excipients and contaminants	Amino acid supplement (0.3%) Phosphate-buffered saline Polysorbate 20 (0.05 mg/mL) Residual MRC-5 cellular proteins (≤5 mcg/mL) Formalin (≤0.1 mg/mL) Neomycin (≤40 ng/mL)	Formaldehyde (≤0.8 mcg/mL) Nonviral protein (<0.1 mcg/mL) DNA (<4 × 10^{-6} mcg/mL) Bovine albumin (≤0.0001 mcg/mL) Sodium borate (70 mcg/mL) Sodium chloride (0.9%) Neomycin (<10 parts per billion)

Latex	Tip cap (and plunger for one presentation) of prefilled syringe contains latex	Vial stopper and tip cap and plunger of prefilled syringe contain latex
Labeled indications	Prevention of hepatitis A	Prevention of hepatitis A
Labeled ages	≥12 months	≥12 months
Dose:[d]		
Pediatric (1 to 18 years)	0.5 mL	0.5 mL
Adult (≥19 years)	1.0 mL	1.0 mL
Route of administration	Intramuscular	Intramuscular
Labeled schedule	0, 6 to 12 months	0, 6 to 18 months
Recommended schedule	12 to 18, 19 to 23 months of age Catch-up, high-risk	12 to 18, 19 to 23 months of age Catch-up, high-risk
How supplied (number in package):		
Pediatric/adolescent formulation	1-dose vial (10) Prefilled syringe (5, 10)	1-dose vial (10) Prefilled syringe (6)
Adult formulation	1-dose vial (10) Prefilled syringe (1, 5, 10)	1-dose vial (1, 10) Prefilled syringe (6)
Cost per dose, pediatric ($US, 2011):		
Public	14.25	14.25
Private	28.74	30.37

Continued

TABLE 13.1 — *Continued*

Trade name	Havrix[a,b]	Vaqta[b]
Abbreviation	HepA	HepA
Cost per dose, adult ($US, 2011):		
Public	20.82	—
Private	63.10	76.71
Reference package insert	July 2011	December 2010

[a] Havrix is also available in combination with HepB (Twinrix; GlaxoSmithKline).
[b] Havrix and Vaqta are considered interchangeable.
[c] The units used to measure antigen content for these vaccines are different and cannot be directly compared.
[d] The patient's age at the time of the dose determines which formulation is used.

sion rates of 96.8% to 100%, and 2 doses given 6 months apart resulted in seroconversion rates of 100%. In adult studies, 1 dose (1440 ELISA units) resulted in seroconversion rates of >96%, and 100% were seropositive 1 month after a booster dose. In children immunized with 2 doses 6 months apart beginning at 11 to 13 months of age, the vaccine response rate was 99%. Persistence of antibody was evaluated in a study of 1016 subjects who had received a 3-dose schedule as adults; 10 years out, 98.3% still had protective levels of antibody.[13]

The efficacy of Vaqta was evaluated in a study of 1037 healthy seronegative children 2 to 16 years of age in Monroe County, New York, a small community with a historically high infection rate.[14] A single dose of vaccine (25 units) or placebo was administered. Beyond the immediate postvaccination period, there were no cases of hepatitis A in the vaccine group and 21 confirmed cases in the placebo group, for an efficacy of 100%. After this study, a subset of vaccinees received a booster dose of vaccine. No cases of hepatitis A occurred among these individuals during 9 years of follow-up.[15] In Butte County, CA, a mass immunization campaign in children 2 to 12 years of age between 1995 and 2000 resulted in a 93.5% decline in cases in the entire county population (**Figure 1.8**).[16]

In studies of children 12 to 23 months of age, seroconversion rates were 96% and 100%, respectively, for 1 or 2 doses of Vaqta (25 units). In studies of children 2 to 18 years of age, seroconversion rates were 97% and 100%, respectively, for 1 or 2 doses (25 units), and in adult studies, seroconversion rates were 95% and 99.9%, respectively, for 1 or 2 doses (50 units).

Safety

Reactions are usually mild and subside within 24 hours. Injection-site reactions, including erythema, swelling, pain, or tenderness, occur in 20% to 50% of patients. Systemic reactions, including low-grade fever, malaise, and fatigue, are reported in <10% of vaccinees. No serious adverse events have been reported.

- *Contraindications*
  - Severe allergic reaction (eg, anaphylaxis) to previous dose of vaccine or any vaccine component (risk of recurrent allergic reaction)
- *Precautions*
  - Moderate or severe acute illness (difficulty distinguishing illness from vaccine reaction)
  - Pregnancy (theoretical risk to the fetus or attribution of birth defects to vaccination). No deleterious effects have been demonstrated from HepA administration during pregnancy, and the risk of adverse fetal effects from an inactivated vaccine is extremely low.

Recommendations

■ Pre-exposure Prophylaxis

All children should be vaccinated against hepatitis A during the second year of life. The first dose of HepA is usually given at 12 to 18 months of age and the second at 19 to 23 months of age. Vaccination for children 2 to 18 years of age should continue in areas that had catch-up programs in place based on the 1999 recommendations; catch-up vaccination for children 2 to 18 years of age in other communities is optional. Anyone who wants protection from hepatitis A should be vaccinated.

The following persons are at increased risk for hepatitis A and should be routinely vaccinated:

- Persons traveling to or working in countries with high or intermediate endemicity (see **Table 6.6** for region-specific recommendations)
- Persons (eg, household members) who will be in close contact with an adoptee from an endemic country during the first 60 days after arrival (Dose 1 should be given at least 2 weeks before arrival)
- Men who have sex with men (the risk is thought to relate to fecal-oral contact)
- Injection and noninjection illegal drugs users (transmission probably occurs through percutaneous and fecal-oral routes)
- Persons who work with HAV-infected primates or with HAV in a research laboratory
- Persons who have clotting-factor disorders (outbreaks presumably due to blood from donors who were viremic at the time of donation were reported in the early 1990s)
- Persons who have chronic liver disease, including those who are waiting for or have received a liver transplant (these persons are particularly susceptible to severe disease)

Vaccination should be considered for juveniles in correctional facilities. For most travelers to endemic areas, vaccination is now preferred over immune globulin (see *Chapter 6: Vaccination in Special Circumstances—Travel*).

Routine vaccination is *not* considered necessary for the following based on occupation alone:

- HCP
- Persons attending or working in child care centers
- Caretakers in institutions for the developmentally challenged
- Persons working in correctional facilities
- Persons working in waste management
- Food service workers, unless recommended by state or local authorities

■ Postexposure Prophylaxis

In the past, prophylaxis with immune globulin was recommended for susceptible persons after exposure to hepatitis A. However, immune globulin is expensive, relatively painful, difficult to obtain, and only offers transient protection. A randomized, double-blind trial published in 2007[17] and experience from other countries suggest that postexposure vaccination also is effective. The recommendations below are for *unimmunized persons* exposed to hepatitis A (persons who received at least 1 dose of vaccine at least 1 month before exposure are considered immune). Prophylaxis should be initiated as soon as possible after exposure, but preferably within 2 weeks (efficacy beyond 2 weeks is questionable). Only monovalent HepA should be used in the following situations:

- *12 months to 40 years of age*: Vaccination is preferred.
- *>40 years of age*: Immune globulin (0.02 mL/kg intramuscularly) is preferred but vaccine can be given if immune globulin is not available. If the person has other reasons to be vaccinated with HepA, he or she should receive a dose of the vaccine simultaneously (at a separate site) and receive the second dose at the appropriate interval.
- *<12 months of age, immunocompromised persons, those with chronic liver disease, and those in whom vaccination is contraindicated*: Immune globulin (0.02 mL/kg intramuscularly) should be given. Immunocompromised persons and those with chronic liver disease should receive a dose of the vaccine simultaneously (at a separate site) and receive the second dose at the appropriate interval.

The following situations constitute a high risk of infection and warrant postexposure prophylaxis (if the person was not previously immunized):

- Household and sexual contacts of a case (consider also for persons with ongoing close personal contact such as occurs with regular babysitting)
- Persons who have shared illicit drugs with a case
- Staff members and attendees at day care centers and day care homes if there has been one or more case in employees or attendees, or if two or more cases occur in the households of attendees. If the center does not have children who are in diapers, prophylaxis should be given only to classroom contacts of the index case. If three or more families are affected, prophylaxis should be considered for members of households that have children in diapers who attend the center.
- Other food handlers at an establishment where there is an index case in a food handler. Prophylaxis of patrons should be considered if the index case could have contaminated food because of diarrhea and poor hygienic practices, and only if

the patrons can be identified and treated within 2 weeks of exposure. Institutional cafeterias might represent a higher risk to patrons than other establishments. In a common-source outbreak, prophylaxis should not be given once cases begin to occur, since by then the 2-week window for effective prophylaxis will have been exceeded.

- Prophylaxis is indicated in the school or hospital setting only if transmission from an index case has been demonstrated.

REFERENCES

1. Fiore AE. *Clin Infect Dis*. 2004;38:705-715.
2. Daniels D, et al. *MMWR*. 2009;58(SS-3):1-27.
3. Mutsch M, et al. *Clin Infect Dis*. 2006;42:490-497.
4. CDC. *MMWR*. 1996;45(RR-15):1-30.
5. CDC. *MMWR*. 1999;48(RR-12):1-37.
6. Armstrong GL, et al. *Pediatrics*. 2007;119:e22-e29.
7. Wasley A, et al. *MMWR*. 2008;57(SS-2):1-24.
8. CDC. *MMWR*. 2006;55(RR-7):1-23.
9. Viral hepatitis surveillance—United States, 2009. Centers for Disease Control and Prevention Web site. http://www.cdc.gov/hepatitis/Statistics/2009Surveillance/index.htm. Accessed January 18, 2011.
10. Weinbaum C, et al. *MMWR*. 2003;52(RR-1):1-36.
11. CDC. *MMWR*. 2007;56:1080-1084.
12. CDC. *MMWR*. 2009;58:1006-1007.
13. Rendi-Wagner P, et al. *Vaccine*. 2007;25:927-931.
14. Werzberger A, et al. *N Engl J Med*. 1992;327:453-457.
15. Werzberger A, et al. *Vaccine*. 2002;20:1699-1701.
16. Averhoff F, et al. *JAMA*. 2001;286:2968-2973.
17. Victor JC, et al. *N Engl J Med*. 2007;357:1685-1694.

14 Hepatitis B

The Pathogen

Hepatitis B virus (HBV) is a nonenveloped, partially double-stranded DNA virus in the Hepadnaviridae family. The virus infects hepatocytes but is not directly cytopathic; instead, damage occurs through the action of cytotoxic T-cells directed against virus-infected cells.[1] Immune tolerance leads to persistent infection in some individuals; hallmark features include low-grade chronic hepatitis and HBsAg (a surface protein of the virion that is overproduced) in the serum, as well as an increased lifetime risk of hepatocellular carcinoma. One factor that contributes to carcinogenesis is chronic inflammation, with attendant regeneration, fibrosis, and the accumulation of cellular mutations.[2] Another factor is the random integration of HBV DNA into the host chromosome, resulting in mutations that either inactivate tumor suppressor genes or activate oncogenes. Finally, much attention has focused on the viral X protein, which can upregulate the expression of host cell oncogenes. 14

Clinical Features

The incubation period ranges from 6 weeks to 6 months and averages 120 days.[3] The clinical course of acute infection is indistinguishable from that of other types of viral hepatitis. While infants and children are usually asymptomatic, clinical signs and symptoms occur in about 50% of adults. The prodromal phase usually lasts 3 to 10 days and is characterized by the insidious onset of malaise, anorexia, nausea, vomiting, right upper-quadrant abdominal pain, fever, headache, myalgia, rash, arthralgia, arthritis, and dark urine. The icteric phase, which usually lasts from 1 to 3 weeks, is characterized by jaundice, elevated hepatic transaminases, light or gray-colored stools, liver tenderness, and hepatomegaly (splenomegaly is less common). During convalescence, malaise and fatigue may persist for weeks to months, while jaundice, anorexia, and other symptoms disappear.

Most acute HBV infections in adults result in complete recovery, with disappearance of HBsAg from the blood and the production of HBsAb (antibody directed against HBsAg), which provides for lasting immunity. However, 90% of infants, 30% of young children, and <5% of adults with acute infection become persistently infected (so-called *chronic carriers*). Premature death from cirrhosis, liver failure, or hepatocellular carcinoma occurs in

25% of those who become persistently infected in childhood and in 15% of those who become persistently infected after childhood.

Epidemiology and Transmission

Humans are the only natural hosts and transmission occurs by contact with contaminated secretions, including semen, vaginal secretions, blood, and saliva; through percutaneous inoculation (eg, accidental needlesticks or sharing of needles with infected people); or by maternal-neonatal transmission (the risk is about 10% if the mother is a chronic carrier). Almost half of the world's population lives in areas where ≥8% of the population is persistently infected; in China, southeast Asia, most of Africa, most of the Pacific Islands, parts of the Middle East, and the Amazon basin, 8% to 15% of the population are chronic carriers, with infection commonly having occurred at birth or in early childhood. The lifetime risk of infection in these areas exceeds 60%. An estimated 2 billion people worldwide have been infected with HBV and 350 million are chronic carriers.

In 2009, 60% of patients in the United States with acute hepatitis B reported no known risk factor for infection; 32% reported multiple sex partners, 16% engaging in injection-drug use, 7% having had sex with a case, and 2% having had household contact with a case.[4] Nineteen percent were men who have sex with men.

Immunization Program

While acute hepatitis B can cause significant morbidity and even death, a major rationale for immunization is to prevent chronic carriage. This is because chronic carriers are often asymptomatic, can infect others over long periods of time, and are at increased risk for developing cirrhosis and primary hepatocellular carcinoma. Data from Hawaii[5] and China[6] show that universal childhood immunization, including a birth dose, can dramatically decrease the prevalence of chronic carriage, and data from Taiwan demonstrate that universal HepB immunization can decrease the incidence of hepatocellular carcinoma.[7] This makes HepB the first vaccine proven to prevent a human cancer.

Selective vaccination of high-risk populations in the 1980s failed to impact disease burden.[8] Universal infant vaccination, first recommended in 1991,[9] aimed to prevent perinatal transmission; arguably, transmission cannot occur if the mother is HBsAg-negative, but many pregnant women are not tested and those who test negative early in pregnancy may develop infection close to delivery (it is even possible that the mother's HBsAg status may be inaccurately reported). Recommendations for prevention of hepatitis B in children were updated in 2005[10] and for adults in

2006.[11] Recommendations for immunization of HCP were published in 2001[12] and updated in 2011,[13] and recommendations for control of hepatitis B in correctional facilities were published in 2003.[14] In October 2011, diabetics were added to the list of adults who should routinely be vaccinated, based on an increased risk of transmission from percutaneous blood glucose monitoring and the fact that chronic nonalcoholic liver disease can contribute to increased morbidity.[15]

As a result of the incremental immunization program in the United States, the estimated number of acute hepatitis B cases fell from 59,000 in 1990 to 9000 in 2009.[4] The prevalence of HBV infection among children 6 to 19 years of age fell from 1.9% in 1988-1994 to 0.6% in 1999-2006, and chronic carriage decreased by 79%; among young adults 20 to 49 years of age, the prevalence fell from 5.9% to 4.6%.[16]

The long incubation period allows for postexposure prophylaxis through vaccination. However, even an accelerated vaccination series requires a minimum of 4 months to complete, and the series cannot be completed in neonates until 24 weeks of age. Therefore, passive immunization with hepatitis B immune globulin (HBIG) is a necessary adjunct to active vaccination for immediate protection after exposure.

Vaccines

Characteristics of the hepatitis B vaccines licensed in the United States are given in **Table 14.1**. Both are inactivated subunit vaccines consisting of HBsAg expressed in yeast using recombinant DNA technology.

HBIG is used in conjunction with vaccination for postexposure prophylaxis. Available products in the United States include *Nabi-HB* (Biotest Pharmaceuticals), *HepaGam B* (Cangene), and *HyperHEP B S/D* (Talecris). They consist of IgG derived from pooled plasma of human donors who have high levels of HBsAb; they are therefore polyclonal (contain a variety of antibodies, including antibodies to other organisms). Various procedures are used to purify the immune globulin and reduce the potential for transmission of blood-borne pathogens, including cold ethanol fractionation, anion-exchange chromatography, solvent-detergent treatment, and filtration. The products are formulated for IM administration.

Efficacy and/or Immunogenicity

Engerix-B was found to be 95% effective in preventing perinatal infection when given without immune globulin on a 0-, 1-, and 2-month schedule to newborns of mothers who were chronic

TABLE 14.1 — Hepatitis B Vaccines

Trade name	Engerix-B[a]	Recombivax HB[b]
Abbreviation	HepB	HepB
Manufacturer/distributor	GlaxoSmithKline	Merck
Type of vaccine	Inactivated, engineered subunit	Inactivated, engineered subunit
Composition:	HBsAg	HBsAg
Expression system	Yeast (*S cerevisiae*)	Yeast (*S cerevisiae*)
Antigen content:		
Pediatric/adolescent formulation	10 mcg/0.5 mL	5 mcg/0.5 mL
Adult formulation	20 mcg/mL	10 mcg/mL
Dialysis formulation	—	40 mcg/mL
Adjuvant	Aluminum hydroxide (0.25 mg/0.5 mL aluminum)	Aluminum hydroxide (0.25 mg/0.5 mL aluminum)
Preservative	None	None
Excipients and contaminants	Yeast protein (≤5%) Sodium chloride (9 mg/mL) Disodium phosphate dihydrate (0.98 mg/mL) Sodium dihydrogen phosphate dihydrate (0.71 mg/mL)	Yeast protein (≤1%) Formaldehyde (<15 mcg/mL)
Latex	Tip cap (and plunger for one presentation) of prefilled syringe contains latex	Vial stopper and tip cap and plunger of prefilled syringe contain latex

Labeled indications	Prevention of hepatitis B	Prevention of hepatitis B
Labeled ages	All ages	All ages
Dose:		
Pediatric/adolescent formulation (≤19 years)	0.5 mL[c]	0.5 mL
Adult formulation (≥20 years)	1 mL[c]	1 mL[d]
Hemodialysis formulation	2 simultaneous adult doses of 1 mL each[e,f]	1 mL[f]
Route of administration	Intramuscular[g]	Intramuscular[g]
Labeled schedule:	0, 1, 6 months[h]	0, 1, 6 months[h]
Hemodialysis patients	0, 1, 2, and 6 months; periodic boosters[i]	0, 1, 6 months; periodic boosters[i]
Alternate dosing for 11 to 15 years of age	—	Adult formulation at 1 and 4 to 6 months[d]
Recommended schedule	0, 1 to 2, 6 to 18 months of age Catch-up, high-risk	0, 1 to 2, 6 to 18 months of age Catch-up, high-risk
How supplied (number in package):		
Pediatric/adolescent formulation	1-dose vial (10) Prefilled syringe (5, 10)	1-dose vial (1, 10) Prefilled syringe (6)
Adult formulation	1-dose vial (10) Prefilled syringe (1, 5, 10)	1-dose vial (1, 10) Prefilled syringe (1, 6)
Hemodialysis formulation	—	1-dose vial (1)
Cost per dose, pediatric ($US, 2011):		
Public	10.35	10.50
Private	21.37	23.20

Continued

TABLE 14.1 — *Continued*

Trade name	Engerix-B[a]	Recombivax HB[b]
Abbreviation	HepB	HepB
Cost per dose, adult ($US, 2011):		
Public	27.33	24.04
Private	52.50	58.95
Reference package insert	December 2010	July 2011

[a] Engerix-B is also available in combination with DTaP and IPV (Pediarix; GlaxoSmithKline) and with HepA (Twinrix; GlaxoSmithKline).
[b] Recombivax HB is also available in combination with Hib (Comvax; Merck).
[c] Adolescents 11 to 19 years of age may receive the adult formulation.
[d] An adult dose (10 mcg/mL) may be constituted by 2 separate injections of the pediatric (5 mcg/0.5 mL) formulation at the same site or by combining 2 pediatric doses in the same syringe.
[e] There is no specific hemodialysis formulation. The 40 mcg/2 mL dose can be constituted by 2 separate injections of the adult (20 mcg/mL) formulation at the same site or by combining 2 adult doses in the same syringe.
[f] Hemodialysis patients need higher doses to respond.
[g] May be administered subcutaneously in patients who are at risk of hemorrhage with intramuscular injections (eg, hemophiliacs). However, reactogenicity may be increased and immunogenicity decreased.
[h] Other dosing regimens are contained in the package insert.
[i] Booster doses are given when annual testing shows that HBsAb levels have fallen below 10 mIU/mL. Annual testing with periodic booster doses may be indicated for other immunocompromised persons, such as those with HIV infection, hematopoietic stem-cell transplant recipients, and those receiving chemotherapy.

carriers. Ninety-seven percent of neonates given the vaccine at 0, 1, and 6 months of age achieved a protective level of antibody (≥10 mIU/mL). Seroprotection rates of 98% were seen in children 6 months to 10 years of age and 97% in adolescents after a 3-dose schedule. Studies in adolescents and adults demonstrate seroprotection rates of >95% after 3 doses, although responses are somewhat lower in those >40 years of age.

Recombivax HB was found to be 95% effective in preventing perinatal transmission among high-risk infants who were given concomitant HBIG. Protective levels of antibody were achieved with 3 doses of vaccine in 100% of infants, 99% of children, and 99% of adolescents. Response rates in adults were 98% in those 20 to 29 years of age, 94% in those 30 to 39 years of age, and 89% in those ≥40 years of age. Seroprotection rates in adolescents who received the 2-dose regimen were 99%.

Although antibody levels after receipt of HepB in infancy wane with time, immune memory remains intact at least into adolescence, when it may be needed the most.[17] Protection lasts as well. A study from The Gambia, for example, showed that 50% of persons followed for ≥15 years had antibody levels that fell below 10 mIU/mL. Despite this, efficacy was 83% against infection and 97% against chronic carriage.[18] In a 2010 meta-analysis that looked at 34 cohorts with a total of 9356 vaccinated subjects, the cumulative incidence of breakthrough HBV infection 5 to 20 years after vaccination was <1%.[19]

Safety

The most common adverse reaction following vaccination is pain at the injection site, reported in 13% to 29% of adults and 3% to 9% of children. Mild systemic complaints, such as fatigue, headache, and irritability, have been reported in 11% to 17% of adults and up to 20% of children. Low-grade fever is seen in 1% of adults and in up to 6% of children. It should be noted that well over 1 billion doses of HepB have been given worldwide since the 1980s, and serious systemic adverse events and allergic reactions have rarely been reported. There is no evidence that HepB causes or exacerbates multiple sclerosis (see *Chapter 7: Addressing Concerns About Vaccines—Do Vaccines Cause Multiple Sclerosis [MS]?*)

- *Contraindications*
  - Severe allergic reaction (eg, anaphylaxis) to previous dose of vaccine or any vaccine component (risk of recurrent allergic reaction; this includes reactions to baker's yeast)
- *Precautions*
  - Moderate or severe acute illness (difficulty distinguishing illness from vaccine reaction)

– Infant weight <2000 g, unless the mother is HBsAg-positive (risk of poor response to vaccination)

Patients with selective IgA deficiency may be at increased risk for anaphylactic reactions to HBIG because it may contain minute amounts of IgA.

Recommendations

■ Universal Infant, Child, and Adolescent Immunization

All infants should be vaccinated against hepatitis B. The usual schedule for HepB is a dose at birth (before hospital discharge), 1 to 2 months of age, and 6 to 18 months of age (6 to 12 months of age for high-risk groups such as Alaska Natives, Pacific Islanders, and immigrants from areas like Asia and Africa). Only monovalent vaccine may be used before 6 weeks of age. Infants who receive subsequent doses as DTaP-HepB-IPV or HepB-Hib-OMP may receive an extra dose at 4 months of age; this does not increase reactogenicity or impair the immune response. The birth dose should be implemented by *standing order* and should be deferred only by a physician's order, with a copy of the mother's *recent* negative HBsAg test result on the infant's chart. If the birth dose is deferred, the first dose of HepB should be administered before 2 months of age. The birth dose *should not be deferred* if the mother is HBsAg-positive *(see below)*, had any behavioral risk factors for HBV infection during pregnancy, or if the infant is unlikely to return for follow-up. However, the birth dose *should be deferred* for preterm infants weighing <2000 g whose mothers are HBsAg-negative. These infants should be vaccinated at 1 month of age or at hospital discharge, whichever comes first (babies are assumed to be medically stable and gaining weight consistently if discharged before 1 month of age).

All children and adolescents ≤18 years of age who were not vaccinated as infants should receive the HepB series. Routine postvaccination testing for HBsAb is not recommended. Engerix-B and Recombivax HB are considered interchangeable except for the 2-dose schedule in adolescents, for which only Recombivax HB is approved.

■ Adult Vaccination

Vaccination is recommended for the following:

- Sex partners of persons who are HBsAg-positive
- Persons with more than one sex partner in the past 6 months
- Persons seeking evaluation or treatment for a sexually transmitted disease
- Men who have sex with men
- Injection drug users
- Household contacts of HBsAg-positive persons

- Residents and staff of facilities for developmentally disabled persons
- Health care and public safety workers at risk for infection through exposure to blood or blood-contaminated body fluids, including hospital, institutional, and laboratory employees, students, contractors, physicians, emergency medical technicians, paramedics, and volunteers
- Patients with end-stage renal disease, including those on hemodialysis and peritoneal dialysis (vaccination of patients with renal failure is encouraged before they require hemodialysis)
- Patients with chronic liver disease
- Persons with HIV infection
- Persons 19 to 59 years of age with diabetes (optional for persons ≥60 years of age)
- Travelers to regions where the prevalence of chronic infection is ≥2%
- Inmates undergoing medical evaluation at a correctional facility, as well as staff who may have contact with blood or body fluids
- Anyone who wants protection from hepatitis B

Standing orders for HepB administration should be implemented in settings where high-risk individuals are seen, including sexually transmitted disease and HIV clinics, drug abuse treatment centers, correctional facilities, facilities that care for men who have sex with men, kidney disease programs, and facilities for the developmentally disabled. Prevaccination testing might reduce costs by avoiding vaccination of persons who are already immune, and is recommended for the following groups: persons born in areas where the prevalence of chronic infection is ≥8%; household, sex, and needle-sharing contacts of HBsAg-positive persons; HIV-infected persons; and other populations in whom the prevalence of chronic infection exceeds 20%. The preferred test is for antibody to hepatitis B core antigen, since this identifies all people with previous infection. Testing for HBsAb can be used, but must be done along with testing for HBsAg, since chronic carriers may have negative tests for HBsAb.

Testing for HBsAb 1 to 2 months after vaccination is recommended for the following groups: health care and public safety workers at high risk for exposure to blood or body fluids; chronic hemodialysis patients; HIV-infected and other immunocompromised persons; and sex partners of HBsAg-positive persons. Levels ≥10 mIU/mL are considered protective. Patients with antibody levels <10 mIU/mL should receive a second 3-dose series of HepB, followed by repeat testing. If the result is still <10 mIU/mL, the person should be tested for HBsAg, since chronic carriage is a reason for nonresponse to vaccination. If they are negative for HBsAg, they are considered primary nonresponders; these persons may respond to intradermal vaccination, although neither HepB product is labeled for this route of administration. Periodic (eg, annual) testing for HBsAb after vaccination is only recommended for dialysis patients and other immunocompromised persons, including those with HIV infection, hematopoietic stem-cell transplant recipients, and persons receiving chemotherapy.

The recommendation to test HIV-infected and immunocompromised persons after vaccination makes the most sense if the individual is at high risk of being exposed to hepatitis B. This might be the case for a person who acquired HIV from injecting drug use, for example, but not for an otherwise healthy congenitally infected person who is at low risk of exposure to hepatitis B.

Postexposure Prophylaxis for Infants of HBsAg-Positive and HBsAg-Unknown Mothers

All pregnant women should be tested for HBsAg early in each pregnancy. Women who were not screened prenatally, those who are at high risk for infection, and those with clinical hepatitis should be tested at the time of delivery. A copy of the test results should be provided to the birthing hospital and the newborn's health care provider.

Infants born to mothers who are HBsAg-positive should receive HepB and HBIG (0.5 mL intramuscularly) at separate sites within 12 hours of birth. The vaccine series should be completed with Dose 2 at 1 to 2 months of age and Dose 3 at 6 months of age. For preterm infants weighing <2000 g, both vaccine and HBIG should be given as well, but the vaccine dose should not count toward the complete series (responses are not reliable); the first valid dose is given at 1 month of age, the second at 2 to 3 months, and the third at 6 months. Both term and preterm infants of HBsAg-positive mothers should be tested for HBsAg and HBsAb 1 to 2 months after the last dose in the series. Those with protective levels of antibody and a negative HBsAg test need no further medical management. Those without protective levels of antibody who are HBsAg-negative should receive a second 3-dose vaccine series and should be tested again 1 to 2 months after completion. Those who are HBsAg-positive should receive appropriate medical management.

Infants born to mothers whose HBsAg status is unknown or not documented at the time of delivery should be vaccinated within 12 hours of birth, and the mother should be tested. If she is HBsAg-positive, the baby should receive HBIG before 7 days of age and should complete the HepB series at 6 months of age. If she is HBsAg-negative, the HepB series should be completed by 6 to 18 months of age. If the mother is not tested, the baby should complete the HepB series by 6 months of age, but HBIG should not be given—unless the baby is preterm and weighs <2000 g. In this situation, if the mother's status will not be known within 12 hours of birth, both vaccine and HBIG should be given and the infant should be followed as if born to an HBsAg-positive mother.

■ Postexposure Prophylaxis in Other Settings

Recommendations for the management of potential occupational and nonoccupational exposures to HBV are given in **Tables 14.2** and **14.3**, respectively.

REFERENCES

1. Liaw Y-F, et al. *Lancet*. 2009;373:582-592.
2. Azam F, et al. *Ann Hepatol*. 2008;7:125-129.
3. Ganem D, et al. *N Engl J Med*. 2004;350:1118-1129.
4. Viral hepatitis surveillance—United States, 2009. Centers for Disease Control and Prevention Web site. http://www.cdc.gov/hepatitis/Statistics/2009Surveillance/PDFs/2009HepSurveillanceRpt.pdf. Accessed January 21, 2012.
5. Perz JF, et al. *Pediatrics*. 2006;118:1403-1408.
6. Liang X, et al. *J Infect Dis*. 2009;200:39-47.
7. Chang MH, et al. *N Engl J Med*. 1997;336:1855-1859.
8. Shepard CW, et al. *Pediatr Infect Dis J*. 2005;24:755-760.
9. CDC. *MMWR*. 1991;40(RR-13):1-20.
10. Mast EE, et al. *MMWR*. 2005;54(RR-16):1-31.
11. Mast EE, et al. *MMWR*. 2006;55(RR-16):1-33.
12. CDC. *MMWR*. 2001;50(RR-11):1-52.
13. Shefer A, et al. *MMWR*. 2011;60(RR-7):1-45.
14. Weinbaum C, et al. *MMWR*. 2003;52(RR-1):1-36.
15. Sawyer MH, et al. *MMWR*. 2011;60:1709-1711.
16. Wasley A, et al. *J Infect Dis*. 2010;202:192-201.
17. Boxall EH, et al. *J Infect Dis*. 2004;190:1264-1269.
18. van der Sande MA, et al. *J Infect Dis*. 2006;193:1528-1535.
19. Poorolajal J, et al. *Vaccine*. 2010;28:623-631.

TABLE 14.2 — Management of Potential Occupational Exposures to Hepatitis B[a]

Vaccination Status of Exposed Person	Response to Vaccination[b]	HBsAg Status of Source Individual		
		Positive	**Negative**	**Unknown**[c]
Not vaccinated or incompletely vaccinated (<3 doses)	—	Give HBIG[d] and initiate or complete HepB series[e]	Initiate or complete HepB series[e]	Initiate or complete HepB series[e]
Vaccinated	Responder[f]	No treatment	No treatment	No treatment
	Nonresponder[f]	Patients who *have not* received a second complete 3-dose HepB series: 1 dose of HBIG[d] and initiate second 3-dose HepB series[e]	No treatment	If high-risk, assume HBsAg-positive and treat accordingly[g]
		Patients who *have* received a second complete 3-dose HepB series: 2 doses of HBIG[d] separated by 1 month	No treatment	If high-risk, assume HBsAg-positive and treat accordingly[g]
	Antibody level unknown—test exposed person for HBsAb:			
	Adequate response[f]	No treatment	No treatment	No treatment
	Inadequate response[f]	Give HBIG[d] and a booster dose of HepB[e,h]	No treatment	Give booster dose of HepB[e,i]

[a] Percutaneous exposures include needle sticks, lacerations, and bites. Permucosal exposures include splashes of blood, any fluid containing visible blood, other potentially infectious fluid (including semen; vaginal secretions; CSF; synovial, pleural, peritoneal, pericardial, or amniotic fluids; tracheal secretions; and saliva), or tissue onto any mucosal surface, including the conjunctival, oral, and buccal mucosa.

[b] Testing for HBsAb 1 to 2 months after vaccination is recommended for health care and public safety workers at high risk for exposure to blood or body fluids.

[c] Efforts should be made to test the source individual for HBsAg.

[d] The dose is 0.06 mL/kg given intramuscularly. HBIG should be given as soon as possible after exposure, preferably within 24 hours. Intervals exceeding 7 days are unlikely to be of benefit after percutaneous exposure.

[e] In cases where the source is HBsAg-positive or -unknown, the first dose should be given as soon as possible, preferably within 24 hours. In cases where the source is HBsAg-negative, the HepB series should be initiated or completed because of occupational risk of exposure in the future.

[f] An adequate response is ≥10 mIU/mL of HBsAb 1 to 2 months postvaccination.

[g] HBIG is given in this situation because the exposed person, for whatever reason, did not respond to previous doses of the vaccine, and therefore might remain vulnerable if only vaccine were given (as is recommended for previously unvaccinated persons exposed to an unknown, but presumed high-risk, source—it is assumed they will respond to vaccination).

[h] Test for HBsAb in 4 to 6 months. If the level is inadequate, give 2 more doses to complete a second 3-dose series.

[i] Test for HBsAb in 1 to 2 months. If the level is inadequate, give 2 more doses to complete a second 3-dose series.

Adapted from Centers for Disease Control and Prevention. *Epidemiology and Prevention of Vaccine-Preventable Diseases*. 12th ed. Atkinson W, et al, eds. Washington, DC: Public Health Foundation, 2011.

TABLE 14.3 — Management of Potential Nonoccupational Exposures to Hepatitis B[a]

Status of Exposed Individual	Source HBsAg Status[b]	Management
Not vaccinated or incompletely vaccinated (<3 doses)	Negative	Catch-up vaccination
	Positive	Initiate or complete HepB series[c] Give HBIG[d]
	Unknown	Initiate or complete HepB series[c]
Vaccinated[e]	Negative	No treatment
	Positive	Give a booster dose of HepB[c]
	Unknown	No treatment

[a] Percutaneous exposures include needle sticks (needle sharing), lacerations, and bites. Permucosal exposures include splashes of blood, any fluid containing visible blood, other potentially infectious fluid (including semen; vaginal secretions; CSF; synovial, pleural, peritoneal, pericardial, or amniotic fluids; tracheal secretions; and saliva), or tissue onto any mucosal surface, including the conjunctival, oral, and buccal mucosa.

[b] Efforts should be made to test the source individual for HBsAg. Needles and syringes discarded in public places, presumably by injection drug users, pose a risk of transmission since HBV can survive on environmental surfaces for up to 7 days. However, the risk depends on the prevalence of hepatitis B in the drug-abusing population and the amount of blood in the needle. There is no consensus opinion regarding the use of HBIG in these situations.

[c] The first dose should be given as soon as possible, preferably within 24 hours.

[d] The dose is 0.06 mL/kg given intramuscularly. HBIG should be given as soon as possible after exposure, preferably within 24 hours. Intervals exceeding 7 days after percutaneous exposure and 14 days after sexual exposure are unlikely to be of benefit.

[e] Written documentation of a complete 3-dose series of HepB should be provided.

Adapted from CDC. *MMWR*. 2006;55(RR-16):1-33.

15 Human Papillomavirus

The Pathogen

Human papillomavirus is a small, nonenveloped, double-stranded DNA virus in the Papillomaviridae family that is tropic for epithelial surfaces.[1] The virion capsid is composed of major and minor late proteins, L1 and L2. The oncogenic human papillomavirus types—most notably 16 and 18, but including types 33, 45, 31, 58, 52, as well as others—are a *necessary* but not *sufficient* cause of cervical cancer. In other words, the virus *must* be present for cervical cancer to develop, but the majority of women who acquire the virus do not develop cancer. Approximately 90% of new infections clear within 2 years, and it is only the remaining 10% of persistent infections that can lead to cancer. It is important to note that certain biologic factors put young women at particularly high risk for infection, persistence, and neoplasia. The most important of these involves the *cervical transformation zone*, an area of metaplasia where the columnar epithelium of the endocervix meets the squamous epithelium of the exocervix. In young girls, the squamocolumnar junction is located outside the cervical opening; during puberty, it regresses into the cervical opening. The area traversed during this regression is thin, friable, and vulnerable to damage; the basal cell layer, which is the site of viral replication and persistence, is easily exposed. The *anal transformation zone*, where the columnar epithelium of the rectum meets the squamous epithelium of the anus, is thought to play an important role in the pathogenesis of human papillomavirus-associated anal cancer.[2]

In basal cells, viral DNA replication and early cell differentiation occur together, but expression of the viral proteins E6 and E7 prevents further cell differentiation and causes delayed cell-cycle arrest. This, along with the virus' mechanisms for evading host immune surveillance,[3] results in vertical expansion of the dividing cell population. Integration of viral DNA into the host genome causes overexpression of E6 and E7, leading to further unchecked cell proliferation and the accumulation of germ-line mutations, which ultimately lead to invasive cancer.

Some human papillomavirus types—most notably 6 and 11—cause anogenital warts rather than cancer, although they may cause low-grade cervical dysplasia that eventually regresses.

Clinical Features

Human papillomavirus is one of the few human viruses unequivocally linked to cancer.[1] *Squamous cell carcinoma of the cervix* comprises 75% of cervical cancers in the United States; the remainder are *adenocarcinomas*. Human papillomavirus 16 and 18 cause approximately 70% of squamous cell carcinomas and 80% of adenocarcinomas. Most human papillomavirus infections are asymptomatic and self-limited. In a minority of women, persistent cervical infection leads to progressive dysplasia, referred to as *cervical intraepithelial neoplasia* grades 1 (CIN 1) through 3 (CIN 3). Approximately 60% of CIN 1 cases spontaneously regress and <1% lead to cancer. On the other hand, only 30% to 40% of CIN 2 or 3 lesions regress, and >12% develop into cancer. The Pap test is used to detect dysplasia early so treatment can be initiated. The duration of time from the first intraepithelial lesion to invasive cancer is 15 to 20 years. Human papillomavirus also causes *vaginal and vulvar intraepithelial neoplasia* (VaIN and VIN) that can progress to cancer; up to 50% of vulvar and vaginal cancers are caused by human papillomavirus.

Human papillomavirus also causes *anal intraepithelial neoplasia* (AIN), which can progress to *anal cancer*—in fact, up to 90% of anal cancers are caused by the virus.[4] It is also estimated that human papillomavirus causes 50% of *penile cancers*, 20% of *oropharyngeal cancers*, and may be an important factor in causing other squamous cell carcinomas of the head and neck[5] as well as bladder cancer[6]. For most of these tumors, types 16 and 18 predominate.

Approximately 90% of *anogenital warts* are caused by types 6 and 11. These are typically small, soft, raised flesh-colored growths; some develop into large, cauliflower-like clusters called *condyloma acuminata*. In women, warts can be seen anywhere from the cervix to the vagina, urethra, inguinal region or upper thighs. In males, the most common site is the shaft of the penis, and lesions may occur on the anus in both sexes. Most individuals are asymptomatic, but some experience itching, burning, pain, bleeding, and tenderness. *Recurrent respiratory papillomatosis*, defined by wart-like lesions that develop on the larynx, nasopharynx, oropharynx, trachea and/or esophagus, is also caused by types 6 and 11. This is seen most commonly in infants and children <5 years of age and is acquired from the mother during vaginal delivery. Infants may present with hoarseness, weak cry, stridor, feeding difficulties, and failure to thrive. Airway obstruction can result from enlarged lesions, and multiple surgical laser procedures are often necessary. Malignancy can develop, albeit rarely.

Epidemiology and Transmission

Human papillomavirus is only transmitted among humans. Direct *skin-to-skin* or *skin-to-mucosa* contact is required; generally, this means sexual activity where there is direct contact with the genitalia, anus, and/or mouth. Direct transfer of virus from the hands can occur. Anal infection is common among women with genital neoplasia, even in the absence of a history of anal sex.[7] In addition, one study found anal infection in 11% of men who have sex with women who denied ever having had anal sex with a man.[8] These data suggest the possibilities of transmission through anodigital sexual behavior, vaginal secretions, or autoinoculation. A meta-analysis that included data on approximately 1 million women with normal cervical cytological findings found the overall prevalence of cervical human papillomavirus infection to be nearly 12%.[9]

Not surprisingly, the overall risk of infection correlates directly with sexual activity. Studies in female college students demonstrate that over half acquire human papillomavirus infection within 4 years of their first sexual intercourse,[10] and the prevalence of human papillomavirus infection among women 20 to 24 years of age in the United States approaches 50%.[11] Estimates of the prevalence of infection in men vary widely, but some are as high as 70%,[12] and the dominant risk factors for virus acquisition are the lifetime number of female sexual partners, as well as male anal-sexual partners.[13,14] The prevalence of antibody to the four human papillomavirus types contained in HPV4 is as high as 42% among women 30 to 39 years of age and 18% among men 50 to 59 years of age.[15]

Worldwide there are 530,000 new cases of cervical cancer and 275,000 cervical cancer deaths each year—virtually all of these caused by human papillomavirus.[16] In the United States, an estimated 6.2 million new infections occur every year. The annual disease burden from cervical disease alone includes approximately 11,000 new cancers, 300,000 high-grade cervical dysplasias, 1,250,000 low-grade cervical dysplasias, and 4000 deaths, and genital warts are present in 1% of the sexually active population.[17] The rate of anal cancer in the United States doubled between the 1970s and the 1990s,[18] and the burden of anal disease caused by human papillomavirus is especially high in men who have sex with men and persons infected with HIV.

All told, human papillomavirus is estimated to cause 22,000 cancers each year in the United States, 7000 of which occur in males.[19]

HPV4, which provides protection against cervical cancer caused by types 16 and 18, as well as genital warts caused by types 6 and 11, was licensed in 2006 and recommended for universal use in girls and young women.[17] The major rationale for a universal recommendation was prevention of cervical cancer due to types 16 and 18. Other benefits were anticipated, including prevention of anogenital warts due to types 6 and 11, reductions in the direct and indirect costs associated with cervical cancer screening and follow-up of abnormal Pap tests, fewer cases of recurrent respiratory papillomatosis, and reductions in the incidence of anal, penile, and oral cancers. HPV2, which provides protection against cervical cancer caused by types 16 and 18, was licensed in 2009 for females 10 to 25 years of age (in 2011, the lower age was revised to 9). In the same year, HPV4 was granted an indication for prevention of genital warts in males 9 to 26 years of age. Recommendations incorporating these changes were published in 2010, including use of HPV2 in females and a permissive statement about use of HPV4 in males.[20,21]

In 2010, the indications for HPV4 were revised again to include prevention of AIN grades 1, 2, and 3 caused by types 6, 11, 16 and 18 as well as anal cancer caused by types 16 and 18 in both males and females. This, along with recognition of the true disease burden in males and the likelihood that immunizing males would further reduce the disease burden in women, led to a routine recommendation for males in 2011.[19]

In 2003, the Youth Risk Behavior Survey showed that 62% of high school seniors in the United States were sexually active.[22] Seven percent of high school students had sexual intercourse before 13 years of age, and 14% had ≥4 lifetime partners. Since the benefits of vaccination are best realized before sexual debut, adding HPV to the routine adolescent health care visit at 11 to 12 years of age makes sense. Moreover, protection lasts >5 years, and antibody levels achieved by young adolescents are actually higher than those achieved by older people. For those who plan to abstain from sex and ultimately enter a monogamous relationship, vaccination still makes sense because the sexual history of the eventual partner may not be known and exposure through involuntary sexual contact is always a possibility.

Vaccination does not lead to clearance of persistent human papillomavirus infection nor does it prevent neoplasia in those who are already infected with a particular virus type. However, sexually active persons or those known to be infected with human papillomavirus can still benefit from vaccination due to protection against the types with which they are not infected.

At the beginning of the HPV program, it was estimated that vaccination of an entire cohort of girls at 12 years of age would reduce the lifetime risk of cervical cancer by 20% to 66%. Models that included only direct effects placed the cost per QALY saved at slightly more than $20,000 (2001 dollars)[23]; models that incorporated herd immunity effects yielded estimates as low as $3000 (2005 dollars) per QALY saved.[24] Subsequent estimates have been as high as $43,600 per QALY saved for routine vaccination of all girls at 12 years of age (2006 dollars).[25] Catch-up programs were estimated to be more expensive—from $97,300 per QALY saved for vaccination of all girls through 18 years of age to $152,700 for all females through 26 years of age.

Initial models predicted that inclusion of boys in a universal vaccination program would not be cost-effective, even when transmission dynamics and other human papillomavirus–related conditions in both males and females are considered.[26] However, subsequent studies suggested that male vaccination would be cost effective, at least when female vaccination rates are low and all potential health benefits are included. For example, the incremental cost per QALY gained by adding male vaccination to a female-only program is as low as $23,600 (2008 dollars) when coverage among 12-year-old girls is only 20%; it increases to $184,300 if 75% of girls are vaccinated.[27]

Vaccines

Characteristics of the human papillomavirus vaccines licensed in the United States are given in **Table 15.1**. Both are produced by recombinant DNA techniques, much the same way as HepB. They are composed exclusively of the L1 major capsid protein of the virus, which self-assembles into virus-like particles that do not contain genetic material and are incapable of replicating, causing infection, or inducing disease. HPV2 contains a novel adjuvant (see *Chapter 1: Introduction to Vaccinology—The Germinal Center Reaction*).

Efficacy and/or Immunogenicity

Prelicensure efficacy studies of HPV4 involved >20,000 women between 16 and 26 years of age. These studies necessarily used CIN 2 or 3 and adenocarcinoma in situ as outcomes, since invasive cervical cancer was not a feasible or ethical end point. Two large phase 3 studies were conducted: FUTURE (**F**emales **U**nited **T**o **U**nilaterally **R**educe **E**ndo/Ectocervical Disease) I,[28] which enrolled 5442 women, and FUTURE II,[29] which enrolled 12,167. Licensure was based on pooled efficacy data from these trials as well as from two smaller phase 2 studies. Ninety-four percent of the women were sexually active at enrollment, 73% were human papillomavirus-naïve, and the median follow-up period ranged from 2.3 to 4 years.

TABLE 15.1 — Human Papillomavirus Vaccines

Trade name	Gardasil	Cervarix
Abbreviation	HPV4	HPV2
Manufacturer/distributor	Merck	GlaxoSmithKline
Type of vaccine	Inactivated, engineered subunit	Inactivated, engineered subunit
Composition:	Virus-like particles composed of self-assembled L1 major capsid protein molecules	Virus-like particles composed of self-assembled L1 major capsid protein molecules
Expression system	Yeast (*Saccharomyces cerevisiae*)	Insect (*Trichoplusia ni*) cells using a Baculovirus vector
Antigen content:		
Type 6 L1 protein	20 mcg	—
Type 11 L1 protein	40 mcg	—
Type 16 L1 protein	40 mcg	20 mcg
Type 18 L1 protein	20 mcg	20 mcg
Adjuvant	Aluminum hydrophosphate sulfate (0.225 mg aluminum)	AS04 (3-*O*-desacyl-4'-monophosphoryl lipid A (a derivative of bacterial lipopolysaccharide, 50 mcg) adsorbed to aluminum hydroxide (0.5 mg)
Preservative	None	None
Excipients and contaminants	Sodium chloride (9.56 mg) L-histidine (0.78 mg) Polysorbate 80 (50 mcg) Sodium borate (35 mcg) Yeast protein (<7 mcg)	Sodium chloride (4.4 mg) Sodium dihydrogen phosphate dihydrate (0.624 mg) Residual insect cell and viral protein (<40 ng) Residual bacterial cell protein (<150 ng)

Latex	None	Tip cap (and plunger for one presentation) of prefilled syringe contains latex
Labeled indications:		
Prevention of diseases caused by types 16 and 18 (females)	Cervical cancer Vulvar cancer Vaginal cancer	Cervical cancer Cervical intraepithelial neoplasia grades 1, 2, and 3 Adenocarcinoma in situ
Prevention of diseases caused by types 6, 11, 16, and 18 (females)	Cervical intraepithelial neoplasia grades 1, 2, and 3 Cervical adenocarcinoma in situ Vulvar intraepithelial neoplasia grades 2 and 3 Vaginal intraepithelial neoplasia grades 2 and 3	—
Prevention of anal cancer caused by types 16 and 18	Males and females	—
Prevention of anal intraepithelial neoplasia grades 1, 2, and 3 caused by types 6, 11, 16 and 18	Males and females	—
Prevention of genital warts caused by types 6 and 11	Males and females	—
Labeled ages	9 to 26 years (females and males)	9 to 25 years (females)

Continued

TABLE 15.1 — *Continued*

Trade name	Gardasil	Cervarix
Abbreviation	HPV4	HPV2
Dose	0.5 mL	0.5 mL
Route of administration	Intramuscular	Intramuscular
Labeled schedule	0, 2, 6 months	0, 1, 6 months
Recommended schedule[a]	11 to 12 years of age Catch-up, high-risk 0, 1 to 2, 6 months	11 to 12 years of age Catch-up, high-risk 0, 1 to 2, 6 months
How supplied (number in package)	1-dose vial (1, 10) Prefilled syringe (6)	1-dose vial (10) Prefilled syringe (1, 5, 10)
Cost per dose ($US, 2011):		
Public	108.72	96.08
Private	130.27	128.75
Reference package insert	April 2011	July 2011

[a] The series should be completed with the same product, but vaccination should not be deferred if the same product is unknown or not available.

The primary efficacy analyses included women who received all 3 doses of vaccine, had no major protocol deviations, and remained human papillomavirus-negative through 1 month after Dose 3 (so-called *per-protocol* analyses). Efficacy against types 16- or 18-related CIN 2 or 3 or adenocarcinoma in situ (AIS) was 98%. Efficacy was 100% against types 16- or 18-related VIN 2 or 3 and VaIN 2 or 3. Efficacy against any grade of CIN or AIS caused by any of the 4 types was 96% and efficacy against genital warts was 99%. Among women who were already infected with one of the human papillomavirus types in the vaccine, efficacy against the remaining types was excellent.

Additional analyses were performed to estimate the impact that a vaccine program would have in practice, where not all women will complete the full series of shots, some will already be infected with one or more human papillomavirus type at the time they start vaccination, and some will become infected right after the first shot. Among women who received at least 1 vaccine dose (a so-called *intention-to-treat* population) and were human papillomavirus-naïve at baseline, efficacy against CIN 2 or 3 or AIS caused by any human papillomavirus type was 43% and against CIN of any grade or AIS was 30%; considering all women regardless of baseline status, the respective efficacies were 18% and 19%. The majority of cases in these analyses occurred

in women who were infected at the time of first vaccination and thus represent *prevalent*, not *incident*, disease.

Cross-protection is a component of the overall impact of HPV4 on disease rates. In an intention-to-treat analysis of human papillomavirus-naïve women, HPV4 demonstrated 25% efficacy against infection with types 31, 33, 45, 52, or 58 (considered as a group) and 29% against CIN of any grade or AIS caused by those types.[30] Among all women regardless of baseline status, the respective efficacies were 18% and 19%.[31] Efficacy against infection with type 31 among human papillomavirus-naïve women was 46%.

Nearly 100% of vaccinated persons develop antibodies to all four types after 3 doses of HPV4, and antibody levels are higher than those seen after natural infection. Licensure for use in girls 9 to 15 years of age was based on immunogenicity bridging studies that demonstrated noninferiority of antibody responses compared with those in women 16 to 26 years of age. In fact, the antibody levels in young adolescents a year and a half postvaccination were 2- to 3-fold higher than those in the older women.[32,33]

HPV4 was tested in a phase 3 study involving 4065 boys and men.[34] Among those who were human papillomavirus-naïve at baseline, per-protocol efficacy was 90% against external genital lesions caused by vaccine types and 86% against persistent infection. In intention-to-treat analyses, efficacy was 66% against lesions caused by vaccine types and 48% against persistent infection. HPV4 was studied in 602 healthy men who have sex with men; here, per-protocol efficacy against AIN of any degree due to vaccine types was 78%, and efficacy in the intention-to-treat analysis was 50%.[35] Protection against AIN and anal cancer in women is inferred from studies showing similar immunogenicity in women and men.

Efficacy of HPV2 in preventing high-grade cervical lesions (CIN 2 or 3) or AIS was assessed in two studies that enrolled nearly 20,000 females 15 to 25 years of age. The first study enrolled 1113 women who were naïve for human papillomavirus infection; follow-up at a mean of 5.9 years was available for 776 subjects.[36-38] Efficacy against type 16- or 18-related CIN 2 or 3 or AIS was 100%, as was efficacy against 12-month persistent infection with type 16 or 18. In the second study, referred to as PATRICIA (**PA**pilloma **TRI**al Against **C**ancer **I**n Young **A**dults), 18,665 women were enrolled regardless of baseline human papillomavirus status and were randomized to receive HPV2 or HepA at 0, 1, and 6 months.[39,40] Before vaccination, 73.6% of subjects were naïve to human papillomavirus 16 and/or 18, and the mean follow-up period after the first dose was 39 months. Among women who were human papillomavirus-naïve at baseline and were vaccinated according to protocol, efficacy against human papillomavirus 16- or 18-related CIN 2 or 3 or AIS was approximately 93%. Among all women who received at least 1 dose of vaccine, regardless of current infection with or prior exposure to human papillomavirus 16 or 18 and including all cases starting on Day 1, efficacy against type 16- or 18-related CIN 2 or 3 or AIS was 52.8%; the majority of cases that occurred were due to *prevalent* infection at the time of vaccination rather than *incident* infection after vaccination. Among all women who received at least 1 dose of vaccine, regardless of current infection with or prior exposure to any human papillomavirus type and including all cases starting on Day 1, efficacy against CIN 2 or 3 or AIS related to any human papillomavirus type was 30.4%. This approximates what might be expected in the general population. Efficacy against incident infection with types 16 and 18 remained high at 95% over 7 years after initial vaccination.[41] Efficacy of 84% against anal infection with types 16 and 18 was demonstrated in a trial involving about 4000 women in Costa Rica.[42]

Among women who were vaccinated according to protocol, efficacy against CIN 2 or 3 or AIS caused by 12 non-vaccine types (considered as a group) was 54.0%. When lesions that contained type 16 and/or 18 DNA were excluded in the outcomes analysis, efficacy against CIN 2 or 3 or AIS caused by these types was 37.4%; arguably, if the vaccine did not protect against any of these other types, this number should have been 0%. Among women who were vaccinated according to protocol and were type 31 DNA-negative through month 6, efficacy against CIN 2 or 3 or AIS caused by type 31 was 89.4% when lesions also containing 16 and 18 were excluded.

Virtually all subjects develop antibodies to human papillomavirus 16 and 18 after 3 doses of HPV2 as measured by ELISA as well as a pseudovirion-based neutralization assay. Persistent responses were seen in 98% when measured 76 months postvaccination. The immune response in girls 10 to 14 years of age was noninferior to older women, allowing the assumption that similar disease protection will ensue. In a head-to-head trial involving 1106 women 18 to 45 years of age, geometric mean titers of neutralizing antibody to type 16 were 2.3 to 4.8-fold higher in HPV2 recipients than in HPV4 recipients; for type 18, they were 6.8 to 9.1-fold higher.[43] It is not known whether higher antibody titers predict better or longer-lasting protection.

Safety

Before licensure, safety data were collected from approximately 12,000 HPV4 recipients, about 5100 of whom kept detailed diaries for 2 weeks after each dose. Pain at the injection site occurred in 84%, compared with 75% of controls who received an aluminum-containing placebo and 49% who received a saline placebo (despite anecdotal accounts and media hype regarding pain, a survey study showed that HPV4 vaccination was less painful than other adolescent vaccinations[44]). Swelling and erythema were reported in about 25% of vaccinees, and fewer than 3% of local reactions were believed to be severe. Approximately 5% of female vaccinees reported a temperature of ≥100°F (≥38°C) after any dose, and temperatures ≥102°F (≥38.9°C) occurred in <1%. The rates of fever, other systemic adverse events, serious adverse events, and new medical conditions arising within 4 years were similar in vaccinees and placebees. There were 10 deaths among vaccinees and 7 among placebees, none of which were considered to be vaccine related (causes of death included motor vehicle accidents, intentional drug overdose or suicide, thromboembolic disease, sepsis, cancer, arrhythmia, and asphyxia).

In a postlicensure review of safety data from clinical trials, there were six serious adverse events (vaginal hemorrhage, bronchospasm, gastroenteritis, ulcerative colitis, hypertension and headache, and injection site reaction) thought to be possibly, probably, or definitely related to vaccine among vaccinees (N=11,778) and 2 (hypersensitivity and chills/headache/fever) among placebees (N=9686).[45] There were 11 deaths among vaccinees and 7 among placebees, none of which were related to the study vaccine. New autoimmune phenomena were reported in 2.4% of both groups. Between licensure and the close of 2008, >23 million doses of HPV4 had been distributed; 12,424 VAERS reports had been received, only 6% of which were considered serious (21% of these were headache, 16% nausea, 15% dizziness, 13% vomiting, 13% fever, 13% fatigue, and 13% syncope).[46] There were 32 deaths, with a mean time from the last vaccination to event onset of 39 days (range 2 to 288) and no common pattern. Causes of death included diabetes, viral illness, illicit drug use, and heart failure. Reporting rates for GBS (0.2 per 100,000 doses distributed), transverse myelitis (0.04 per 100,000), and motor neuron disease (0.009 per 100,000) were extremely low. The reporting rate for syncope was 8.2 per 100,000; 90% of cases occurred on the day of vaccination, and >50% of these occurred within 15 minutes. There were 56 reports of venous thromboembolic events; in 90% of the 31 that could be reviewed, known risk factors for such events were present. In 2011, a Vaccine Safety Datalink study of over 600,000 doses of HPV4 found no statistically significant increased risk of GBS, stroke, venous thromboembolism, and other serious events.[47]

In prelicensure trials, local reactions (pain, 91.8%; redness, 48.0%; swelling, 44.1%) occurred more frequently among HPV2 recipients than placebees; the majority of reactions were mild or moderate in intensity. Approximately half of vaccinees experienced fatigue, headache, and myalgia. In a pooled safety analysis, serious adverse events were reported in 5.3% of 16,142 vaccinees and 5.9% of 13,811 placebees during a follow-up period of 7.4 years. In a database of studies including 57,323 females, there were 20 deaths among HPV2 recipients and 17 among control recipients. The causes of death were as expected for the patient population under study. In the largest randomized controlled trial in women 15 to 25 years of age, new-onset autoimmune disease was seen in 78 (0.8%) of 9319 vaccinees compared with 77 (0.8%) of 9325 HepA controls. Postmarketing studies of HPV2 safety in the United States are not available.

- *Contraindications*
  - Severe allergic reaction (eg, anaphylaxis) to previous dose of vaccine or any vaccine component (risk of recurrent allergic reaction; for HPV4, this includes reactions to baker's yeast)
- *Precautions*
  - Moderate or severe acute illness (difficulty distinguishing illness from vaccine reaction)
  - Pregnancy (theoretical risk to the fetus or attribution of birth defects to vaccination). No deleterious effects have been demonstrated from HPV administration during pregnancy, and the risk of adverse fetal effects from an inactivated vaccine is extremely low.

Recommendations

All adolescent boys and girls should be vaccinated against human papillomavirus. The usual schedule is 3 doses of HPV (given at 0, 1 to 2, and 6 months) at 11 to 12 years of age (the series may be started as early as 9 years of age). There is no preference for HPV2 or HPV4 for prevention of cervical cancer in females, but only HPV4 should be used in males. All previously unvaccinated females 13 to 26 and males 13 to 21 years of age also should be vaccinated, whether or not they are sexually active (HPV2 may be used off-label in females 26 years of age). Vaccination of males 22 to 26 years of age is optional, unless they are immunocompromised or are men who have sex with men, in which case routine vaccination is recommended. Screening for human papillomavirus infection before vaccination is not needed, and vaccine should be given regardless of personal history of human papillomavirus infection, cervical, vaginal, or vulvar dysplasia, genital warts, and Pap test results. Vaccination of men and women >26 years of age is not recommended, but if a person turns 27 after initiation of the vaccine series, the series may be completed.

Routine cytologic screening of women for cervical cancer should continue even if they are vaccinated. New guidelines from the American College of Obstetricians and Gynecologists, issued in November 2009,[48] include the following: 1) no screening <21 years of age, regardless of sexual history; 2) screening every 2 years from 21 to 29 years of age; 3) screening every 3 years from 30 to 65 or 70 years of age, provided there have been 3 consecutive negative tests (exceptions include women with HIV infection, compromised immunity, history of CIN 2 or CIN 3, or in utero exposure to diethylstilbestrol; and 4) discontinuation of screening in women 65 to 70 years of age who have had ≥3 consecutive negative tests and no abnormal tests in the preceding 10 years (exceptions include women with multiple sexual partners).

There are no national guidelines for cytological screening for anal cancer.

REFERENCES

1. Schiffman M, et al. *Lancet*. 2007;370:890-907.
2. Palefsky J. *Curr HIV/AIDS Rep*. 2008;5:78-85.
3. Einstein MH, et al. *Lancet Infect Dis*. 2009;9:347-356.
4. Joseph DA, et al. *Cancer*. 2008;113(Suppl 10):2892-2900.
5. Kreimer AR, et al. *Cancer Epidemiol Biomarkers Prev*. 2005;14: 467-475.
6. Li N, et al. *J Infect Dis*. 2011;204:217-223.
7. Park IU, et al. *Gyn Oncol*. 2009;114:399-403.
8. Nyitray AG, et al. *J Infect Dis*. 2010;201:1498-1508.

9. Bruni L, et al. *J Infect Dis*. 2010;202:1789-1799.
10. Winer RL, et al. *Am J Epidemiol*. 2003;157:218-226.
11. Dunne EF, et al. *JAMA*. 2007;297:813-819.
12. Dunne EF, et al. *J Infect Dis*. 2006;194:1044-1057.
13. Lu B, et al. *J Infect Dis*. 2009;199:362-371.
14. Giuliano AR, et al. *Lancet*. 2011;377:932-940.
15. Markowitz LE, et al. *J Infect Dis*. 2009;200:1059-1067.
16. GLOBOCAN 2008 database. International Agency for Research on Cancer Web site. http://globocan.iarc.fr. Accessed February 22, 2012.
17. Markowitz LE, et al. *MMWR*. 2007;56(RR-2):1-24.
18. Johnson LG, et al. *Cancer*. 2004;101:281-288.
19. Dunne EF, et al. *MMWR*. 2011;60:1705-1708.
20. CDC. *MMWR*. 2010;59:626-629.
21. CDC. *MMWR*. 2010;59:630-632.
22. Grunbaum JA, et al. *MMWR*. 2004;53(SS-2):1-96.
23. Sanders GD, et al. *Emerg Infect Dis*. 2003;9:37-48.
24. Elbasha E, et al. *Emerg Infect Dis*. 2007;13:29-41.
25. Kim JJ, et al. *N Engl J Med*. 2008;359:821-832.
26. Kim JJ, et al. *BMJ*. 2009;339:b3884.
27. Chesson HW, et al. *Vaccine*. 2011;29:8443-8450.
28. Garland SM, et al. *N Engl J Med*. 2007;356:1928-1943.
29. The FUTURE II Study Group. *N Engl J Med*. 2007;356:1915-1927.
30. Brown DR, et al. *J Infect Dis*. 2009;199:926-935.
31. Wheeler CM, et al. *J Infect Dis*. 2009;199:936-944.
32. Block SL, et al. *Pediatrics*. 2006;118:2135-2145.
33. Reisinger KS, et al. *Pediatr Infect Dis J*. 2007;26:201-209.
34. Giuliano AR, et al. *N Engl J Med*. 2011;364:401-411.
35. Palefsky JM, et al. *N Engl J Med*. 2011;365:1576-1585.
36. Harper DM, et al. *Lancet*. 2004;364:1757-1765.
37. Harper DM, et al. *Lancet*. 2006;367:1247-1255.
38. The GlaxoSmithKline HPV-007 Study Group. *Lancet*. 2009;374:1975-1985.
39. Paavonen J, et al. *Lancet*. 2007;369:2161-2170.
40. Paavonen J, et al. *Lancet*. 2009;374:301-314.
41. Carvalho ND, et al. *Vaccine*. 2010;28:6247-6255.
42. Kreimer AR, et al. *Lancet Oncol*. 2011;12:862-870.
43. Einstein MH, et al. *Human Vaccines*. 2009;5:705-719.
44. Reiter PL, et al. *Vaccine*. 2009;27:6840-6844.
45. Block SL, et al. *Pediatr Infect Dis J*. 2010;29:95-101.
46. Slade BA, et al. *JAMA*. 2009;302:750-757.
47. Gee J, et al. *Vaccine*. 2011;29:8279-8284.
48. American College of Obstetricians and Gynecologists. *Obstet Gynecol*. 2009;114:1409-1420.

16 Influenza

The Pathogen

Influenza virus, which belongs to the Orthomyxoviridae family, is enveloped and has a segmented, single-stranded RNA genome. Two major surface proteins are involved in infectivity and generation of protective immune responses.[1] Hemagglutinin (H) mediates attachment, and antibodies directed against it block attachment and fusion, neutralize infectivity, and are protective against infection. Neuraminidase (N) mediates release from cells, and antibodies against it limit the spread of infection and reduce disease severity. Proteolytic cleavage of the H molecule is required for infectivity. H and N types for influenza A viruses are designated by numbers—since 1977, the predominant circulating strains have been A(H1N1) and A(H3N2). The H and N molecules undergo minor changes from year to year that result in slight variation in antigenicity, termed *antigenic drift*. This accounts for the fact that a person's experience with influenza in the prior year does not prevent infection with the current year's strain, although severity of illness might be mitigated, depending on how much drift has occurred. Occasionally, a major change occurs, resulting in strains that express novel H or N molecules to which few people have immunity—this is termed *antigenic shift*. Influenza B viruses do not change as much from year to year because they have a limited host range (humans and seals) and they mutate at a slower rate.

Antigenic shift can occur when an animal (usually a pig) is simultaneously infected with an animal strain of influenza A (usually an avian strain) and a human strain (pigs are in a position to be exposed to both). Through *ressortment*, the human strain may package the RNA segment encoding the avian H or N molecule, creating a human virus with the avian H or N type. If this reassortant is capable of spreading from person-to-person, a pandemic may ensue. A global reservoir of influenza viruses (and gene segments) exists in aquatic birds.[2] These viruses are adapted to the avian enteric tract and do not cause disease. However, when they enter the pig along with human influenza strains, new strains can emerge that spread from person-to-person and cause disease. Pigs are good "mixing vessels" because their respiratory epithelial cells express both alpha 2,3-linked sialic acid residues, to which avian influenza viruses bind (via the H molecule), as well as alpha 2,6-linked sialic acid residues, to which human influenza viruses bind.

Pandemic strains can also emerge if animal influenza viruses adapt directly to humans. This is what happened in 1918, leading to the "mother of all influenza pandemics."[3] The A(H1N1) Spanish flu killed 50 million people worldwide; more Americans died from influenza in 1918 than were killed during World Wars I and II and the Korean, Vietnam, Gulf, Afghanistan, and Iraq wars—*combined*.[4] The adaptation of this virus to human-to-human transmission was facilitated by a single amino acid change in the H molecule; the exceptional virulence was due to its ability to cause dysregulation of the host inflammatory response.[5] All interpandemic influenza A *epidemics* since 1918 have been caused by descendants of the 1918 strain that underwent antigenic drift; the 1957 H2N2 "Asian" flu and the 1968 H3N2 "Hong Kong" flu pandemics were caused by descendants of the 1918 virus that underwent antigenic shift.

The 2009 A(H1N1) pandemic was caused by a reassortant that derived from a number of exchange events between circulating viruses.[6] In particular, the H gene came from classic swine influenza and the N gene from Eurasian swine influenza (both of which are descendants of the 1918 virus); other genes came from a human H3N2 strain and an avian strain. Antibodies against the novel 2009 virus were found in very few children and in only 6% to 9% of adults under 65 years of age, suggesting that the virus had not circulated among humans for several generations.[7] Antibody *was*, however, detected in about a third of adults over 60 years of age, suggesting that a similar virus may have circulated years ago, or that a previous version of the seasonal vaccine may have had shared antigenic determinants. The H of 2009 A(H1N1) is only about 70% homologous at the amino acid level with previous seasonal H1 viruses; it is not surprising, therefore, that vaccination with recent seasonal vaccines did not induce protective responses.

The influenza A(H5N1) strain that emerged in Southeast Asia in 2005 (bird flu) is entirely of avian origin (ie, not the product of reassortment).[8] Its ability to spread to humans appears to have resulted from a change in its H molecule, allowing binding to alpha 2,6-linked sialic acid residues. Its increased virulence may be explained by the presence of multiple basic amino acids in the region of the connecting peptide that links the two H subunits—this allows for cleavage by ubiquitous intracellular proteases, thus enhancing infectivity and expanding tissue tropism. Other virulence factors also may be involved.

Influenza virus infects columnar epithelial cells of the respiratory tract, causing necrosis, edema, and inflammation. Systemic symptoms are probably caused by circulating interleukin-6 and interferon-alpha induced by the infection. Influenza A virus infects all age groups and causes the most severe disease. Influenza B is milder and occurs more often in children.

Clinical Features

The incubation period is 1 to 4 days. Symptoms include abrupt onset of fever, myalgia, headache, sore throat, photophobia, tearing, rhinitis, and nonproductive cough. Older children may experience nausea and vomiting, and infants may present with a sepsis-like syndrome. Fever is usually 101° to 102°F (38.3° to 38.9°C) and may be accompanied by prostration. Uncomplicated illness lasts from 3 to 7 days, and while recovery is usually rapid, some patients may have lingering cough and fatigue for several weeks.

Secondary bacterial infection (eg, pneumonia, sinusitis, and otitis media) is the most common complication of influenza. The risk of complications and hospitalization with influenza is highest among persons ≥65 years of age, the very young, and those with certain underlying medical conditions. The virus itself may cause pneumonia, encephalitis, myocarditis, and myositis. Pregnant women, young children, and persons with morbid obesity were at particular risk for complications during the 2009 pandemic.[9]

Bird flu typically manifests as febrile pneumonia that progresses rapidly to respiratory failure. Clinical features include dyspnea, sore throat, headache, elevated transaminases, leukopenia, and thrombocytopenia. Mortality rates are extremely high, ranging from 39% to 88% in various studies, and young adults are disproportionately affected. Death usually occurs during the second week of illness.

Epidemiology and Transmission

Influenza virus is transmitted from person-to-person through large-particle respiratory droplets that are expelled during coughing or sneezing. Maximum communicability occurs from 1 day before the onset of illness to 5 days after. Disease activity typically peaks between December and March in temperate climates (the disease peaks between April and September in temperate regions of the Southern Hemisphere and occurs throughout the year in tropical areas; because of this, traveling with large tourist groups that include persons from these areas increases the risk of infection during the summer). During 1976 to 2006, peak influenza activity in the United States occurred most frequently in January (19% of seasons) and February (45% of seasons).[10] However, peak activity occurred in March, April, or May in 19% of seasons. During average interpandemic years, anywhere from 5% to 15% of the population may become infected, and up to half of these infections will result in medical attention. Illness rates are highest among school-aged children, sometimes as high as 30%. Among adults, influenza illness results in an average of 2 lost workdays per episode.

School-aged children are at low risk for complications, but they play a key role in spreading the virus throughout the community. This was demonstrated in a classic study in Houston showing that school absenteeism during the influenza season preceded workplace absenteeism by several weeks.[11] In fact, during the 2009 pandemic a tight correlation was seen between the date of school opening and the beginning of influenza activity in communities.[12] Routine vaccination of school children in Japan between the 1960s and early 1980s resulted in dramatic reductions in excess (influenza-related) mortality among the elderly and other high-risk groups.[13]

Annual hospitalization rates for laboratory-confirmed influenza are around 20 per 100,000 for children 2 to 5 years of age, but as high as 240 to 720 per 100,000 for infants <6 months of age.[14] The rate of hospitalization for infants is similar to the rate for children with high-risk conditions and is comparable to that for adults ≥65 years of age. The annual outpatient burden of influenza may be as high as 100 clinic visits and 30 emergency department visits per 1000 children.

During the 1980s and 1990s in the United States, influenza resulted in an average of 226,000 hospitalizations and 36,000 deaths[15,16]; a more recent estimate encompassing 1976 through 2007 placed the average number of deaths at about 24,000, ranging from 3349 in 1986-1987 to 48,614 in 2003-2004.[17] Although the number of deaths in US children is small (153 in the 2003-2004 season), it is notable that nearly two thirds occur in children without underlying medical conditions. It is estimated that over 100,000 children die each year from influenza worldwide.[18]

In April 2009, two children in southern California were found to be infected with a new strain of influenza A(H1N1).[19] By June, the WHO announced that the criteria for an influenza pandemic had been met,[20] and by March 2010 in the United States alone there had been an estimated 60 million cases, 270,000 hospitalizations, and 12,270 deaths.[21] Most cases (35 million), hospitalizations (158,000), and deaths (9420) had occurred among persons 18 to 64 years of age. The same strain of A(H1N1) has persisted seasonally since then.

Between May 2005 and December 2007, bird flu was reported in 340 humans, most of whom lived in Southeast Asia, Eurasia, and Africa. The median age of affected persons was around 18 years, and the vast majority of patients were <40; this is strikingly different from seasonal influenza, which disproportionately affects the young and the old, but it is reminiscent of the 1918 pandemic. Humans are infected directly from birds—risk factors include handling of sick or dead poultry; slaughtering, defeathering, or preparing sick poultry for consumption; eating undercooked poultry products; and other close contact with birds, such as ducks. Some cases may have been acquired through contaminated fomites, and whereas there is no evidence of sustained human-to-human transmission, limited transmission might have occurred from very close contact with severely affected persons.

Immunization Program

The first influenza vaccines became available in 1945. Between then and 2008, the focus was on protecting individuals from complications, hospitalization, and death related to influenza. High-risk groups were identified and recommended for annual immunization, and increasing emphasis was placed on immunizing close contacts of those individuals. Immunization of all adults ≥65 years of age was recommended until 2000, when the recommendation was broadened to include all adults ≥50 years of age. In 2002, immunization of all children 6 to 23 months of age was "encouraged"[22]; in 2004, this was changed to a strong recommendation.[23] In 2006, all children 24 to 59 months of age were added to the routine vaccination list.[24]

In 2008, an unprecedented step was taken—going beyond protecting individuals to protecting the general community. The recommendation was made to extend routine childhood immunization to include all children 6 months to 18 years of age.[25] As noted earlier, there is good reason to believe that preventing influenza in school-aged children will change the epidemiology of influenza transmission in the community. In 2009, there was a subtle but important change in the language surrounding universal childhood immunization, from "if feasible" to, essentially, "just do it."[26] Finally, in 2010 it was decided to recommend yearly influenza immunization for all persons ≥6 months of age.[27] Recommendations for seasonal influenza vaccination are updated in the summer of each year.

Studies among working adults suggest that influenza immunization reduces health care provider visits and lost workdays by nearly half.[28] A study in 2001 looked at the direct and indirect costs of both vaccination and disease, assuming that vaccination occurred in a low-cost setting, such as the workplace.[29] This analysis demonstrated that routine vaccination of healthy working adults would result in an average cost saving of $13.66 per person vaccinated (1998 dollars). The cost of immunization per quality-adjusted life year (QALY) saved is estimated to be $980 (2000 dollars) for persons ≥65 years of age and $28,000 for persons 50-64 years of age.[30] The cost per QALY saved in healthy children 6 to 23 months of age is estimated to be around $12,000 (2003 dollars), and for adolescents around $119,000.[31] The additional benefits that would accrue from the herd immunity effects of immunizing all school-aged children are difficult to assess.

Recommendations for influenza vaccination of HCP were updated in 2006[32] and 2011.[33]

Vaccines

Characteristics of the influenza vaccines licensed in the United States are given in **Table 16.1**, and differences between LAIV and IIV are summarized in **Table 16.2**.

Influenza vaccines are made using the very same reassortment process that leads to pandemic strains.[34] In the case of IIV, the circulating wild-type viruses are reassorted with a strain that is well adapted to growth in embryonated hen's eggs (allantoic fluid provides the protease necessary for cleavage of the H molecule that is necessary for infectivity). The reassortants have the backbone of the adapted strain and therefore grow efficiently to bulk levels; however, they express the H and N of the wild-type strain and therefore yield useful vaccine antigens. Reassortants can also be made using *reverse genetics*, whereby the relevant genes are harvested and introduced into cells to produce viruses. Vaccine viruses are inoculated into large numbers of hen's eggs; progeny virions are concentrated from allantoic fluid, chemically inactivated, and disrupted ("split"); the H and N proteins are then purified and formulated into a final product. Standard dose, intramuscular formulations of IIV have been around for many years. In 2009, a high-dose formulation (Fluzone High-Dose) was licensed for use in older persons ≥65 years of age, and in 2011, an intradermal IIV (Fluzone Intradermal) was licensed for use in persons 18 to 64 years of age. Intradermal delivery is not only convenient but also allows for antigen sparing, given the abundance of dendritic cells in the dermis that can process antigen (see *Chapter 1: Introduction to Vaccinology—The Germinal Center Reaction*).

In the case of LAIV, the wild-type strains are reassorted with a master donor virus (MDV) that is *attenuated*, *cold-adapted* (replication is efficient at 25°C), and *temperature-sensitive* (replication is restricted at 37°C to 39°C). The reassortants have the backbone of MDV and can therefore be produced in bulk (MDV also grows well in embryonated eggs); because they carry the H and N of the wild-type viruses, they engender protective immune responses to the circulating strains. The vaccine viruses are grown in hen's eggs; progeny viruses are concentrated from allantoic fluid, suspended in stabilizing buffer, and packaged for intranasal administration. LAIV replicates in the nasopharynx but is incapable of replicating lower in the respiratory tract.

There is an influenza A (H5N1) IIV licensed in the United States. Manufactured by Sanofi Pasteur and approved in 2007, the vaccine is based on a laboratory strain of influenza A that was modified to carry the genes encoding the H and N of the human isolate A/Vietnam/1203/2004 (H5N1, clade 1). The H gene was mutated to prevent cleavage of the mature protein, reducing pathogenicity and allowing the vaccine to grow efficiently in embryonated eggs. Licensure was based on demonstrated immunogenicity. The vaccine is not commercially available but has been purchased by the federal government for inclusion in the National Stockpile for distribution by public health officials, if necessary.

Efficacy and/or Immunogenicity

Each years' influenza vaccines are licensed based on immunogenicity, not efficacy. The accepted correlate of protection is a hemagglutination inhibition titer of ≥1:40 (this test measures the ability of serum to compete with the binding of influenza virus to red blood cells); 50% of individuals who achieve this level of antibody are presumed to be protected.[35] Practically speaking, vaccine-induced immunity to influenza is good for only 1 year because antibody wanes and the vaccine strains chosen for a given year may not be a good match with the prevailing strains. For example, during the 2007 to 2008 influenza season, the circulating A(H3N2) and B viruses (A/Brisbane/10/2007-like and B/Florida/04/2006-like, respectively) were substantially different from the strains in the vaccine (A/Wisconsin/67/2005-like and B/Malaysia/2506/2004-like, respectively). Effectiveness against medically attended influenza A infection was 58% but no effectiveness against influenza B was seen.[36]

16

Efficacy (eg, reduction in laboratory-confirmed cases in studies) and effectiveness (eg, reduction in symptomatic cases when the vaccine is used in the real world) may differ markedly. For example, a systematic review in 2005 found that efficacy of LAIV in children >2 years of age was 79% but effectiveness was 38%; for IIV, the respective numbers were 65% and 28%.[37] A 2012 meta-analysis highlighted gaps in the evidence base regarding the protective effects of influenza vaccine among children 2 to 17 years of age and adults ≥65 years of age.[38] Overall efficacy of IIV among adults 18 to 64 years of age was 59%, with LAIV showing consistently better protection (83%) among young children compared with IIV.

■ IIV

Most vaccinees develop serum hemagglutination inhibition and neutralizing antibodies. Children 6 months to 8 years of age require 2 doses in the same season to ensure protective responses. In a study among children conducted between 1985 and 1990, annual vaccination with IIV reduced laboratory-confirmed influenza A by 77% to 91%.[39] A 1-year placebo-controlled study yielded efficacy estimates of 56% among healthy children 3 to 9 years of age and 100% among adolescents,[40] and a retrospective study of 30,000 young children showed approximately 50% effectiveness against medically-attended, clinically diagnosed

TABLE 16.1 — Influenza Vaccines, 2011-2012 Season[a]

Trade Name	Manufacturer/ Distributor	Type	Presentation	Preservative	Labeled Ages	Dose/ Administration	Latex
Afluria	CSL Biotherapies/ Merck	IIV	Prefilled syringe (10)	None	≥5 years[b]	0.5 mL intramuscular	No
			10-dose vial (1)	Thimerosal (24.5 mcg mercury)	≥5 years[b]	0.5 mL intramuscular	No
Fluarix	GlaxoSmithKline	IIV	Prefilled syringe (10)	None	≥3 years	0.5 mL intramuscular	Yes
FluLaval	ID Biomedical/ GlaxoSmithKline	IIV	10-dose vial (1)	Thimerosal (25 mcg mercury)	≥18 years	0.5 mL intramuscular	No
FluMist[c]	MedImmune	LAIV	Prefilled sprayer (10)	None	2 to 49 years[d]	0.1 mL per nostril[d]	No
Fluvirin	Novartis	IIV	Prefilled syringe (10)	None	≥4 years	0.5 mL intramuscular	Yes
			10-dose vial (1)	Thimerosal (25 mcg mercury)	≥4 years	0.5 mL intramuscular	No
Fluzone	Sanofi Pasteur	IIV	Prefilled syringe (10)	None	6 months to 2 years	0.25 mL intramuscular	Yes
			Prefilled syringe (10)	None	≥3 years	0.5 mL intramuscular	Yes
			1-dose vial (10)	None	≥3 years	0.5 mL intramuscular	No
			10-dose vial (1)	Thimerosal (25 mcg mercury)	≥6 months	0.25 mL or 0.5 mL intramuscular	No
Fluzone High-Dose	Sanofi Pasteur	IIV	Prefilled syringe (10)	None	≥65 years	0.5 mL intramuscular	Yes

Fluzone Intradermal	Sanofi Pasteur	IIV	Prefilled micro-injector (10)	None	18 to 64 years	0.1 mL intradermal[e]	No

[a] "IIV" stands for "inactivated influenza vaccine" (other publications may refer to this as "TIV," for "trivalent [inactivated] influenza vaccine). "LAIV" stands for "live-attenuated influenza vaccine." All vaccines for the 2011-2012 season are 3-valent and contain antigens from the strains that are predicted to circulate during the season (for 2010-2011 and 2011-2012, the strains were A/California/7/2009 (H1N1)-like, A/Perth/16/2009 (H3N2)-like, and B/Brisbane/60/2008-like). For IIV, the standard hemagglutinin content is 15 mcg/0.5 mL from each of the strains that make up the vaccine, except for Fluzone High-Dose, which contains 60 mcg/0.5 mL from each strain and Fluzone Intradermal, which contains 9 mcg/0.1 mL from each strain. LAIV contains $10^{6.5-7.5}$ fluorescent focus units of each live-attenuated, cold-adapted, temperature-sensitive reassortant strain per 0.2 mL. None of the vaccines contain adjuvants. The dose of IIV is 0.25 mL at 6 months to 2 years of age and 0.5 mL at ≥3 years of age. See the respective package inserts for the list of excipients and contaminants. Influenza vaccines are interchangeable in the sense that one product (any inactivated influenza vaccine or live influenza vaccine) can be used 1 year and another product the next year. Although no data are available regarding 2 consecutive doses of different products in the same year, it is assumed that this is acceptable. The public and private cost of influenza vaccines is generally in the range of 10 to 20 $US (2011).

[b] Afluria should not be used in children 6 months to 8 years of age because of increased febrile reactions, unless there is no other vaccine available and the patient is at high risk for influenza complications.

[c] In February 2012, a 4-valent version of FluMist (FluMist Quadrivalent) was licensed. In addition to the B strain from the Yamagata lineage contained in the standard 3-valent vaccines, FluMist Quadrivalent contains a B strain from the Victoria lineage.

[d] FluMist is only indicated for use in healthy, nonpregnant persons. If the patient sneezes after administration, the dose should not be repeated. Individuals who are too old to receive LAIV themselves or who have medical contraindications other than severe immunosuppression may administer the vaccine.

[e] Fluzone Intradermal is administered using a prefilled microinjector system that delivers a measured dose into the dermis of the skin.

Adapted from Grohskopf L, et al. *MMWR*. 2011;60:1128-1132, as well as the respective package inserts.

TABLE 16.2 — Differences Between Live and Inactivated Influenza Vaccines

Characteristic	Live	Inactivated
Route of administration	Intranasal spray	Intramuscular injection
Type of vaccine	Live attenuated, engineered	Inactivated, purified subunits
Labeled age indication	2 to 49 years of age	≥6 months of age[a]
Minimal interval between doses	4 weeks	4 weeks
Simultaneous administration with other vaccines	Yes	Yes
Minimum interval for any inactivated vaccine not given on the same day	None	None
Minimum interval for any live vaccine not given on the same day	4 weeks[b]	None
Can the vaccine be used in the following situations?		
Persons with medical conditions that place them at increased risk for complications of influenza	No	Yes
Persons with asthma or children 2 to 4 years of age with wheezing in the past year	No	Yes
Close contacts of immunosuppressed persons who *do not* require a protected environment	Yes	Yes
Close contacts of immunosuppressed persons who *do* require a protected environment	No	Yes
Close contacts of persons at high risk but who are not severely immunosuppressed	Yes	Yes

[a] Approved ages vary by product (see **Table 16.1**).
[b] The concern here is the potential for interference between the replicating vaccine viruses.

Adapted from Fiore AE, et al. *MMWR*. 2010;59(RR-8):1-62.

pneumonia or influenza.[41] Effectiveness of 56% was seen in a study of children 6 months to 5 years of age conducted from 2005 to 2007.[42] IIV may reduce episodes of otitis media in children by as much as 30%.

Randomized controlled trials demonstrate efficacy against laboratory-confirmed influenza illness of 70% to 90% among healthy adults <65 years of age.[26] Whereas estimates of efficacy drop to 50% to 77% when the vaccine and circulating strains are not well matched, protection against hospitalization appears to be preserved. Efficacy against illness is lower among adults ≥65 years of age, but protection against influenza-related death may be as high as 80%. In a study among 2575 adults ≥65 years of age, the geometric mean titer of antibody against influenza A strains was almost twice as high for those receiving high-dose IIV compared with standard dose IIV, and the seroprotection rate for A(H1N1) was 13% higher.[43] Efficacy of maternal immunization in preventing hospitalization of infants due to influenza exceeds 90%.[44]

Antibody responses to intradermal IIV are noninferior to IIV given intramuscularly, despite the lowered antigen content of the former.[45]

■ LAIV

Immunologic correlates of protection after administration of live influenza vaccine have not been established but probably include antibodies in nasal secretions. LAIV was evaluated in a placebo-controlled study between 1996 and 1998 involving 1602 healthy children 15 to 71 months of age.[46] Efficacy against culture-confirmed influenza was 89% for those who received 1 dose and 94% for those who received 2 doses. In the second year, despite a poor match with the circulating A(H3N2) strain, efficacy was 86%. Efficacy against pneumonia, other lower respiratory tract disease, and influenza-associated otitis media was also demonstrated. In a multinational trial conducted during the 2004-2005 influenza season, 3916 children <5 years of age were randomized to receive LAIV and 3936 to receive IIV.[47] Culture-confirmed influenza illness caused by any strain was reduced by 55% in recipients of LAIV compared with recipients of IIV; for matched strains, the reduction was 45% and for mismatched strains it was 58%, suggesting that LAIV provides broader cross-protection. Additional prelicensure, placebo-controlled trials involving >4000 children demonstrated efficacy of 73% to 93% for culture-confirmed influenza due to any strain. A meta-analysis published in 2009 suggested that LAIV was 46% more effective than IIV in preventing influenza illness due to matched strains among young children receiving 2 doses in one season[48]; the relative efficacy among older children receiving one dose was 35%. A pooled analysis of clinical trials suggested that LAIV was 85% efficacious at preventing acute otitis media related to influenza compared with placebo and 54% compared with IIV.[49] The efficacy of LAIV and IIV are more comparable in adults.[50]

A multicenter placebo-controlled trial among 4561 healthy, working adults was conducted during 1997-1998, a season when the A(H3N2) strain in the vaccine was not well matched with the circulating strain.[51] Febrile illnesses were not reduced among vaccinees, but severe febrile illnesses and febrile upper respiratory tract illnesses were (19% and 24% reduction, respectively). There were also reductions in days of illness (23% for febrile illnesses, 27% for severe febrile illnesses), days of work lost (18% for severe febrile illnesses, 28% for febrile respiratory tract illnesses), and days with health care provider visits (25% for severe febrile illnesses, 41% for febrile upper respiratory tract illnesses). Use of prescription antibiotics and over-the-counter medications was reduced.

Safety

IIV

Inactivated influenza vaccine cannot cause influenza. Less than one third of vaccinees develop local redness or induration for 1 to 2 days at the site of injection. Fever, chills, headache, and malaise, although infrequent, most often affect children who have had no previous exposure to the antigens contained in the vaccine. These reactions generally begin 6 to 12 hours after vaccination and persist for only 1 to 2 days. Immediate reactions, presumably allergic, may consist of hives, angioedema, allergic asthma, or systemic anaphylaxis. These are rare and probably result from hypersensitivity to a vaccine component, most likely residual egg protein. If influenza vaccines have any association with GBS, it is on the order of one case per million vaccinees, well below the background rate in the population (see *Chapter 7: Addressing Concerns About Vaccines—Do Vaccines Cause Guillain-Barré Syndrome?*).

In a retrospective study of 45,000 children 6 to 23 months of age, vaccination was not associated with any adverse medically attended outcome,[52] and no serious medically attended events were associated with IIV in a Vaccine Safety Datalink study involving approximately 66,000 children 24 to 59 months of age.[53] Some studies in adults show similar rates of systemic symptoms, such as fever, malaise, myalgia, and headache, between vaccinees and placebees. There is no evidence that IIV has any deleterious impact on HIV infection.

High-dose IIV is somewhat more reactogenic than standard-dose.[43] Pain is reported by 36% of vaccinees and erythema by 15%; reactions are generally mild and resolve within 3 days. High fever is more common than standard-dose vaccine but experienced by only 1% of vaccinees. Erythema occurs in about 75%

and swelling in about 25% of adults who receive intradermal IIV; about half of subjects say the intradermal injection is less painful than the intramuscular.[45]

During the 2000 to 2001 season in Canada, a discrete oculo-respiratory syndrome was reported with IIV.[54] Symptoms were mild and self-limited, began within 24 hours of injection, and included hoarseness, sore throat, difficulty swallowing, cough, sore and/or itchy eyes, bilateral conjunctival erythema, facial edema, and nasal congestion. Microaggregates of unsplit virus were implicated as the cause.

■ LAIV

Children report rhinorrhea or congestion (20% to 75%), headache (2% to 46%), fever (up to 26%), vomiting (3% to 13%), abdominal pain (2%), and myalgias (up to 21%). Symptoms are more often associated with the first dose and are self-limited. In a randomized trial in 8352 children 6 to 59 months of age, rhinorrhea among first-time vaccinees was reported in 57% of LAIV recipients and in 46.3% of IIV recipients.[47] Temperature >100°F (37.8°C) was reported in 5.4% of LAIV and in 2% of IIV recipients. Among children <24 months of age, 3.2% of LAIV recipients and 2.0% of IIV recipients had medically significant wheezing after 1 dose.

Adult vaccinees report rhinorrhea (44%, vs 27% in placebees), headache (40% vs 38%), sore throat (28% vs 17%), tiredness (26% vs 22%), muscle aches (17% vs 15%), cough (14% vs 11%), and chills (9% vs 6%).

Serious adverse events are rare. Shedding of vaccine virus is common among children, with up to 80% shedding at least one strain from 1 to 21 days postvaccination. However, the risk of horizontal transmission is very low—the estimated probability of a young child acquiring a vaccine virus from a vaccinated child in the day care setting is 0.6% to 2.4%. Up to 50% of adults may have viral antigen in nasal secretions for the first 7 days after vaccination. Person-to-person transmission among adults has not been assessed.

- IIV

  Contraindications

  - Severe allergic reaction (eg, anaphylaxis) to previous dose of vaccine or any vaccine component, including eggs (risk of recurrent allergic reaction). Persons who are able to eat lightly cooked (eg, scrambled) eggs without reaction are not likely to be allergic (tolerance to baked goods containing eggs is not a reliable predictor). Whereas skin and/or blood testing for IgE against egg proteins can confirm egg allergy, this is not necessary in persons without a history of severe allergy or anaphylaxis. Mild or local manifestations of allergy to eggs or feathers are not contraindications to vaccination. Persons who experience only hives after egg exposure may be vaccinated with IIV (but not LAIV), as long as the provider is familiar with the potential manifestations of egg allergy and the patient can be observed for 30 minutes. Persons who report more serious reactions that fall short of anaphylaxis (eg, angioedema, respiratory distress, lightheadedness, or emesis) should be referred to a physician with expertise in allergic conditions for further risk assessment.

Precautions

– Moderate or severe acute illness (difficulty distinguishing illness from vaccine reaction)
– Personal history of GBS within 6 weeks of a prior dose of influenza vaccine (risk of recurrent GBS; family history not relevant)

• LAIV

Contraindications

– Severe allergic reaction (eg, anaphylaxis) to previous dose of vaccine or any vaccine component, and any reported allergy to eggs (risk of recurrent allergic reaction)
– Underlying medical conditions that place patients at high risk for complications and serve as an *indication* for influenza vaccination, including asthma (or equivalent), chronic cardiopulmonary disease (except hypertension), diabetes, renal dysfunction, hemoglobinopathy, immunodeficiency, or immunosuppression (risk of exacerbating underlying condition or causing influenza-like disease)
– Children or adolescents receiving aspirin or other salicylates (risk of Reye syndrome)
– Pregnancy (theoretical risk to the fetus of live-virus vaccine or attribution of birth defects to vaccination)
– Household or health care contacts of severely immunosuppressed individuals, eg, hematopoietic stem-cell transplant recipients who are confined to protective environments with regulated airflow, filtration, etc (risk of transmission of live virus to immunosuppressed person). Individuals who receive LAIV should avoid contact with severely immunosuppressed patients for 7 days; contact with patients who have lesser degrees of immunosuppression is acceptable. HCP who work in the neonatal intensive care unit may receive LAIV.
– Receipt of influenza antivirals within 48 hours before or 2 weeks after vaccination (risk of decreased viral replication and poor immune response)

Precautions

– Moderate or severe acute illness (difficulty distinguishing illness from vaccine reaction)

– Personal history of GBS within 6 weeks of a prior dose of influenza vaccine (risk of recurrent GBS; family history not relevant)
– Severe nasal congestion (interference with delivery of vaccine). Use of nasal steroids is *not* a contraindication or precaution *per se*, but there are the theoretical risks of reduced immunogenicity and increased side effects. In addition, if the patient is being treated for nasal congestion, one should consider whether or not vaccine delivery to the nasal mucosa might be affected.

Recommendations

Influenza vaccine is given annually, usually beginning in October in the United States (in truth, vaccinations can begin as soon as vaccine is available). It is never too late in the season to vaccinate. In general, vaccination efforts should continue well into March. There is no preference for LAIV or IIV in otherwise healthy persons in any age group for which the vaccines are labeled, and there is no preference for any particular version of IIV in any target group.

Every person ≥6 months of age should receive yearly influenza immunization. IIV may be used for anyone without a contraindication; LAIV should only be used for healthy persons 2 to 49 years of age. While asthma is a contraindication for LAIV, there are children in the 2- to 4-year age group who have had episodes of wheezing but who have not (yet) been diagnosed with asthma. The following screening question for parents has been suggested: "In the past 12 months, has a health care provider ever told you that your child had wheezing or asthma?" If the answer is yes, or if there is a wheezing episode documented in the medical record in the past 12 months, the child should receive IIV instead of LAIV.

Children <9 years of age who are receiving influenza vaccine for the first time need 2 doses separated by ≥4 weeks in the same season. If the child reaches 9 years of age before the second dose is given, the second dose is not necessary. Because the vaccine strains did not change between 2010-2011 and 2011-2012, children who received at least one dose in 2010-2011 only need one dose for the 2011-2012 season. Those who were not vaccinated in 2010-2011, and those whose influenza immunization history in the 2010-2011 season is unknown, need 2 doses.

Within the context of a universal immunization program, the following groups that are at high risk of complications or high risk of spreading influenza should be given priority:

- Adults ≥50 years of age, regardless of underlying conditions (IIV only)
- Children 6 months to 4 years of age (IIV from 6 to 23 months of age, either IIV or LAIV from 2 to 4 years of age)

- Women who are or will be pregnant during influenza season, regardless of trimester (IIV only). There is no preference for products that are thimerosal free (see *Chapter 6: Vaccination in Special Circumstances—Pregnancy and Breast-Feeding* and *Chapter 7: Addressing Concerns About Vaccines—Did the Thimerosal Used as a Preservative in Vaccines Cause Autism?*)
- Patients with chronic conditions involving the following systems (IIV only):
  - Pulmonary (eg, emphysema, chronic bronchitis, and asthma)
  - Cardiovascular, except for hypertension (eg, congestive heart failure)
  - Metabolic diseases (eg, diabetes mellitus)
  - Renal (eg, nephrotic syndrome, hemodialysis)
  - Hepatic (eg, cirrhosis)
  - Hematologic (eg, sickle cell disease, other hemaglobinopathies)
  - Immunologic (eg, immunosuppressive medications, congenital immunodeficiency, HIV infection)
  - Neurologic (eg, cognitive dysfunction, spinal cord injury, seizure disorder, neuromuscular disorder that compromises respiratory function or handling of secretions)
- Persons 6 months to 18 years of age on long-term aspirin therapy who may be at risk of Reye syndrome (IIV only)
- Household contacts of, and persons who provide care for, children <5 years of age (especially <6 months), adults ≥50 years of age, and persons with any of the high-risk conditions listed earlier (IIV or LAIV, except that LAIV should not be used for those who have contact with severely immunosuppressed patients)
- HCP, including physicians, nurses, residents, students, medical emergency response workers, and other workers in hospitals and clinics (IIV or LAIV, except that LAIV should not be used for those who have contact with severely immunosuppressed patients). Mandatory influenza immunization for HCP is discussed in *Chapter 3: Standards, Principles, and Regulations—Mandates.*
- Residents and employees of assisted-living residences, chronic or long-term care facilities, correctional facilities, nursing homes, and similar residential institutions (IIV or LAIV)
- Persons who provide essential community services (IIV or LAIV)
- Students living in dormitories (IIV or LAIV)
- Travelers ((IIV or LAIV; see *Chapter 6: Vaccination in Special Circumstances—Travel*)

REFERENCES

1. Lambert LC, et al. *N Engl J Med.* 2010;363:2036-2044.
2. Morens DM, et al. *N Engl J Med.* 2009;361:225-229.
3. Taubenberger JK, et al. *Emerg Infect Dis*. 2006;12:15-22.
4. Johnson NPAS, et al. *Bull Hist Med.* 2002;76:105-115.
5. Kobasa D, et al. *Nature*. 2007;445:319-323.
6. Trifonov V, et al. *New Engl J Med.* 2009;361:115-119.
7. CDC. *MMWR*. 2009;58:521-524.
8. Writing Committee of the Second World Health Organization Consultation on Clinical Aspects of Human Infection with Avian Influenza A (H5N1) Virus, et al. *N Engl J Med.* 2008;358:261-273.
9. Writing Committee of the WHO Consultation on Clinical Aspects of Pandemic (H1N1) 2009 Influenza. *N Engl J Med.* 2010;362:1708-1719.
10. CDC. *MMWR.* 2007;56(RR-6):1-54.
11. Glezen WP, et al. *N Engl J Med.* 1978;298:587-592.
12. Chao DL, et al. *J Infect Dis*. 2010;202:877-880.
13. Reichert TA, et al. *N Engl J Med.* 2001;344:889-896.
14. Poehling KA, et al. *N Engl J Med.* 2006;355:31-40.
15. Thompson WW, et al. *JAMA*. 2003;289:179-186.
16. Thompson WW, et al. *JAMA.* 2004;292:1333-1340.
17. Thompson MG, et al. *MMWR*. 2010;59:1057-1062.
18. Nair H, et al. *Lancet*. 2011;378:1917-1930.
19. CDC. *MMWR*. 2009;58:400-402.
20. Sekkides O. *Lancet Infect Dis*. 2010;10:663.
21. CDC estimates of 2009 H1N1 cases and related hospitalizations and deaths from April 2009 through March 13, 2010, by age group. Centers for Disease Control and Prevention Web site. http://www.cdc.gov/h1n1flu/pdf/graph_March%202010.pdf. Accessed February 19, 2012.
22. CDC. *MMWR.* 2002;51(RR-3):1-32.
23. CDC. *MMWR.* 2004;53(RR-6):1-40.
24. CDC. *MMWR.* 2006;55(RR-10):1-42.
25. CDC. *MMWR.* 2008;57(RR-7):1-60.
26. CDC. *MMWR.* 2009;58(RR-8):1-52.
27. Fiore AE, et al. *MMWR*. 2010;59(RR-8):1-62.
28. Nichol KL, et al. *N Engl J Med.* 1995;333:889-893.
29. Nichol KL. *Arch Intern Med.* 2001;161:749-759.
30. Maciosek MV, et al. *Am J Prev Med.* 2006;31:72-79.
31. Prosser LA, et al. *Emerg Infect Dis*. 2006;12:1548-1558.
32. Pearson ML, et al. *MMWR*. 2006;55(RR-2):1-16.
33. Shefer A, et al. *MMWR*. 2011;60(RR-7):1-45.
34. Treanor J. *N Engl J Med.* 2004;351:2037-2040.

35. Food and Drug Administration. Guidance for industry: clinical data needed to support the licensure of seasonal inactivated influenza vaccines. http://www.fda.gov/BiologicsBloodVaccines/GuidanceComplianceRegulatoryInformation/Guidances/Vaccines/ucm074794.htm. Accessed February 19, 2012.
36. CDC. *MMWR*. 2008;57:393-398.
37. Jefferson T, et al. *Lancet*. 2005;365:773-780.
38. Osterholm MT, et al. *Lancet Infect Dis*. 2012;12:36-44.
39. Neuzil KM, et al. *Pediatr Infect Dis J*. 2001;20:733-740.
40. Clover RD, et al. *J Infect Dis*. 1991;163:300-304.
41. Ritzwoller DP, et al. *Pediatrics*. 2005;116:153-159.
42. Staat MA, et al. *Vaccine*. 2011;29:9005-9011.
43. Falsey AR, et al. *J Infect Dis*. 2009;200:172-180.
44. Benowitz I, et al. *Clin Infect Dis*. 2010;51:1355-1361.
45. Frenck RW, et al. *Vaccine*. 2011;29:5666-5674.
46. Belshe RB, et al. *J Pediatr*. 2000;136:168-175.
47. Belshe RB, et al. *N Engl J Med*. 2007;356:685-696.
48. Rhorer J, et al. *Vaccine*. 2009;27:1101-1110.
49. Block SL, et al. *Pediatr Infect Dis J*. 2011;30:203-207.
50. Jefferson TO, et al. *Cochrane Database Syst Rev*. 2007;(2):CD001269.
51. Nichol KL, et al. *JAMA*. 1999;282:137-44.
52. Hambidge SJ, et al. *JAMA*. 2006;296:1990-1997.
53. Glanz JM, et al. *Arch Pediatr Adolesc Med*. 2011;165:749-755.
54. Boulianne N, et al. *Can Commun Dis Rep*. 2001;27:85-90.

17 Japanese Encephalitis

The Pathogen

Japanese encephalitis (JE) virus is a mosquito-borne flavivirus with a single-stranded RNA genome surrounded by a protein nucleocapsid and a lipid envelope. It is antigenically related to West Nile virus and St. Louis encephalitis virus.

Clinical Features

Only 1 in 250 to 1 in 1000 infections with JE virus results in symptomatic illness.[1] The incubation period is 5 to 15 days. The most common clinical syndrome is *acute encephalitis*, followed by *aseptic meningitis* and *undifferentiated febrile illness*. Symptoms begin abruptly with fever, lethargy, headache, abdominal pain, nausea, and vomiting. Mental status changes, including disorientation, personality change, agitation, delirium, and abnormal movements are seen, classically resembling parkinsonism, with tremor, ataxia, choreoathetosis, cogwheel rigidity, mask-like facies, and extrapyramidal signs; progression to confusion, delirium, and coma are common.[2] Mutism is a presenting sign in some cases. Up to 75% of patients present with or develop seizures. One third of patients develop cranial nerve palsies and some develop generalized or asymmetric muscular weakness, flaccid or spastic paralysis, and clonus, and some cases resemble polio.

Analysis of the CSF shows moderate lymphocytic pleocytosis and moderately elevated protein. Imaging studies may show diffuse white matter edema, abnormal signal in the thalamus, and hemorrhage. Hyponatremia due to inappropriate secretion of antidiuretic hormone is a frequent complication. The case fatality rate is 20% to 30%; recovery may take months to years, and 30% to 50% of survivors have neurologic or psychiatric sequelae, including memory loss, motor and cranial nerve paresis, movement disorders, chronic seizures, cortical blindness, and behavioral disorders. JE virus may cause intrauterine infection and miscarriage when it is acquired in the first or second trimester of pregnancy.

Epidemiology and Transmission

JE is endemic throughout China, Southeast Asia, the Indian subcontinent, Indonesia, the Philippines, and Australia; approximately half of the world's population is potentially at risk.[3] In temperate areas, transmission generally occurs from May through September with periodic seasonal epidemics. In subtropical Asia, transmission is hyperendemic and the season is longer, from March through October. In tropical Asia, transmission occurs year-round without noticeable seasonable epidemics. In areas where the virus is endemic, almost all individuals will have been infected by early adulthood.

The virus is spread by *Culex* mosquitoes, which breed in ground pools (eg, rice paddies and ditches) in rural areas. These mosquitoes feed on aquatic birds and other animals that remain asymptomatic despite infection. Domestic pigs in particular have sustained viremia and serve as host to many feeding mosquitoes. Humans, horses, and domestic animals are incidental hosts. The risk of transmission is highest in rural areas, and the incidence of disease correlates with abundance of mosquitoes, proximity of pigs and birds, rainy season, and irrigation of agricultural fields. Most cases occur in children 2 to 10 years of age. Persons who travel extensively in or move to endemic areas acquire symptomatic infection at a rate of 1 per 50,000 persons per month.[4] The risk of disease in short-term travelers to developed or urban areas is <1 per million; the risk for travelers to rural areas during the season of risk is somewhere between 1 in 5000 to 1 in 20,000 travelers per week. The risk of infection increases with travel during the transmission season, exposure to rural areas, extended period of travel or residence, and outdoor activities, especially in the evenings when mosquitoes are active. Despite the known risks, only around 10% of at-risk travelers are vaccinated.[5]

Immunization Program

Residing in air-conditioned or screened-in areas, avoiding outdoor activities, and using permethrin-treated mosquito nets, insect repellents, and protective clothing can reduce the risk of infection. Societal changes, such as urbanization, less agriculture, use of pesticides, centralized pig rearing, and improved standards of living, may also contribute to lower disease rates. Since 1996, childhood immunization programs in China, Taiwan, Japan, and Korea have resulted in marked decreases in the number of reported cases. However, there are still 30,000 to 50,000 annual cases worldwide, mostly among children.

Until 2009, the only vaccine available in the United States was an inactivated, whole-virus vaccine derived from mouse brain (JEV-MB; JE-Vax, Sanofi Pasteur). The vaccine was highly immunogenic but was also reactogenic, and there were reports of a possible association with acute disseminated encephalomyelitis (ADEM), an autoimmune disease of the central nervous system. JEV-MB was not manufactured after 2006 and stockpiled vaccine was no longer available as of February 2011. A new Vero cell culture-derived vaccine (JE-VC; Ixiaro, Novartis) was approved for use in adults in 2009 and is now the only available vaccine (JEV-MB was still used in children until 2011). Recommendations for use of JEV were published in 1993[6] and were updated in 2010.[7] Guidelines for booster dosing[8] and use of JEV-VC in children[9] were published in 2011.

Vaccines

Characteristics of the JEV licensed in the United States are given in **Table 17.1**. This is an inactivated, whole-virus vaccine, made much the same way as the original Salk vaccine.[10]

Efficacy and/or Immunogenicity

JEV-MB was tested in a placebo-controlled trial involving over 21,000 children in Thailand, where the efficacy of a 2-dose regimen was found to be 91%. Studies in the United States demonstrated that 3 doses were necessary, and the standard regimen became doses at 0, 7, and 30 days, with a booster dose in 2 years if exposure was anticipated. Immunogenicity of JEV-VC (2 doses) was compared with JEV-MB (3 doses) in a blinded, randomized controlled trial involving 867 adults.[11] The proportion of subjects who achieved a plaque reduction neutralization titer of ≥1:10 (a recognized correlate of protection) after 2 doses was 96.4%, compared with 93.8% in the control group, and the respective geometric mean titers were comparable. Licensure of JEV-VC was thus based on immunogenicity that was noninferior to JEV-MB.

Protective levels of antibody were found in 58% of adults in one study 12 months after a 2-dose primary series of JEV-VC; by 24 months, fewer than half had protective levels, but all responded to a booster dose.[12] In another study, high titers of antibody persisted for at least a year after a booster dose.[13]

Safety

In a pooled analysis of over 4000 subjects from 10 phase 3 trials, local reactions occurred in about half of vaccines, including pain (33%), tenderness (33%), redness (9%), hardening (8%), swelling (5%), and itching (4%).[14] Three percent of subjects reported at least one severe local reaction. Systemic adverse events felt to be vaccine-related included headache (19%), myalgia (13%), fatigue (10%), flu-like illness (9%), and nausea (5%). There were no vaccine-related serious adverse events. Post-marketing reports suggest that hypersensitivity reactions such as

TABLE 17.1 — **Japanese Encephalitis Vaccine**[a]

Trade name	Ixiaro
Abbreviation	JEV-VC (Vero cell-derived)
Manufacturer/distributor	Intercell Biomedical/Novartis
Type of vaccine	Inactivated, whole agent
Composition:	
Virus strain	SA_{14}-14-2
Propagation	Vero cells
Inactivation	Formaldehyde
Adjuvant	Aluminum hydroxide (0.25 mg)
Preservative	None
Excipients and contaminants	Formaldehyde (≤200 ppm) Bovine serum albumin (≤100 ng/mL) Host cell DNA (≤200 pg/mL) Sodium metabisulphite (≤200 ppm) Host cell proteins (≤300 ng/6 mcg protein) Protamine sulfate (≤1 mcg/mL)
Latex	None
Labeled indications	Prevention of JE
Labeled ages	≥17 years
Dose	0.5 mL
Route of administration	Intramuscular
Labeled schedule	0, 28 days Booster dose if exposure is anticipated and >1 year have elapsed since primary series
Recommended schedule	Same See text regarding vaccination of children <17 years of age Persons ≥17 years of age previously vaccinated with JEV-MB and in need of a booster should receive 2 doses
How supplied (number in package)	Prefilled syringe (1)
Cost per dose ($US, 2011):	
Public	—
Private	216.30
Reference package insert	September 2010

[a] Mouse brain-derived vaccine (JEV-MB; JE-Vax, Sanofi Pasteur) was not manufactured after 2006, but stockpiled vaccine was available until February 2011.

urticaria and swelling of the upper airway are less common after JEV-VC than was reported after JEV-MB.[14]

- *Contraindications*
  - Severe allergic reaction (eg, anaphylaxis) to previous dose of vaccine or any vaccine component (risk of recurrent allergic reaction)
- *Precautions*
  - Moderate or severe acute illness
  - Pregnancy (theoretical risk to the fetus or attribution of birth defects to vaccination). No deleterious effects have been demonstrated from JEV administration during pregnancy, and the risk of adverse fetal effects from an inactivated vaccine is extremely low.

Recommendations

Vaccination is not recommended for short-term travelers who will be restricted to urban areas or who are traveling outside of transmission season. Factors that should be considered in the decision to vaccinate include the incidence of JE in the location of intended stay, the conditions of housing, nature of activities, duration of stay, and the possibility of unexpected travel to high-risk areas. In general, persons spending a month or longer in epidemic or endemic areas during the transmission season, especially if travel will include rural areas, should be vaccinated (see *Chapter 6: Vaccination in Special Circumstances—Travel*). Depending on the epidemic circumstances, vaccination should be considered for persons spending <30 days who are at particularly high risk, such as those engaging in extensive outdoor activities (eg, camping, hiking, fishing) in rural areas and those whose accommodations lack air conditioning, screens, or bed nets. Vaccination also should be considered for travel to areas with ongoing outbreaks and those who have uncertain or nonspecific itineraries. The vaccine series should be completed at least 1 week before potential exposure, and travelers should take personal precautions to reduce exposure to mosquito bites. Current CDC advisories should be consulted with regard to disease activity in specific locales.

Children <17 years of age may be vaccinated (off-label recommendation). Alternatives to off-label vaccination include enrollment in a clinical trial[15] or having the child vaccinated at an international travelers' health clinic in Asia.

Laboratory workers with potential exposure to infectious JE virus should be vaccinated. Periodic monitoring for neutralizing antibodies and/or administration of booster doses may be indicated.

REFERENCES

1. Thongcharoen P. *Southeast Asian J Trop Med Public Health.* 1989;20:559-573.
2. Ooi MH, et al. *Clin Infect Dis*. 2008;47:458-468.
3. Erlanger TE, et al. *Emerg Infect Dis*. 2009;15:1-7.
4. Shlim DR, et al. *Clin Infect Dis*. 2002;35:183-188.
5. Duffy M, Reed C, Edelson P, et al. Survey of US travelers to Asia to assess compliance with recommendations for Japanese encephalitis vaccine [presentation]. International Conference on Emerging Infectious Diseases; March 16-19, 2008, Atlanta, GA.
6. CDC. *MMWR*. 1993;42(RR-1):1-15.
7. Fischer M, et al. *MMWR*. 2010;59(RR-1):1-27.
8. CDC. *MMWR*. 2011;60:661-663.
9. CDC. *MMWR*. 2011;60:664-665.
10. Beasley DWC, et al. *Expert Opin Biol Ther*. 2008;8:95-106.
11. Tauber E, et al. *Lancet*. 2007;370:1847-1853.
12. Dubischar-Kastner K, et al. *Vaccine*. 2010;28:5197-5202.
13. Eder S, et al. *Vaccine*. 2011;29:2607-2612.
14. Schuller E, et al. *Vaccine*. 2011;29:8669-8676.
15. Update on Japanese encephalitis (JE) vaccine for U.S. children. Centers for Disease Control and Prevention Web site. http://www.cdc.gov/ncidod/dvbid/jencephalitis/children.htm. Accessed January 21, 2012.

18 Measles, Mumps, Rubella

The Pathogens

Measles

Measles (rubeola) virus is an enveloped, single-stranded RNA virus in the Paramyxoviridae family.[1] There is only one serotype. Two proteins—the hemagglutinin, which mediates attachment, and the fusion protein, which facilitates cell-to-cell spread—are important in generating neutralizing antibodies. The virus infects the nasopharyngeal epithelium and then spreads to regional lymph nodes, where replication leads to widespread dissemination, including the reticuloendothelial system, viscera, respiratory tract, and skin. Pathologic changes include lymphoid hyperplasia, mononuclear cell infiltration of infected tissues, and multinucleated giant cells. Virus-induced immune suppression leads to secondary bacterial and viral infection, including pneumonia and gastroenteritis.

Mumps

Mumps virus is an enveloped, single-stranded RNA virus in the Paramyxoviridae family.[2] While the virus is not classified into serotypes, there are 12 known genotypes (A through L) that vary in geographic distribution. A surface hemagglutinin-neuraminidase and fusion protein mediate, respectively, adsorption to cells and fusion with the cell membrane. Initial infection occurs in the nasopharyngeal epithelium and then spreads to regional lymph nodes, where replication leads to plasma viremia and dissemination via mononuclear cells. The virus is tropic for glandular epithelia, including the salivary glands (especially the parotids), pancreas, ovaries, and testes, where infection can lead to atrophy of the germinal epithelium. Pathologic changes include interstitial edema and lymphocytic infiltration. The virus also may spread to the central nervous system (CNS), where it infects the choroidal epithelium and ependymal lining of the ventricles, resulting in aseptic meningitis, and, in some cases, encephalitis.

Rubella

Rubella virus is an enveloped, single-stranded RNA virus in the Togavirus family.[3] Neutralizing antibodies are directed predominately against E1, a major surface glycoprotein with hemagglutinin and fusion activity. There is only one serotype, although the virus is classified into genotypes I and II based on E1 sequences. Infection occurs in the nasopharyngeal epithelium and then spreads to regional lymph nodes, where replication leads to viremia and dissemination to the respiratory tract, skin, lymph nodes, body fluids, and, in pregnant women, the placenta. While postnatal infection is relatively benign, infection of the fetus leads to progressive, generalized vasculitis, affecting organ development. A characteristic feature of early fetal infection is cell necrosis without an inflammatory response, consistent with the virus' ability to induce apoptosis and the immaturity of the fetal immune system. Another characteristic is persistent viral replication, thought to be related to immune tolerance.

Clinical Features

Measles

Measles is characterized by a several-day prodrome of malaise, fever, anorexia, *cough, coryza*, and *conjunctivitis*.[1] Temperature usually increases for 5 or 6 days and can be as high as 104°F (40°C). *Koplik's spots*—small white lesions on the buccal mucosa that resemble grains of sand on a moist, red background—appear between the second and fourth days. After this, a characteristic *rash* appears around the ears and hairline and spreads downward and outward to cover the face, trunk, and extremities over the next 3 to 4 days. Initially erythematous, maculopapular, and splotchy, the rash tends to become confluent as it spreads, especially on the face and neck, lasts about 5 days and resolves in the order of appearance.

Complications, including diarrhea, middle ear infection, and bronchopneumonia, occur in up to 40% of patients. *Encephalitis* occurs in approximately 1 out of every 1000 cases, and survivors often have permanent brain damage. Death, usually from pneumonia or acute encephalitis, occurs in 1 to 2 out of every 1000 cases; the risk is greater for infants, young children, and adults than it is for older children and adolescents. *Subacute sclerosing panencephalitis* is a rare, fatal degenerative disease of the CNS that appears years after measles infection (1 in 10,000 to 100,000 patients) and is caused by persistent infection with a mutant form of the virus.

In developing countries, measles is often more severe, with case-fatality rates as high as 25%. Measles can be severe in persons with vitamin A deficiency, as well as in immunocompromised persons, particularly those who have leukemia, lymphoma, or HIV infection.

Mumps

About two-thirds of infections are symptomatic, and 95% of those with symptoms develop *parotitis*, usually characterized by fever, headache, malaise, myalgia, anorexia, and bilateral swelling of the parotid glands.[2] Parotitis occurs more commonly among children and subclinical infection is more common among adults. The disease is usually self-limited but complications do occur.

Orchitis, characterized by abrupt onset of testicular swelling, warmth, and tenderness accompanied by high fever, vomiting, headache, and malaise, is the most common complication in adult males, occurring in up to 30% of cases. Half of patients are left with some degree of testicular atrophy, but sterility is unusual. *Oophoritis* develops in 5% of postpubertal women. *Aseptic meningitis* is common, occurring asymptomatically in half of patients and associated with headache and stiff neck in up to 10%. Adults are at greater risk for this complication than children, and boys are more often affected than girls. *Encephalitis* is rare, occurring in 0.1% of infections. Mumps was a leading cause of acquired *sensorineural deafness* in the prevaccine era, with an estimated incidence of one per 20,000 cases.

■ Rubella

Rubella is characterized by nonspecific signs and symptoms including transient, erythematous, and sometimes pruritic *rash*, postauricular or suboccipital lymphadenopathy, arthralgia, and low-grade fever.[3] Twenty-five percent to 50% of infections are subclinical, and while up to 60% of postpubertal women develop *arthritis*, the disease is generally considered benign and self-limited—unless you are a fetus.

Maternal-fetal transmission rates approach 100% in the first trimester, and fetal damage is almost universal. Whereas transmission is common later in gestation, fetal damage is rare. Manifestations of *congenital rubella syndrome* (CRS) at birth include deafness, cataracts, micro-ophthalmia, cardiac defects, and CNS abnormalities. Late effects, most notably type 1 diabetes, may occur.

Epidemiology and Transmission

■ Measles

Humans are the only natural hosts. In temperate climates, measles usually occurs in late winter and spring. Transmission is primarily person-to-person via large respiratory droplets. Airborne transmission has been documented in closed areas (such as office examination rooms) after the presence of an infected person. Measles is one of the most contagious diseases known to man, with secondary household attack rates exceeding 90%. In 1999, decades after the first measles vaccine was introduced, there were nearly 1 million deaths worldwide; by 2008, after a call to action by the World Health Assembly, that number had fallen to 164,000. Eradication is considered feasible, but there are many obstacles.[1]

It is estimated that before the introduction of the first vaccine in 1963, there were 3 to 4 million cases of measles each year in the United States. That number had fallen to about 1500 by 1983.[4] However, between 1989 and 1991, there were almost 56,000 reported cases and 123 deaths.[5] This resurgence was primarily due to pockets of low vaccine coverage in the population. Another contributing factor was the fact that infants <1 year of age were more susceptible than in previous eras—their mothers had vaccine-induced immunity rather than natural immunity, and their transplacental antibody inheritance was lower. Primary vaccine failure after one dose, which occurs in 2% to 5% of children, also may have contributed.

Renewed efforts to vaccinate young children and the institution of a second dose at school entry reversed the resurgence, such that by 2000, measles was considered to be no longer endemic in the United States.[6] This is not to say that importation-related outbreaks do not continue to occur. For example, from January through July of 2008, 131 measles cases were reported; 17 were directly imported from other countries and 99 were epidemiologically linked to imported cases. Eleven percent of the patients were hospitalized. Among the 123 US residents who got measles, 80% were under 20 years of age and 91% were either unvaccinated or had unknown vaccination status.[7] Measles was seen again in 2011—118 cases were reported in the first 19 weeks, and, as in 2008, most cases were associated with importation and unvaccinated status.[8] These experiences underscore the importance of maintaining immunization rates at home as well as immunizing travelers.[9] It sounds cliché, but—quite literally—measles is just a plane flight away.

■ Mumps

Humans are the only natural hosts. Incidence peaks in winter and spring, but disease has been reported throughout the year. Transmission occurs through airborne droplet nuclei or direct contact with saliva. Contagiousness is similar to that of influenza and rubella but less than that for measles and chickenpox. The infectious period is from 3 days before to 4 days after the onset of active disease.

In 1968, just after licensure of the first vaccine, there were 185,691 cases of mumps in the United States.[1] By 2006, despite a resurgence among teenagers in the late 1980s that was reversed by the recommendation for a second dose of MMR, the number of cases had fallen to below 500.[10] However, 2006 saw a multistate outbreak with nearly 7000 cases, mostly among college students and other young adults, many of whom had received 2 doses of the vaccine.[11] Another large outbreak in the New York area began in June 2009.[12] The index case was an 11-year-old boy who had acquired mumps in the United Kingdom and attended a tradition-observant Jewish summer camp after returning to the United States. By January 2010, 1521 cases had been reported, most of which had occurred in the same Jewish community; 75% of case patients had received 2 doses of vaccine.

■ Rubella

Humans are the only natural hosts. In temperate climates, rubella occurs in late winter and early spring. There is no carrier state per se, but infants with CRS may shed large quantities of virus for up to a year. Rubella is only moderately contagious and spreads from person-to-person via airborne droplet nuclei shed from the respiratory tract. Transmission by subclinical cases, which constitute 20% to 50% of all infections, can occur. The disease is most contagious when the rash is erupting, but virus may be shed from 7 days before to 7 days after rash onset. Between 1964 and 1965, there were >12 million cases of rubella in the United States and 20,000 babies were born with CRS.[13] After vaccination was initiated in 1969, the number of cases declined dramatically, such that by 2004, rubella was considered to be no longer endemic in the United States.[14] Disease, however, is still seen, especially in immigrants from Latin America.

Immunization Program

The rationale for measles and mumps immunization is to prevent complications and death in children and adults. The rationale for rubella immunization is to prevent infection in pregnant women, thereby preventing CRS. The first live-attenuated measles vaccine was licensed in 1963; mumps vaccine was licensed in 1967, and rubella vaccine in 1969. The MMR was licensed in 1971; in 1979, a rubella vaccine grown in human diploid fibroblasts (RA 27/3) was licensed and replaced the duck embryo-passaged strain that was in MMR (hence the trade name M-M-R_{II}). Since 1980, MMR has been the preferred vaccine against these diseases. A single dose was recommended for all children at 15 months of age until 1989, when the measles resurgence discussed above prompted recommendations for a routine second dose at 4 to 6 years of age.[15] In 1998, the age for the first dose was changed to 12 to 15 months, and the preference for MMR (as opposed to the corresponding component vaccines) was reiterated.[4] MMRV was licensed in 2005, and, in the context of a general preference for combination vaccines, was preferred over separate MMR plus VAR (see *Chapter 29: Combination Vaccines*).[16]

In 2006, in response to the mumps resurgence discussed above, the 2-dose requirement was extended to mumps immunization (practically speaking, this had already occurred because of the 2-dose measles recommendation and the use of MMR).[17] In 2008, because of concerns over febrile seizures (see *Chapter 7: Addressing Concerns About Vaccines—Can Vaccines Cause Febrile Seizures?*), the general preference for MMRV was retracted.[18] In 2010, the ACIP clarified that while either MMR plus VAR or MMRV could be used for the first dose when given at 12 to 47 months of age, the former was preferred unless the parents expressed a preference for the combination.[19] Differing slightly from this position, the AAP maintained that either option was acceptable, as long as the caregivers were fully informed about the risks and benefits (ie, febrile seizures with MMRV, extra injection with MMR plus VAR).[20] MMRV is generally preferred for the second dose. Recommendations for HCP, including the definition of evidence of immunity, were updated in 2011.[21]

Use of MMR in the United States has been remarkably successful, leading to the elimination of endemic transmission of measles and rubella and drastically reducing the annual number of reported cases of mumps. However, since 1998 these successes have been threatened by the false belief that MMR vaccine causes autism (see *Chapter 7: Addressing Concerns About Vaccines—Does MMR Cause Autism?*).

Vaccines

Characteristics of the MMR vaccine licensed in the United States are given in **Table 18.1**. This vaccine is a mixture of live-attenuated strains of measles, mumps, and rubella viruses. Each was attenuated by serial passage in tissue culture, much the same way as the Sabin polio vaccine.

Efficacy and/or Immunogenicity

■ Measles

Antibodies develop in approximately 95% of children vaccinated at 12 months of age and 98% of children vaccinated at 15 months of age. Studies show that >99% of persons who receive 2 doses of vaccine (separated by at least 1 month) at ≥1 year of age develop serologic evidence of measles immunity. Although vaccine-induced antibody titers are lower than those following natural disease, immunity is probably lifelong in most people. Individuals who lose antibody over time have demonstrable anamnestic responses to revaccination, indicating that they are most likely still protected. A small percentage of vaccinated individuals may lose protection after several years.

■ Mumps

More than 97% of vaccinees develop protective antibody titers. In postlicensure studies conducted between 1973 and 1989, efficacy of a single dose was 75% to 91%, and efficacy of 2 doses during the 2006 US outbreak was estimated at 76% to 88%.[22] A study published in 2008 showed that 94% of university students and staff had antibody to mumps virus after having received 2 doses of vaccine.[23] The level of antibody was lower among those vaccinated ≥15 years earlier compared with those vaccinated in the preceding 5 years, but seronegative subjects mounted anamnestic responses after repeat vaccination. Whereas antibody titers have been shown to wane with time,[24] cellular responses have been shown to persist beyond 15 years.[25]

The continued occurrence of mumps outbreaks has raised concerns about vaccine efficacy and persistence of immunity.[26] It is possible that 2 doses of the current vaccine may not be enough to overcome contagion in high-density communal living situations. Moreover, as 2-dose coverage rates exceed 90%, the herd immunity threshold (see *Chapter 1: Introduction to Vaccinology—Herd Immunity*) may be higher than once thought and not achievable with current recommendations.[27]

■ Rubella

At least 95% of vaccinees ≥12 months of age develop protective antibody titers. Vaccine-induced rubella antibodies have persisted in >90% of vaccinees at least 15 years after receipt of the RA 27/3 vaccine. Lifelong protection against clinical reinfection, asymptomatic viremia, or both usually results from a single dose of vaccine early in childhood. In some cases, vaccinees exposed to natural rubella develop an asymptomatic increase in antibody titer (reinfection with wild-type rubella virus has been observed in persons with previous natural rubella). However, infection of vaccinees is rarely associated with viremia or pharyngeal shedding, and, among vaccinated women, the risk of CRS from rubella infection during pregnancy is extremely low.

Safety

Five to 15% of vaccinees develop fever ≥103°F (39.4°C) and about 5% develop a mild measles-like rash, usually within 7 to 10 days. Transient lymphadenopathy sometimes occurs, and parotitis has been reported rarely. Arthralgia, reported in up to 25% of susceptible adult women given MMR, is attributed to the rubella component; persistent or recurrent joint symptoms are rare (the incidence of joint problems after immunization is lower than that after natural infection).

One case of immune thrombocytopenic purpura, defined as a platelet count ≤50,000 per microliter with clinical bleeding, occurs for every 40,000 doses; this is much less than the incidence after natural measles or rubella.[28] Severe bleeding is rare and the vast majority of patients recover completely.[29] The risk of febrile seizures is increased 2- to 3-fold in the second week after vaccination, but there is no association with subsequent seizures or neurodevelopmental disabilities.[30] Most allergic reactions are minor and consist of a wheal and flare or urticaria at the injection site, and anaphylactic reactions are extremely rare. The vaccine does not contain significant amounts of egg protein and can safely

TABLE 18.1 — Measles, Mumps, and Rubella Vaccine[a]

Trade name	M-M-R_{II}
Abbreviation	MMR
Manufacturer/distributor	Merck
Type of vaccine	Live-attenuated, classical
Composition	Measles virus, Moraten strain (derived from the Edmonston B strain), propagated in chick embryo cells, at least 1000 $TCID_{50}$ Mumps virus, Jeryl Lynn strain (actually consists of two distinct strains), propagated in chick embryo cells, at least 12,500 $TCID_{50}$ Rubella virus, RA 27/3 strain, propagated in human diploid lung fibroblast (WI-38) cells, at least 1000 $TCID_{50}$
Adjuvant	None
Preservative	None
Excipients and contaminants	Sorbitol (14.5 mg) Sodium phosphate Sucrose (1.9 mg) Sodium chloride Hydrolyzed gelatin (14.5 mg) Recombinant human albumin (≤0.3 mg) Fetal bovine serum (<1 ppm) Neomycin (25 mcg) Buffer and media ingredients
Latex	None
Labeled indications	Prevention of measles, mumps, and rubella
Labeled ages	≥12 months
Dose	0.5 mL
Route of administration	Subcutaneous
Labeled schedule	12 to 15 months Revaccination before school entry
Recommended schedule	12 to 15 months, 4 to 6 years of age
How supplied (number in package)	1-dose vial (10), lyophilized, with diluent
Cost per dose ($US, 2011):	
Public	18.99
Private	52.07
Reference package insert	December 2010

Continued

TABLE 18.1 — *Continued*

[a] The components of MMR (Attenuvax [measles], Mumpsvax [mumps], Meruvax II [rubella], and M-M-Vax [measles and mumps]) are licensed by Merck as separate vaccines, but as of 2008, are no longer available in the United States. MMR is also available in combination with VAR (MMRV; ProQuad, Merck).

be given to patients with allergies to eggs, chickens, and feathers without prior skin testing and without incremental dosing.

The viruses in MMR are not transmitted from person-to-person after vaccination and therefore the vaccine can be given to contacts of immunosuppressed and pregnant individuals.

- *Contraindications*
  - Severe allergic reaction (eg, anaphylaxis) to previous dose of vaccine or any vaccine component (risk of recurrent allergic reaction; this includes reactions to gelatin and neomycin)
  - Severe immunodeficiency or immunosuppression (risk of disease caused by live virus)
  - Pregnancy (theoretical risk to the fetus of live-virus vaccine or attribution of birth defects to vaccination). ACIP recommends that vaccinated women avoid pregnancy for 1 month; the package insert says 3 months (ACIP recommendations are usually followed in practice).
- *Precautions*
  - Moderate or severe acute illness (difficulty distinguishing illness from vaccine reaction)
  - History of thrombocytopenia or thrombocytopenic purpura (risk of recurrent thrombocytopenia)
  - Recent receipt of antibody-containing blood product (risk of impaired response to vaccine)
  - Active, untreated tuberculosis (risk of exacerbation of tuberculosis; initiate antituberculosis therapy before vaccinating). Measles vaccine virus replication can suppress the response to a tuberculin skin test (TST) and may cause false negative results in an interferon-gamma release assay (IGRA). If testing for tuberculosis is warranted, the preferred option is to place the TST or perform an IGRA on the same day as measles vaccination (any immunosuppression would occur later, at the peak of viral replication). Otherwise, the tuberculosis test should be delayed ≥4 weeks. Note that the package insert states that persons with active, untreated tuberculosis should not be vaccinated.
  - MMRV: personal, sibling or parent history of seizures (risk of febrile seizure)

Recommendations

All persons who do not have evidence of immunity to measles, mumps, and rubella should be vaccinated with MMR. The criteria for immunity to these diseases are given in **Table 18.2**. For children, the first dose is usually given at 12 to 15 months of age and the second dose at 4 to 6 years of age. The second dose may be given any time ≥28 days following the first dose. High-risk adults who lack evidence of immunity should receive 2 doses of MMR separated by ≥28 days (those who have a history of 1 dose in the past should have a second dose). Low-risk adults who lack evidence of immunity should receive at least 1 dose. Women who might become pregnant and who lack evidence of immunity should receive 1 dose of MMR (pregnancy should be deferred at least 1 month after vaccination). Rubella vaccine may be given after anti-Rho(D) immune globulin administration, but testing for seroconversion should be performed 6 to 8 weeks later.

During measles outbreaks, when the likelihood of exposure is high, measles vaccine can be given to infants as young as 6 months of age. Doses given before the first birthday, however, *do not count* in the series, and these children should receive 2 subsequent doses according to the usual schedule. Persons who lack evidence of immunity and are planning travel to areas where measles or mumps are endemic (this includes developed countries like the United Kingdom) should receive 2 doses of MMR (separated by ≥28 days) before leaving. Infants 6 to 12 months of age who will be traveling anywhere outside the United States (even places like Canada, but not including US territories like Puerto Rico, the Virgin Islands, American Samoa, etc.) should receive 1 dose, but should be revaccinated according to the routine schedule when they reach 12 months of age (vaccination of infants <6 months of age is not necessary because most will be protected by maternal antibodies).

Measles vaccine given within 72 hours of exposure to measles may prevent infection, but this is not true for mumps and rubella vaccines. Immunocompromised individuals who are exposed to measles should receive intramuscular immune globulin, 0.5 mL/kg (maximum 15 mL), within 6 days of exposure. The AAP recommends immune globulin prophylaxis for *all* HIV-infected children and adolescents exposed to measles, regardless of vaccination status, degree of symptoms, and level of immune suppression (the dose for asymptomatic HIV-infected persons is 0.25 mL/kg, maximum 15 mL); the ACIP specifies prophylaxis only for *symptomatic* HIV infection. Susceptible household contacts of measles cases, especially those <1 year of age, should receive immune globulin as well (0.25 mL/kg, maximum 15 mL). Immune globulin is not recommended for postexposure prophylaxis against rubella or mumps.

REFERENCES

1. Moss WJ, et al. *Lancet*. 2012;379:153-164.
2. Hviid A, et al. *Lancet*. 2008;371:932-944.
3. Banatvala JE, et al. *Lancet*. 2004;363:1127-1137.
4. Watson JC, et al. *MMWR*. 1998;47(RR-8):1-57.
5. The National Vaccine Advisory Committee. *JAMA*. 1991;266:1547-1552.
6. CDC. *MMWR*. 2004;53:713-716.
7. CDC. *MMWR*. 2008;57:893-896.
8. CDC. *MMWR*. 2011;60:666-668.
9. Cocoros NM, et al. *MMWR*. 2011;60:398-401.
10. McNabb SJN, et al. *MMWR*. 2007;54:2-92.
11. Dayan GH, et al. *N Engl J Med*. 2008;358:1580-1589.
12. High P, et al. *MMWR*. 2010;59:125-129.
13. CDC. *MMWR*. 2005;54:279-282.
14. Reef SE, et al. *Clin Infect Dis*. 2006;43(suppl 3):S126-S132.
15. CDC. *MMWR*. 1989;38(S-9):1-18.
16. CDC. *MMWR*. 2005;54:1212-1214.
17. CDC. *MMWR*. 2006;55:629-630.
18. CDC. *MMWR*. 2008;57:258-260.
19. CDC.*MMWR*. 2010;59(RR-3):1-12.
20. American Academy of Pediatrics Committee on Infectious Diseases. *Pediatrics*. 2011;128;630-632.
21. Shefer A, et al. *MMWR*. 2011;60(RR-7):1-45.
22. Marin M, et al. *Vaccine*. 2008;26:3601-3607.
23. Date AA, et al. *J Infect Dis*. 2008;197:1662-1668.
24. LeBaron CW, et al. *J Infect Dis*. 2009;199:552-560.
25. Vandermeulen C, et al. *J Infect Dis*. 2009;199:1457-1460.
26. Quinlisk MP. *J Infect* Dis. 2010;202:655-656.
27. Kutty PK, et al. *J Infect Dis*. 2010;202:667-674.
28. France EK, et al. *Pediatrics*. 2008;121:e687-e692.
29. Mantadakis E, et al. *J Pediatr*. 2010;156:623-628.
30. Vestergaard M, et al. *JAMA*. 2004;292:351-357.

TABLE 18.2 — Immunity to Measles, Mumps, and Rubella

	Persons to Whom the Criteria Apply		
Criteria[a]	**Measles**	**Mumps**	**Rubella**
Birth before 1957	Everyone except HCP[b]	Everyone except HCP[b]	Everyone except HCP[b] and women who might become pregnant
Personal history of clinical disease	Persons with a history of *physician-diagnosed* disease except HCP[b]	Persons with a history of *physician-diagnosed* disease except HCP[b]	Not considered reliable evidence of immunity in anyone
Personal history of laboratory-confirmed disease	Everyone	Everyone	Everyone
Written history of at least 1 properly administered vaccine dose	Children 1 year of age to school age Low-risk adults	Children 1 year of age to school age Low-risk adults	Anyone ≥1 year of age
Written history of at least 2 properly administered vaccine doses	School age children (grades K-12) High-risk adults (HCP[b], international travelers, students at postsecondary educational institutions)	School age children (grades K-12) High-risk adults (HCP[b], international travelers, students at postsecondary educational institutions)	Not required

Positive virus-specific IgG antibody test[c]	Everyone	Everyone	Everyone

[a] Any one criterion is considered sufficient. Clinical, virologic, and vaccination criteria trump the results of serologic tests. For example, HCP with written documentation of 2 properly administered doses of MMR are considered immune even if their antibody tests are negative.
[b] Vaccination (2 doses of MMR separated by ≥28 days) should be considered for unvaccinated HCP born before 1957 without laboratory evidence of immunity or a history of laboratory-confirmed disease. If there is an outbreak, vaccination should be recommended. A personal history of physician-diagnosed measles or mumps is not sufficient proof of immunity for HCP.
[c] Equivocal results are considered negative.

Adapted from Watson JC, et al. *MMWR*. 1998;47(RR-8):1-57; CDC. *MMWR*. 2006;55:629-630; and Shefer A, et al. *MMWR*. 2011;60(RR-7):1-48.

19 *Neisseria meningitidis*

The Pathogen

N meningitidis is a gram-negative bacterium that typically takes the appearance of intracellular diplococci on Gram stain.[1] The organism produces a polysaccharide capsule that is the basis for classification into serogroups, the most important of which are A, B, C, W-135, and Y. The capsule contributes to virulence by inhibiting complement-mediated lysis, phagocytosis by neutrophils, and the action of antimicrobial peptides (antibodies to the capsular polysaccharide are protective).[2] Pathogenicity is enhanced by the production of endotoxin. *N meningitidis* often colonizes the nasopharynx, and disease results from bacteremia and spread to distant sites such as the meninges. Colonization occurs through the interaction between host cell receptors and bacterial adhesins, which undergo antigenic and phase variation that facilitate evasion of host immunity.[3] Certain genetic polymorphisms, particularly those involving the complement and coagulation systems, contribute to disease outcome.[4]

Clinical Features

Meningococcemia (bloodstream infection with *N meningitidis*) is characterized by the sudden onset of fever, lethargy, myalgia, rash, and vomiting, followed by altered mental status, high fever or hypothermia, tachypnea, and hypotension.[1] Initially, the rash may be macular or maculopapular, but there is rapid transition to petechiae and/or purpura. *Purpura fulminans* is characterized by rapid progression to disseminated intravascular coagulation, hypotension, and shock within hours, despite antimicrobial therapy and supportive measures. Death is common, and survivors may lose extensive areas of skin or extremities due to ischemia. Some individuals experience transient meningococcal bacteremia that resolves spontaneously without treatment.

Meningococcal *meningitis* presents with fever, vomiting, headache, and photophobia. It is distinguished from other forms of pyogenic meningitis by the association with petechial or purpuric rash in two thirds of patients. Neurologic sequelae include deafness, cranial nerve palsies, hydrocephalus, and developmental delay. Meningococcus also causes pneumonia, myocarditis, pericarditis, arthritis, conjunctivitis, endophthalmitis, urethritis, and pharyngitis. Immune-mediated arthritis, cutaneous vasculitis, and pericarditis can occur late in the course of infection, after antibiotic therapy is instituted. *Chronic meningococcemia* occurs rarely and is characterized by recurrent episodes of fever, chills, rash, arthralgias, and headache over a 6- to 8-week period.

Epidemiology and Transmission

Humans are the only natural hosts and transmission occurs by direct person-to-person contact or via respiratory droplets. Asymptomatic carriage of *N meningitidis* is low in infants, around 5%, and increases to almost 25% in young adults.[5] Colonization with invasive strains approaches 50% in closed settings where a case has occurred. The secondary attack rate in households is 3% to 4%, and the risk to household members is 500 to 800 times the risk in the general population (this is why chemoprophylaxis is used for close contacts).

Data from 1998 to 2007 indicate that the highest incidence of invasive meningococcal disease, 5.4 per 100,000, occurs in infants <1 year of age.[6] A second peak, 0.78 per 100,000, occurs in adolescence and young adulthood, when intimate contact with other people increases. The overall incidence of disease decreased 64% from 1998 to 2007, probably the result of natural epidemiological cycles, less smoking and crowding in the population, and increased antibiotic use. Disease occurs predominantly in late winter and early spring, and outbreaks may parallel increases in influenza activity. Risk factors include active and passive smoking, respiratory illness, steroid use, new residence, new school, lower socioeconomic status, and household crowding. Individuals with congenital or acquired immunodeficiency, especially complement deficiency (classically terminal component deficiency), asplenia, antibody deficiency, and HIV infection are also at increased risk. During outbreaks, alcohol use and patronizing bars and nightclubs are implicated as risk factors.

Epidemics caused by serogroup A most commonly occur in the meningitis belt of sub-Saharan Africa, central Asia, the Indian subcontinent, and Saudi Arabia. Such epidemics are rare in developed countries. In the United States, the vast majority of cases are sporadic, but localized outbreaks have increased. In the 1980s, most US cases were due to serogroups B and C, and only 2% were due to serogroup Y. By the 1990s, serogroups B, C, and Y each accounted for about one third of cases.[7] Between 1998 and 2007, serogroup B accounted for 31% of invasive disease overall but 57% of cases <1 year of age; overall, serogroup C accounted for 28% and serogroup Y 34% of cases.[6]

Immunization Program

Prior to the initiation of a universal adolescent immunization program in the United States, up to 2800 cases of invasive disease occurred each year. The overall case-fatality rate was close to

10% and was higher (around 20%) in adolescents than in young children (around 5%).[8] Up to 20% of survivors had some form of permanent disability; that proportion approached 60% in teenage survivors.[9] Half of patients had meningitis, making *N meningitidis* the most common cause of bacterial meningitis in persons 2 to 18 years of age.

Since licensure in 1981, MPSV4 was used in persons with medical conditions that placed them at high risk for meningococcal disease, as well as in persons traveling to endemic areas, laboratory workers, and for outbreak control. The vaccine was never recommended for universal use for a number of reasons, including the limited duration of protection, absence of herd-immunity effects, and the low incidence of disease in the general population. In the late 1990s, studies showed that college freshmen living in dormitories were at increased risk for meningococcal disease, of the order of 2- to 5-fold higher than the general population.[10] Upwards of 80% of these cases were caused by serotypes A, C, W-135, or Y. In 2000, it was recommended that all college students be informed about the risk of meningococcal disease, and that MPSV4 be made available to those who requested it.[11] It was estimated that vaccination of all college freshmen living in dormitories would prevent 16 to 30 cases and one to three deaths, at a cost of $617,000 to $1.85 million per case prevented and $6.8 to $20.4 million per death prevented.

The licensure of MCV4-D in 2005 prompted reassessment of the meningococcal prevention strategy in the United States. Meningococcal conjugate vaccines can engender more effective and longer-lived antibody responses, and reduced nasopharyngeal colonization and resultant herd immunity would be expected. The reality of herd effects was borne out in the experience with serogroup C conjugate vaccines in the United Kingdom, where a universal immunization program for children 12 months to 17 years of age initiated in 1999 resulted in dramatic declines in disease among both vaccinated and unvaccinated persons, as well as decreases in nasopharyngeal carriage.[12,13] It was estimated that a universal MCV4 program in the United States for children 11 years of age plus a catch-up campaign for adolescents would, assuming herd effects, prevent >5000 cases over a 10-year period, at a cost of $532,000 per case prevented and $5.9 million per death prevented.[14]

These estimates make routine MCV4 vaccination more costly per health outcome than the programs for prevention of disease due to *H influenzae* type b and *S pneumoniae*. Nevertheless, recommendations for universal immunization of adolescents at 11 to 12 years of age, with limited catch-up of adolescents at 15 years of age, were released in 2005[14]; the idea was to provide protection against the exposures that would occur in high school (more aggressive catch-up was not recommended because of anticipated supply issues). It was felt that immunization at 11 to 12 years of age would anchor the recommended routine preadolescent health care visit and would lay a foundation for the adolescent vaccination platform, which has since been rounded out with Tdap and HPV. MCV4-D also was recommended as a replacement for MPSV4 in high-risk persons 11 to 55 years of age, and the recommendation for college freshmen living in dormitories was strengthened from "educate" to "vaccinate."

In 2007, when supply was sufficient, catch-up of all adolescents 11 to 18 years of age with MCV4-D was recommended.[15] Also in that year, with extension of the label down to 2 years of age, the recommendation was made to substitute MCV4-D for MPSV4 in high-risk children.[16] In 2008, the decision was made *not* to recommend universal immunization of children 2 to 10 years of age, for the following reasons: 1) it was not clear that immunization at younger ages would provide protection when it would be needed most, ie, at high school entry; 2) the burden of disease in that age group was lower than in infants and adolescents, and a smaller proportion of cases were due to vaccine serogroups; and 3) vaccinating children at 2 years of age would be much less cost-effective than vaccinating children at 11 years of age.[17]

In 2009, the ACIP recommended routine revaccination of persons who remain at high risk.[18] MCV4-CRM was licensed in 2010 for use in persons 11 to 55 years of age, and updated recommendations were issued.[19] Also in 2010, because of studies demonstrating waning immunity, the ACIP recommended a routine one-time booster dose for adolescents, as well as a 2-dose primary series for persons with persistent complement component deficiency, functional or anatomic asplenia, and adolescents with HIV infection who are receiving routine immunization (routine revaccination also was recommended for persons with persistent complement component deficiency and functional or anatomic asplenia).[20] In addition, immunization for college students was recommended whether or not they would be living in dormitories. In January 2011, the license for MCV4-CRM was extended to include children 2 to 10 years of age,[21] and in April 2011, the license for MCV4-D was extended to include a 2-dose primary series for infants 9 to 23 months of age; recommendations for use in high-risk children in that age group were published shortly thereafter.[22]

Vaccines

Characteristics of meningococcal vaccines licensed in the United States are given in **Table 19.1**. One consists of pure polysaccharide and the other two are protein-polysaccharide conjugates, made much the same way as Hib and PCV13.[23] Biologic differences between conjugate and polysaccharide vaccines are discussed in *Chapter 1: Introduction to Vaccinology—The Germinal Center Reaction* and are summarized in **Table 1.3**.

Efficacy and/or Immunogenicity

Serogroup A polysaccharide vaccines are immunogenic in infants as young as 3 months of age, but antibody responses are not comparable to those in adults and efficacy declines within 3 years.[14] Serogroup C polysaccharide is poorly immunogenic in children <18 months of age. Efficacy of serogroup A and C vaccines has been ≥85% in a variety of clinical settings; serogroup Y and W-135 polysaccharides induce bactericidal antibodies, although direct documentation of protection is lacking. Administration of serogroup C vaccine to all US troops beginning in 1972 resulted in the elimination of serogroup C disease in this population. Some studies suggest that multiple doses of serogroup A and C polysaccharides (but not conjugated polysaccharides) can cause immunologic hyporesponsiveness, which means that the response to subsequent doses is reduced[24,25]; the clinical significance of this phenomenon is not known.

Licensure of MCV4-D was based on immunologic noninferiority to MPSV4. In a randomized trial of adolescents who received either MCV4-D or MPSV4, the percentage of subjects in each group achieving a ≥4-fold rise in bactericidal antibody titer was ≥90% for serogroups A, C, and W-135; responses to serogroup Y were lower but similar for both vaccines (about 80%). The percentage of subjects achieving a *rabbit complement assay* serum bactericidal titer (rSBA) of ≥1:128—the presumed protective level with this assay—was >98% for all serogroups for each vaccine. In a similar study of adults, those who received MCV4-D less often had ≥4-fold rises in antibody compared with those who received MPSV4; however, the percentage achieving rSBA titers ≥1:128 were similar and the criteria for noninferiority were met. Again, 4-fold responses for serogroup Y were lower than for other serogroups. Between 2005 and 2008, the effectiveness of MCV4-D was estimated to be 80% to 85% within 3 years of vaccination,[26] but an ongoing case-control study suggests that effectiveness drops to near 50% from 2 to 5 years out from vaccination.[20]

In a study involving children 2 to 3 years of age, antibody responses to each serogroup were higher among MCV4-D recipients than MPSV4 recipients. The percentage of MCV4-D subjects achieving a *human complement assay* serum bactericidal titer (hSBA) of ≥1:8—the presumed protective level for this assay—was 73% for serogroup A, 63% for C, 63% for W-135, and 88% for Y. Similarly, responses were higher among children 4 to 10 years of age who received MCV4-D compared with those who received MPSV4. The percentage of MCV4-D subjects

TABLE 19.1 — *N meningitidis* Vaccines

Trade name	Menactra	Menveo	Menomune—A/C/Y/W-135
Abbreviation	MCV4-D	MCV4-CRM	MPSV4
Manufacturer/distributor	Sanofi Pasteur	Novartis	Sanofi Pasteur
Type of vaccine	Inactivated, engineered subunits	Inactivated, engineered subunits	Inactivated, purified subunits
Composition	Group-specific polysaccharides (4 mcg each) from *N meningitidis* serogroups A, C, Y, and W-135, conjugated to diphtheria toxoid (48 mcg)	Group-specific polysaccharides (serogroup A, 10 mcg; serogroups C, Y, W-135, 5 mcg each) from *N meningitidis*, conjugated to CRM_{197}, a nontoxic mutant diphtheria toxin (32.7 to 64.1 mcg)	Group-specific polysaccharides (50 mcg each) from *N meningitidis* serogroups A, C, Y, and W-135
Adjuvant	None	None	None
Preservative	None	None	10-dose vial: thimerosal (25 mcg mercury)
Excipients and contaminants	Formaldehyde (<2.66 mcg) Sodium phosphate buffered isotonic sodium chloride	Formaldehyde (<0.3 mcg)	Lactose (2.5 to 5 mg)
Latex	None	None	Vial stopper contains latex

Labeled indications	Prevention of invasive meningococcal disease due to serogroups A, C, Y, and W-135	Prevention of invasive meningococcal disease due to serogroups A, C, Y, and W-135	Prevention of invasive meningococcal disease due to serogroups A, C, Y, and W-135
Labeled ages	9 months to 55 years	2 to 55 years	≥2 years
Dose	0.5 mL	0.5 mL	0.5 mL
Route of administration	Intramuscular	Intramuscular	Subcutaneous
Labeled schedule	9 to 23 months: 2 doses separated by 3 months 2 to 55 years: 1 dose	1 dose[a]	1 dose
Recommended schedule	11 to 12, 16 years of age Catch-up, high-risk Revaccination *(see text)*	11 to 12, 16 years of age Catch-up, high-risk Revaccination *(see text)*	High-risk Revaccination *(see text)*
How supplied (number in package)	1-dose vial (5)	1-dose vial (5), lyophilized serogroup A, with diluent containing serogroups C, Y and W-135	Preservative-free formulation: 1-dose vial (1), lyophilized, with diluent Thimerosal-containing formulation: 10-dose vial (1), lyophilized, with diluent

Continued

19

TABLE 19.1 — *Continued*

Trade name	Menactra	Menveo	Menomune—A/C/Y/W-135
Abbreviation	MCV4-D	MCV4-CRM	MPSV4
Cost per dose ($US, 2011):			
Public	82.12	82.12	—
Private	106.49	106.49	107.80
Reference package insert	November 2011	March 2011	January 2009

[a] The package insert states that 2 doses separated by 2 months may be given to children 2 to 5 years of age at continued high risk of meningococcal disease.

achieving an hSBA titer of ≥1:8 was 81% for serogroup A, 79% for C, 85% for W-135, and 99% for Y. In a study of infants who received MCV4-D alone at 9 and 12 months of age, hSBA titers were ≥95% for all serogroups except W-135, which was 86%. Coadministration with PCV7 resulted in diminished antipneumococcal antibody responses.

Licensure of MCV4-CRM was based on immunologic noninferiority to MCV4-D. In a randomized, controlled trial, 2663 subjects received MCV4-CRM and 876 received MCV4-D; the primary end point was seroresponse rates, defined as a postvaccination hSBA titer of ≥1:8 in those with no prevaccination antibody, or a ≥4-fold increase in titer. The seroresponse rate for each serogroup among adolescents who received MCV4-CRM was noninferior to that of MCV4-D recipients. For serogroups A, W-135, and Y, the seroresponse rates were statistically superior (75% vs 66%, 75% vs 63%, and 68% vs 41%, respectively), and the geometric mean titers for all serogroups were statistically superior.[27] Twenty-two months after vaccination, more subjects who received MCV4-CRM had titers ≥1:8 (36% vs 25% for serogroup A, 62% vs 58% for C, 84% vs 74% for W-135, and 67% vs 54% for Y).[28] The seroresponse rate for each serogroup among adults who received MCV4-CRM also was noninferior to that of MCV4-D recipients, and in fact the responses were statistically superior for serogroups C, W-135, and Y. In a study of nearly 3000 children 2 to 10 years of age, MCV4-CRM was noninferior to MCV4-D for all serogroups and was statistically superior for serogroups C, Y, and W-135.[29]

Safety

Among teenagers receiving MPSV4, solicited adverse events include localized pain (29%), redness (6%), and induration (5%), none of which are severe. Systemic symptoms include fatigue (25%), headache (29%), and malaise (17%), and <1% of reactions are severe. Moderate to severe fever is seen in <1% of vaccinees. Solicited adverse events are more common among adults.

Pain is reported in about half of adolescent and adult MCV4-D recipients and is of moderate severity in <15%. Induration or erythema occur in 10% to 20% but is moderate or severe in <5%. Headache occurs in 36% to 41%, fatigue 30% to 35%, malaise 22% to 24%, and fever 2% to 5%. One percent or less of these reactions is considered severe. The reactogenicity of MCV4-CRM is comparable.

- *Contraindications*
  - Severe allergic reaction (eg, anaphylaxis) to previous dose of vaccine or any vaccine component (risk of recurrent allergic reaction; for MCV, this includes reactions to any diphtheria toxoid-containing vaccine, since these vaccines

contain either diphtheria toxoid or CRM_{197}, a mutant diphtheria toxin)

- *Precautions*
  - Moderate or severe acute illness (difficulty distinguishing illness from vaccine reaction)
  - Personal or family history of GBS *is not* considered a contraindication or precaution, even though the MCV4-D package insert lists it as a precaution (the MCV4-CRM package insert states that data are not available to assess the risk). See *Chapter 7: Addressing Concerns About Vaccines—Do Vaccines Cause Guillain-Barré Syndrome?* for a discussion about GBS following receipt of MCV4-D.

Recommendations

All adolescents should be vaccinated against *N meningitidis*. The usual schedule is 1 dose of MCV4 (for HIV-infected adolescents, 2 doses separated by 2 months) at 11 to 12 years of age followed by a one-time booster dose at 16 years of age. Adolescents ≤18 years of age who have not been vaccinated should receive a dose at the earliest opportunity. For those who receive Dose 1 at 13 to 15 years of age, routine (one-time) revaccination is recommended at 16 to 18 years of age. Persons who were first immunized at ≥16 years of age do not need a booster dose. Routine vaccination of persons >21 years of age is not recommended, but vaccination should be offered to anyone wanting to reduce his or her risk of meningococcal disease. There is no preference for MCV4-D or MCV4-CRM.

In all situations where vaccination against *N meningitidis* is called for, MCV4 is preferred over MPSV4 if the individual is 9 months to 55 years of age (only MCV4-D is licensed for use at 9 to 23 months of age). At ≥56 years of age, MPSV4 should be used. In addition to age-based routine use, MCV4 is recommended for the persons or situations listed below:

- Unvaccinated incoming college students ≤21 years of age (incoming college students whose last dose of a meningococcal vaccine was >5 years earlier should receive a booster dose; unvaccinated students, and those who are already in college and whose last dose was >5 years earlier also may be vaccinated)
- Microbiologists routinely exposed to *N meningitidis*
- Military recruits
- Travelers to or residents of countries in which *N meningitidis* is hyperendemic or epidemic
- Outbreak control

Vaccination and revaccination of high-risk persons is discussed in *Chapter 6: Vaccination in Special Circumstances* and is outlined in **Table 6.3**.

REFERENCES

1. Stephens DS, et al. *Lancet*. 2007;369:2196-2210.
2. Lo H, et al. *Lancet Infect Dis*. 2009;9:418-427.
3. Carbonnelle E, et al. *Vaccine*. 2009;27S:B78-B89.
4. Wright V, et al. *Vaccine*. 2009;27S:B90-B102.
5. Christensen H, et al. *Lancet Infect Dis*. 2010;10:853-861.
6. Cohn AC, et al. *Clin Infect Dis*. 2010;50:184-191.
7. Rosenstein NE, et al. *J Infect Dis.* 1999;180:1894-1901.
8. Kaplan SL, et al. *Pediatrics*. 2006;118:e979-e984.
9. Borg J, et al. *Pediatrics*. 2009;123:e502-e509.
10. Bruce MG, et al. *JAMA*. 2001;286:688-693.
11. CDC. *MMWR*. 2000;49(RR-10):1-22.
12. Balmer P, et al. *J Med Microbiol.* 2002;51:717-722.
13. Maiden MCJ, et al. *Lancet*. 2002;359:1829-1830.
14. Bilukha OO, et al. *MMWR*. 2005;54(RR-7):1-21.
15. CDC. *MMWR.* 2007;56:794-795.
16. CDC. *MMWR*. 2007;56:1265-1266.
17. CDC. *MMWR.* 2008;57:462-465.
18. CDC. *MMWR.* 2009;58:1042-1043.
19. CDC. *MMWR*. 2010;59:273.
20. CDC. *MMWR*. 2011;60:72-76.
21. CDC. *MMWR*. 2011;60:1018-1019.
22. CDC. *MMWR*. 2011;60:1391-1392.
23. Snape MD, et al. *Lancet Infect Dis*. 2005;5:21-30.
24. MacDonald NE, et al. *JAMA*. 1998;280:1685-1689.
25. Borrow R, et al. *Vaccine*. 2000;19:1129-1132.
26. MacNeil JR, et al. *Pediatr Infect Dis J*. 2011;30:451-455.
27. Jackson LA, et al. *Clin Infect Dis*. 2009;49:e1-e10.
28. Gill CJ, et al. *Hum Vac*. 2010;6:1-7.
29. Halperin SA, et al. *Vaccine*. 2010;28:7865-7872.

20 Polio

The Pathogen

Poliovirus is small, nonenveloped, single-stranded RNA virus in the Picornaviridae family. Initial replication occurs in the pharynx, lower gastrointestinal tract, and associated lymph nodes. This leads to primary viremia that seeds peripheral sites, including the viscera and skeletal muscle. Most infections are contained at this point and are therefore subclinical. In a minority of individuals, replication at peripheral sites leads to secondary viremia and nonspecific symptoms such as fever and malaise; about 1% of the time the CNS is involved, either through hematogenous spread or axonal transport from muscle. Once in the CNS, poliovirus can cause self-limited aseptic meningitis, but more importantly can replicate in and destroy anterior horn cells of the spinal cord, leading to lower motor-neuron paralysis.

Clinical Features

Approximately 95% of infections are asymptomatic. Minor, nonspecific illness with low-grade fever and sore throat occurs in 4% to 8% of infected people; *aseptic meningitis*, sometimes with paresthesias, occurs in 1% to 2% of patients a few days after these symptoms resolve. The CSF may show mild pleocytosis with lymphocytic predominance. Less than 1% of patients experience rapid onset of *asymmetric flaccid paralysis* and areflexia; the proximal lower extremity muscles are most often involved, and some patients have cranial nerve involvement. Prior to the availability of modern assisted ventilation, most deaths occurred from respiratory failure. In the past, patients who survived the acute illness but failed to recover respiratory muscle function lived out the remainder of their lives in iron lungs; today, tracheostomy and positive-pressure ventilation are used. Somewhat more than half of patients who develop limb paralysis have permanent functional deficits. Adults who contracted paralytic polio during childhood may develop *postpolio syndrome*, characterized by muscle pain and exacerbation of weakness 30 to 40 years later.

Epidemiology and Transmission

Humans are the only natural hosts and transmission occurs by the fecal-oral route, although pharyngeal secretions may be involved. Communicability is greatest shortly before and after onset of clinical illness, but patients may be contagious in the absence of symptoms and fecal excretion may persist for weeks. Immunodeficient patients can excrete the virus for >6 months.

Infection is more common in infants and young children and occurs at an earlier age among children living in poor hygienic conditions. The risk of paralytic disease increases with age. In temperate climates, poliovirus infections are most common during the summer and autumn. In the tropics, the seasonal pattern is variable with a less-pronounced peak of activity.

The last reported indigenous case of polio in the United States occurred in 1979, and the only identified imported case of paralytic polio since 1986 occurred in a child transported here for medical care in 1993. After 1979, all other cases of polio, an average of eight per year between 1980 and 1996, were caused by OPV-derived strains. While OPV has not been used in the United States since 2000, infections with OPV-derived strains still occur. In 2005, four unimmunized children in an Amish community in Minnesota were found to be infected with an OPV-derived strain of poliovirus.[1] The index case was an infant with severe combined immunodeficiency disease, and the other three children were otherwise healthy siblings in a separate household. Genetic analysis suggested that the strain had been imported by someone vaccinated with OPV in another country. Vaccine-derived poliovirus that has reverted to virulence can emerge because of continuous replication in immunodeficient individuals or continuous circulation in unimmunized populations. The latter phenomenon was highlighted during an outbreak of paralytic polio in the Caribbean in 2000 to 2001, which was caused by a strain of OPV that had reverted to virulence in areas of very low vaccine coverage.[2]

Immunization Program

Because of widespread vaccination, worldwide eradication of polio is now on the horizon. In the United States, the annual number of wild-type cases fell from >18,000 to zero in about 2 decades. In 1988, the World Health Assembly resolved to eradicate polio through the Global Polio Eradication Initiative. As a result, the number of cases worldwide was reduced from 350,000 in 1988 to 1352 in 2010.[3] The number of countries that have never succeeded in interrupting wild poliovirus transmission went from 125 to just 4: Afghanistan, India, Nigeria, and Pakistan. Unfortunately, transmission had been re-established in 3 countries: Angola, Chad, and the Democratic Republic of the Congo.

In 2006 alone, Global Polio Eradication Initiative partners immunized 375 million children in 36 countries with 2.1 billion doses of vaccine, and the technical feasibility of polio eradication was affirmed.[4] We may soon be living in a world free of circulating wild-type polioviruses.[5] After global eradication, however, it will be difficult to decide when or if polio immunization should be discontinued. Live-attenuated vaccine strains could still be circulating. In addition, reservoirs of wild-type virus could still exist (eg, in laboratories that have frozen stool specimens from the polio era), and infectious virus that could be used for bioterrorism can be reconstructed from the genetic material of the virus.

OPV was the vaccine of choice for children in the United States since the early 1960s because it induced optimal intestinal immunity, was relatively inexpensive, was painless, required little training to administer, and contributed to immunity at the population level through fecal-oral spread. For these same reasons, OPV continues to be used in the worldwide eradication effort. However, the continued use of OPV, with the attendant five to ten cases of vaccine-associated polio per year, was unjustified in the United States in the absence of wild-type disease. IPV was known to be highly effective, incapable of causing polio, and was used routinely in several countries that controlled or eliminated polio. Accordingly, expanded use of IPV was recommended beginning in 1997,[6] and as of January 2000, the recommendation was made to substitute IPV for OPV in the United States.[7]

In 2009, the ACIP updated the polio recommendations, emphasizing the importance of a dose at ≥4 years of age (regardless of the number of previous doses), extending the minimum interval from Dose 3 to Dose 4 to 6 months, and clarifying the schedule when combination vaccines containing IPV are used.[8]

Vaccines

Characteristics of the polio vaccines licensed in the United States are given in **Table 20.1**. These are inactivated, whole-virus vaccines, made much the same way as the original Salk vaccine.

Efficacy and/or Immunogenicity

Ninety-percent or more of vaccinees develop protective antibody to all three serotypes after 2 doses, and ≥99% are immune after 3 doses. Protection against paralytic disease correlates with the presence of serum antibody. IPV appears to induce less mucosal immunity than does OPV, so persons who receive IPV are more readily infected in the gastrointestinal tract with wild poliovirus. Thus a person immunized with IPV could become infected in an endemic area and shed virus upon return to the United States. The infected person would be protected from paralytic polio, but the wild virus shed in the stool could be transmitted to a contact. The duration of immunity from IPV is not known with certainty but is probably many years after a complete series.

TABLE 20.1 — Polio Vaccine[a]

Trade name	IPOL[b]
Abbreviation	IPV
Manufacturer/distributor	Sanofi Pasteur
Type of vaccine	Inactivated, whole agent
Composition:	
Virus strain and amount	Type 1 (Mahoney), 40 D antigen units Type 2 (MEF-1), 8 D antigen units Type 3 (Saukett), 32 D antigen units
Propagation	Vero (African green monkey kidney) cells
Inactivation	Formalin
Adjuvant	None
Preservative	2-phenoxyethanol (0.5%) Formaldehyde (≤0.02%)
Excipients and contaminants	Neomycin (<5 ng) Streptomycin (<200 ng) Polymyxin B (<25 ng) Calf serum protein (<1 ppm)
Latex	None
Labeled indications	Prevention of poliomyelitis
Labeled ages	≥6 weeks
Dose	0.5 mL
Route of administration	Intramuscular or subcutaneous
Labeled schedule	2, 4, 6 to 18 months, 4 to 6 years of age
Recommended schedule	Same
How supplied (number in package)	10-dose vial (1) Prefilled syringe (10)
Cost per dose ($US, 2011):	
Public	11.97
Private	25.43
Reference package insert	December 2005

[a] An IPV that is very similar to IPOL is available in combination with DTaP and HepB (Pediarix; GlaxoSmithKline). This IPV is not licensed or distributed separately in the United States. Pediarix is usually given at 2, 4, and 6 months of age. The same IPV is available in combination with DTaP (Kinrix; GlaxoSmithKline). Kinrix is indicated for the booster doses of DTaP and IPV at 4 to 6 years of age. The IPV in Pediarix and Kinrix is considered interchangeable with IPOL.

[b] An IPV that is very similar to IPOL (Poliovax; Sanofi Pasteur) is available in combination with DTaP and Hib (Pentacel; Sanofi Pasteur). Pentacel is usually given at 2, 4, 6, and 15 to 18 months of age.

Safety

Minor local reactions, such as pain and redness, may occur following IPV. No serious adverse events have been associated with use of the currently available vaccine.

- *Contraindications*
  - Severe allergic reaction (eg, anaphylaxis) to previous dose of vaccine or any vaccine component (risk of recurrent allergic reaction)
- *Precautions*
  - Moderate or severe acute illness (difficulty distinguishing illness from vaccine reaction)
  - Pregnancy (theoretical risk to the fetus or attribution of birth defects to vaccination). No deleterious effects have been demonstrated from IPV administration during pregnancy, and the risk of adverse fetal effects from an inactivated vaccine is extremely low.

Recommendations

All children should be vaccinated against polio. The primary series of IPV consists of 3 doses, usually given at 2, 4, and 6 to 18 months of age. Dose 4 is given at 4 to 6 years of age, around the time of school entry. The final dose should be given at ≥4 years of age; therefore, if Dose 4 is given at <4 years of age (as would be the case, for example, in a child who receives DTaP-IPV/Hib-T at 2, 4, 6, and 15 months of age), another dose of IPV should be given at 4 to 6 years of age. In the first 6 months of life, the minimum age and minimum intervals should only be used if imminent exposure to polio is expected (as, for example, in the case of an infant traveling to an endemic area).

Routine immunization of US adults ≥18 years of age is not recommended. However, a 3-dose series of IPV (0, 1 to 2, and 6 to 12 months) is recommended for previously unvaccinated adults in the following circumstances (an accelerated schedule consisting of doses at 0, 1, and 2 months can be used if necessary):

- Travel to countries where polio is epidemic or endemic
- Members of a community experiencing wild-type poliovirus disease
- HCP who will come into close contact with patients potentially excreting wild-type poliovirus
- Laboratory workers who will come in contact with specimens that may contain poliovirus

Adults who have received a primary series of at least 3 doses who are at increased risk of exposure to polio should receive a single supplemental dose of IPV (this does not need to be repeated). Those who have had <3 doses (of either OPV or IPV) should complete the primary series of 3 doses using IPV, regardless of the interval since the last dose and the type of vaccine that was previously given.

REFERENCES

1. CDC. *MMWR*. 2005;54:1053-1055.
2. CDC. *MMWR*. 2001;50:855-856.
3. Wild poliovirus (WPV) cases. Global Polio Eradication Initiative Web site. http://www.polioeradication.org/Dataandmonitoring/Poliothisweek.aspx. Accessed January 18, 2012.
4. Global Polio Eradication Initiative. Annual Report 2006. http://www.polioeradication.org/content/publications/AnnualReport2006_ENG.pdf. Accessed February 5, 2010.
5. Senior K. *Lancet Infect Dis*. 2010;10:148-149.
6. CDC. *MMWR*. 1997;46(RR-3):1-25.
7. Prevots DR, et al. *MMWR*. 2000;49(RR-5):1-22.
8. CDC. *MMWR*. 2009;58:829-830.

21 Rabies

The Pathogen

Rabies virus is an enveloped, bullet-shaped, single-stranded RNA virus in the Rhabdoviridae family. The virion surface is covered with glycoprotein (G-protein) spikes, which mediate attachment to the heavily sialated gangliosides on neuronal cells. Attachment also may occur at nicotinic acetylcholine receptors in muscle, facilitating entry into peripheral nerves. The virus moves by retrograde axoplasmic flow from the site of inoculation to neuronal cell bodies, where it replicates and spreads to the brain; from there it may spread further to other organs, such as salivary and lacrimal glands. Gross pathologic changes in the brain include vascular congestion and edema, and the characteristic cellular abnormality is eosinophilic cytoplasmic neuronal inclusions called *Negri bodies*. The clinical severity of the disease is disproportionate to the degree of histopathologic derangement.

Clinical Features

Rabies presents in four sequential stages: the incubation period, prodrome, acute neurologic phase, and coma/death.[1] Two thirds of patients present with a *furious form*, characterized by fluctuating consciousness, phobic spasms, dilated pupils, and hypersalivation. The other one third present with a *paralytic form*, which is differentiated from GBS by the presence of fever, intact sensation, and urinary incontinence. The incubation period is typically a few weeks to 2 months but may be many years. Animal bites to the head usually result in shorter incubation periods than bites to the extremities.

There are no symptoms during the *incubation phase*, but the *prodrome*, which lasts 2 to 10 days, is characterized by fever, headache, malaise, fatigue, anorexia, anxiety, agitation, irritability, insomnia, depression, and pain, pruritus, or paresthesia at the site of the bite. The *acute neurologic phase*, which lasts 2 to 12 days, is characterized by hyperactivity, disorientation, hallucinations, bizarre behavior, aggressiveness, seizures, paralysis, aerophobia, hyperventilation, and cholinergic manifestations, including hypersalivation, lacrimation, mydriasis, and hyperpyrexia. Agitation may be precipitated by tactile, auditory, visual, or other stimuli, and hydrophobia, characterized by painful spasms of the pharynx and larynx, may be precipitated by eating or drinking or even the sight of liquids. Paralysis occurs in 20%

of cases. At the end of the neurologic phase, the patient may become comatose. Death from respiratory or cardiac arrest usually occurs within 7 days, although with supportive care, coma may last for months. There are only a handful of reported survivors, most of whom have neurologic sequelae. Successful treatment of a 15-year-old girl from Wisconsin was reported in 2005; the strategy included therapeutic coma using gamma-aminobutyric acid receptor agonists along with *N*-methyl-D-aspartate receptor antagonists.[2]

Epidemiology and Transmission

All mammals can be infected with rabies, but only carnivorous mammals and bats are considered true reservoirs. Transmission from animals to humans occurs by exposure to saliva, usually through an animal bite, scratch, or contact with mucous membranes. Infection by aerosol has been reported in laboratories that handle the virus and in caves inhabited by bats (here, direct infection of the olfactory apparatus is implicated). Rabies can also be transmitted by allografts. In nature, dogs, wolves, foxes, coyotes, jackals, raccoons, skunks, weasels, bats, and mongooses are most commonly infected. However, in some areas of the world, dogs and cats account for the majority of animal rabies and the greatest number of exposures to humans. In the United States, where domestic animal rabies is well controlled through animal vaccination, most human exposures come from contact with wild animals, such as skunks, raccoons, and bats. Silver-haired bats have become a particular problem because the strains they carry may infect human skin more easily and their bites may be too small to see. Small rodents (eg, squirrels, rats, and mice) and lagomorphs (eg, rabbits and hares) rarely carry rabies.

Most animal exposures in the United States involve dogs, cats, and rodents; the vast majority of these exposures carry a very low risk for rabies transmission, even though postexposure prophylaxis is commonly given.[3] Insectivorous bats are now the most common source of human infection in the United States.[4,5] In at least half of cases, there is no known bite—a bite may simply have been imperceptible or might have occurred during sleep, or transmission might have occurred through bat saliva contacting a mucous membrane or break in the skin.

Oral vaccination of wildlife has proven effective in preventing spread of enzootic disease. Traditional approaches have utilized bait seeded with live-attenuated rabies strains. A recent approach uses a vaccinia recombinant expressing the G protein of rabies virus.

Immunization Program

There are an estimated 50,000 human rabies cases each year worldwide; only one or two of these occur in the United States. The long incubation period makes rabies uniquely suited to postexposure prophylaxis through both vaccination and passive immunization with human rabies immune globulin (HRIG); in this respect, rabies is similar to hepatitis B.[6] The common occurrence of animal contacts combined with the near certainty of death if rabies occurs leads to frequent consideration of postexposure prophylaxis. However, postexposure prophylaxis is considered *urgent*, not *emergent*—in other words, the time frame in which to administer prophylaxis is hours, not minutes, and in some cases may be days (eg, if signs of rabies develop in an animal during quarantine).

Postexposure prophylaxis is cost saving (from the societal perspective) when given to persons bitten by test-positive rabid animals or untested reservoir or vector animals. For other risk situations, the cost-effectiveness of postexposure prophylaxis varies widely. For example, it costs $2.9 million per life saved to administer prophylaxis after a bite from an untested cat, $403 million per life saved after a bite from an untested dog, and $4 billion per life saved after a lick from an untested dog (2004 dollars).[7] Although it still stands, the recommendation to administer postexposure prophylaxis after bedroom exposure to a bat while sleeping (without direct evidence of physical contact) has been called into question—approximately 2.7 million persons would need to be treated in this context to prevent a single case of rabies.[8] About 23,000 courses of postexposure prophylaxis are given each year in the United States, most of which are given without guidance from public health authorities.[9]

Pre-exposure vaccination of persons likely to encounter the virus can simplify postexposure treatment by eliminating the need for HRIG and reducing the number of vaccine doses needed. It also protects people who may have inapparent exposures or whose postexposure therapy might be delayed. Pre-exposure vaccination is particularly important for persons who are at high risk of exposure, but who may be in situations where modern prophylaxis is not available.

Recommendations for prevention of human rabies were published in 1999[10] and updated in 2008.[7] In 2010, based on new data from pathogenesis studies, animal models, clinical observations, and epidemiologic surveillance, the recommended vaccine series was reduced from 5 to 4 doses for otherwise healthy persons.[11]

Vaccines

Characteristics of the rabies vaccines licensed in the United States are given in **Table 21.1**. These are inactivated, whole-virus vaccines, made much the same way as the original Salk vaccine.

HRIG is used in conjunction with vaccination for postexposure prophylaxis. Two preparations, *HyperRAB S/D* (Talecris Biotherapeutics) and *Imogam Rabies—HT* (Sanofi Pasteur), are available in the United States. They consist of IgG derived from pooled plasma of human donors who have been hyperimmunized with RAB; they are therefore polyclonal (contain a variety of antibodies, including antibodies to other organisms). Both products are initially purified by cold ethanol fractionation and then formulated for IM administration.

Efficacy and/or Immunogenicity

Essentially all persons given pre- or postexposure prophylaxis achieve seroprotective concentrations of antibody.[12] Multiple studies have demonstrated that postexposure prophylaxis with cell culture-derived vaccine and HRIG provide absolute protection against rabies—in fact, there has never been a failure of properly administered postexposure prophylaxis in the United States.

Safety

Local reactions to RAB-HDC occur in 60% to 90% of vaccinees, with local pain occurring in 21% to 77%. Mild systemic symptoms, such as fever, headache, dizziness, and gastrointestinal complaints, occur in 7% to 56%. Systemic hypersensitivity, including urticaria, pruritic rash, and angioedema, may be seen in up to 6% of persons receiving booster doses. This is thought to be mediated by IgE antibodies to human albumin that is chemically altered by betapropiolactone.

Local reactions to RAB-PCEC occur in 11% to 57% of vaccinees, with local pain occurring in 2% to 23%. Mild systemic symptoms are seen in 0% to 31%. From 1997 to 2005, the reporting rate to VAERS for adverse events was 30 per 100,000 doses distributed, and for serious adverse events it was 3 per 100,000 doses distributed.[13]

Local reactions to HRIG include pain, tenderness, erythema, and induration. Systemic reactions are reported in 75% to 81% of recipients.

- *Contraindications*
  - In the event of exposure to rabies, there are no contraindications to vaccination or use of HRIG.

- *Precautions*
  - Severe allergic reaction (eg, anaphylaxis) to previous dose of vaccine or any vaccine component (risk of recurrent allergic reaction). This is not listed as a contraindication, as it is for other vaccines, because rabies is considered universally fatal and therefore the risks of recurrent allergic reaction must be weighed against the possibility of exposure.
  - *Immunosuppression*: Immunosuppressive agents should not be administered during postexposure prophylaxis unless absolutely essential. If possible, pre-exposure prophylaxis should be postponed until immunocompromising conditions are resolved. When an immunosuppressed person is given pre- or postexposure prophylaxis, antibody titers should be checked (a rapid fluorescent focus inhibition test that demonstrates complete virus neutralization at a serum dilution of 1:5 is considered to be indicative of protection).
  - Patients with selective IgA deficiency may be at increased risk for anaphylactic reactions to HRIG because it may contain minute amounts of IgA.

Recommendations

Table 21.2 gives recommendations for pre-exposure prophylaxis. **Table 21.3** lists the situations where postexposure prophylaxis should be considered, and **21.4** gives the postexposure regimens. Cell culture-derived rabies vaccines are considered interchangeable, although situations where one would need to complete a series with one vaccine that was initiated with a different vaccine are rare.

REFERENCES

1. Plotkin SA. *Clin Infect Dis*. 2000;30:4-12.
2. Willoughby RE Jr, et al. *N Engl J Med*. 2005;352:2508-2514.
3. Moran GJ, et al. *JAMA*. 2000;284:1001-1007.
4. Messenger SL, et al. *Clin Infect Dis*. 2002;35:738-747.
5. De Serres G, et al. *Clin Infect Dis*. 2008;46:1329-1337.
6. Rupprecht CE, et al. *N Engl J Med*. 2004;351:2626-2635.
7. Manning SE, et al. *MMWR*. 2008;57(RR-3):1-28.
8. De Serres G, et al. *Clin Infect Dis*. 2009;48:1493-1499.
9. Christian KA, et al. *Vaccine*. 2009;27:7156-7161.
10. Arguin PM,et al. *MMWR*. 1999;48(RR-1):1-23.
11. Rupprecht CE, et al. *MMWR*. 2010;59(RR-2):1-9.
12. Rupprecht CE, et al. *Vaccine*. 2009;27:7141-7148.
13. Dobardzic A, et al. *Vaccine*. 2007;25:4244-4251.

TABLE 21.1 — Rabies Vaccines[a]

Trade name	Imovax Rabies	RabAvert
Abbreviation	RAB-HDC	RAB-PCEC
Manufacturer/distributor	Sanofi Pasteur	Novartis
Type of vaccine	Inactivated, whole agent	Inactivated, whole agent
Composition:		
Virus strain	PM-1503-3M	Flury LEP
Propagation	Human diploid (MRC-5) cells	Purified chick embryo cells (fibroblasts)
Inactivation	Beta-propiolactone	Beta-propiolactone
Antigen content	≥2.5 IU	≥2.5 IU
Adjuvant	None	None
Preservative	None	None
Excipients and contaminants	Albumin (<100 mg) Neomycin sulfate (<150 mcg) Phenol red (20 mcg)	Polygeline (processed bovine gelatin) (<12 mg) Human serum albumin (<0.3 mg) Potassium glutamate (1 mg) Sodium EDTA (0.3 mg) Ovalbumin (<3 ng) Neomycin (<1 mcg) Chlorotetracycline (<20 ng) Amphotericin B (<2 ng)
Latex	None	None
Labeled indications	Pre-exposure (primary series and booster dose) and postexposure prophylaxis	Pre-exposure (primary series and booster dose) and postexposure prophylaxis

Labeled ages	All ages	All ages
Dose	1 mL	1 mL
Route of administration	Intramuscular	Intramuscular
Labeled schedule:		
Pre-exposure	0, 7, and 21 or 28 days Periodic booster doses	0, 7, and 21 or 28 days Periodic booster doses
Postexposure (unvaccinated)[b]	0, 3, 7, 14, 28 days	0, 3, 7, 14, 28 days
Postexposure (previously vaccinated)	0, 3 days	0, 3 days
Recommended schedule:		
Pre-exposure	See **Table 21.2**	See **Table 21.2**
Postexposure[b]	See **Table 21.4**	See **Table 21.4**
How supplied (number in package)	1-dose vial (1), lyophilized, with diluent	1-dose vial (1), lyophilized, with diluent
Cost per dose ($US, 2011):		
Public	—	—
Private	204.74	228.70
Reference package insert	December 2005	October 2006

[a] Two vaccines are no longer available in the United States: Rabies Vaccine Adsorbed (BioPort) and Imovax Rabies I.D. (Sanofi Pasteur).
[b] HRIG should also be given to exposed, previously unvaccinated persons (see **Table 21.4**).

TABLE 21.2 — Indications for Pre-exposure Rabies Prophylaxis

Intensity of Exposure	Nature of Exposure[a]	Examples	Vaccination
Continuous	Continuous Possible high concentration of virus May go unrecognized Bite, nonbite, aerosol	Rabies research laboratory workers[b] Rabies biologics production workers	3-dose primary series[c] Serology every 6 months Booster dose if titer[d] <1:5
Frequent	Episodic with recognized source May go unrecognized Bite, nonbite, aerosol	Rabies diagnostic laboratory workers[b] Spelunkers Veterinarians and staff Animal-control and wildlife workers in enzootic areas All persons who frequently handle bats	3-dose primary series[c] Serology every 2 years Booster dose if titer[d] <1:5
Infrequent	Episodic with recognized source Bite or nonbite	Veterinarians, animal-control, and wildlife workers in nonenzootic areas Veterinary students Travelers to enzootic areas where immediate access to medical care is limited	3-dose vaccine series[c]
Rare	Episodic with recognized source Bite or nonbite	General US population (including epizootic areas)	Not necessary

[a] See **Table 21.3** for explanation of types of exposure.
[b] Judgment of relative risk and monitoring of immunization status is the responsibility of the laboratory supervisor.
[c] 1 mL intramuscularly on days 0, 7, and 21 or 28.
[d] Rapid fluorescent focus inhibition test.

Adapted from Manning SE, et al. *MMWR*. 2008;57(RR-3):1-28.

TABLE 21.3 — Indications for Postexposure Rabies Prophylaxis

Animal[a]	Animal Evaluation and Disposition	Recommendations
Dog, cat, ferret	Healthy and quarantined for 10-day observation period[b]	Do not begin prophylaxis routinely Institute prophylaxis at first sign of rabies in the animal[c]
	Rabid or suspected rabid	Institute prophylaxis immediately[c]
	Unknown or not available for observation	Consult public health officials[d]
Skunk, raccoon, fox, other carnivore (eg, coyote, bobcat, wild-animal hybrid), bat	Regard as rabid[e]	Consider immediate prophylaxis[c]
Livestock, horse, small rodent (eg, squirrel, chipmunk, rat, mouse, hamster, guinea pig, gerbil), large rodent (eg, woodchuck or groundhog, beaver), lagomorph (eg, rabbit, hare), other mammal[f]	Consider individually	Consult public health officials[d]

[a] *Bite* exposures occur when there has been any penetration of the skin by teeth. *Nonbite* exposures include scratches, abrasions, open wounds, or mucous membranes contaminated with saliva or other potentially infectious material (eg, brain or neural tissue). Contact between intact skin and saliva does not constitute an exposure; neither does casual petting or handling or contact with blood, urine, or feces. However, any potential contact with a bat deserves evaluation because bat bites are small and can go unrecognized. Exposure is assumed to have occurred if a person in the same room as a bat might have been unaware that a bite or direct contact had occurred. Examples include a sleeping person who awakens to find a bat in the room or finding a bat in the room with an unattended child, mentally disabled person, or intoxicated person (awake or asleep). *Aerosol* exposure is rare but has been reported in laboratories that handle the virus and in caves infested with millions of bats. *Human-to-human* transmission occurs almost exclusively through tissue or organ transplantation.

[b] The animal should be quarantined and observed for 10 days. This usually takes place under the supervision of the local health department, which specifies approved facilities (private or government) and monitors the animal's behavior. If signs of rabies develop (eg, aggressive or combative behavior, irritability, hyperreaction to stimuli, or paralysis), the animal should be euthanized and the brain sent for detection of rabies virus antigens by direct fluorescent antibody test (this is usually done at the state lab).

[c] **Table 21.4** gives the recommended prophylaxis regimens. If prophylaxis is initiated but the animal is found not to have rabies by direct fluorescent antibody testing of the brain, prophylaxis may be discontinued.

[d] The epidemiology of rabies is complex and varies from region to region. Local and state public health officials should be consulted to determine the likelihood of exposure in specific situations.

[e] These animals should be regarded as rabid unless proved negative by immunofluorescence testing of the brain (this is usually done at the state lab). Prophylaxis should be initiated unless the brain is known to be negative or expeditious testing is under way. Prophylaxis should be considered more urgent if the exposure was from an animal species in the area known to carry rabies; if the animal exhibited abnormal behavior or signs of illness, had an unexplained wound, attacked *without provocation* (bites that result from attempts to feed or handle an apparently healthy animal should generally be regarded as *provoked*); or if the person's wounds were severe or involved the head and neck. Every effort should be made by properly trained officials to obtain the animal for euthanization and testing; quarantine for observation is *not* recommended because signs of rabies in wild animals cannot be interpreted reliably.

[f] Bites of small rodents and lagomorphs almost never require prophylaxis. Large rodents, such as woodchucks, could survive an attack by a rabid animal and go on to develop rabies. This should be considered in areas where raccoon rabies is prevalent.

Adapted from Manning SE, et al. *MMWR*. 2008;57(RR-3):1-28, and Rabies exposure: When should I seek medical attention? Centers for Disease Control and Prevention Web site. http://www.cdc.gov/rabies/exposure/index.html. Accessed January 20, 2011.

TABLE 21.4 — Postexposure Rabies Prophylaxis Regimens

Vaccination Status	Treatment[a]	Regimen
Not previously vaccinated	Wound cleansing	Immediately cleanse all wounds thoroughly with soap and water Use a virucidal agent like povidone-iodine solution if available
	HRIG	Administer 20 IU/kg (0.133 mL/kg)[b] Infiltrate the full dose around the wound and give any remaining volume intramuscularly at another site[c] Do not exceed the recommended dose[d] Use separate syringes for HRIG and vaccine
	Rabies vaccine	*Healthy individual*: administer 1 mL intramuscularly on days 0, 3, 7, and 14[e] *Immunosuppressed individual*: administer 1 mL intramuscularly on days 0, 3, 7, 14, and 28[e]
Previously vaccinated[f]	Wound cleansing	Immediately cleanse all wounds thoroughly with soap and water Use a virucidal agent like povidone-iodine solution if available
	HRIG	Not recommended
	Rabies vaccine	Administer 1 mL intramuscularly on days 0 and 3[e]

[a] Postexposure prophylaxis should be initiated regardless of the time that has elapsed since the exposure. State or local health departments should be contacted for patients whose postexposure prophylaxis was initiated outside of the United States, because the regimens and products used may be suboptimal. For bites, the need for tetanus immunization and prophylactic antibiotics should be assessed. Wound closure should be avoided if possible.

[b] HRIG should be given at the same time the vaccine series is initiated. If not given on the day of the first dose of vaccine (day 0), it may be given up to and including day 7. Beyond this it is not indicated because the vaccine is presumed to have induced antibodies by then.

[c] The intramuscular site, if used, should be different from the site where the first dose of vaccine is given. Subsequent doses of the vaccine may be given in the same muscle where the HRIG was given, if that is a preferred site for vaccination.

[d] Exceeding the dose of HRIG may suppress the antibody response to vaccination.

[e] In 2010, the recommended number of doses was reduced from 5 to 4 for otherwise healthy persons (off-label recommendation). The deltoid area is the only acceptable site for adults and older children. The anterolateral thigh can be used for young children (see **Table 4.7**), and the dose is the same as for adults. The gluteal area should never be used. The series does not need to be reinitiated because of minor interruptions of the vaccine schedule—just pick up at the point it was discontinued, maintaining the proper intervals between doses specified in the schedule. If major deviations occur, and for all immunosuppressed individuals, test for antibody after completing the series (a rapid fluorescent focus inhibition test that demonstrates complete virus neutralization at a serum dilution of 1:5 is considered to be indicative of protection).

[f] This includes: 1) persons who received a full pre- or postexposure series of one of the currently licensed cell culture-derived vaccines or of Rabies Vaccine Adsorbed (which is no longer available in the United States); and 2) persons who received another type of rabies vaccine and had a documented antibody response. Serologic testing at the time of exposure is not recommended.

Adapted from Rupprecht CE, et al. *MMWR*. 2010;59(RR-2):1-9.

22 Rotavirus

The Pathogen

Rotavirus is a nonenveloped virus with a wheel-like appearance in the Reoviridae family.[1] The genome is divided into 11 double-stranded RNA segments, most of which encode only one viral protein. Infection of the gastrointestinal tract causes diarrhea by several mechanisms: increased fluid secretion due to the effects of a virus-encoded enterotoxin (NSP4) and stimulation of the enteric nervous system, and increased osmotic load caused by destruction of villus epithelial cells, decreased absorption of salt and water, and decreased disaccharidase activity. Protection against disease is mediated by immune responses to the G protein (G stands for "glycoprotein"), also known as VP7 or the coat protein, and the P protein (P stands for "protease-sensitive"), also known as VP4 or the spike protein. Any given rotavirus strain has a specific G type, designated by a serotype number (as in "G1"), and a P type, designated by a serotype number (as in "P1a") and/or a genotype number in brackets (as in "P[8]"). Certain combinations of G and P types, such as G1P[8] and G2P[4], are found more commonly than others.

Clinical Features

The incubation period is 1 to 4 days.[1] Illness begins abruptly with fever and vomiting, and diarrhea ensues shortly thereafter. There may be >20 daily episodes of vomiting and/or diarrhea during the peak of the illness. Severe vomiting may lead to dehydration even before the diarrhea begins, and associated symptoms include irritability and lethargy. The illness lasts for about a week and appears to be more severe than other forms of gastroenteritis in infants.[2] Risk factors for hospitalization include low birth weight, childcare attendance, and absence of breast-feeding.[3] Common complications of severe rotavirus infection include isotonic dehydration, electrolyte disturbances, metabolic acidosis, and temporary milk intolerance. Rare complications include necrotizing enterocolitis and hemorrhagic gastroenteritis. Immunocompromised patients may develop particularly severe or fatal illness and may shed virus in the stool for months.[4]

Epidemiology and Transmission

Transmission occurs from person-to-person through the fecal-oral route, airborne droplets, and contaminated fomites. Infected children shed as many as 100 billion viral particles per milliliter of stool. Since the infectious dose is around 10,000 particles, it only takes one ten-millionth of a milliliter of stool to transmit the infection. This makes rotavirus one of the more contagious forms of gastroenteritis. Because rotavirus is not spread through contaminated food or water, improvements in sanitation and public hygiene do not affect the incidence of disease; this explains why the proportion of severe gastroenteritis caused by rotavirus is the same in developed countries as it is in developing countries.

Virtually all children experience at least one rotavirus infection by 5 years of age. Before the universal immunization program in the United States, rotavirus caused up to 410,000 annual office visits, 272,000 emergency department visits, 70,000 hospitalizations, and 60 deaths.[5] Rotavirus hospitalizations occurred at a frequency of 22.5 per 10,000 children <3 years of age, emergency department visits at 301 per 10,000, and outpatient visits at 312 per 10,000.[6] The numbers worldwide are staggering—2 million annual hospitalizations and approximately 25 million outpatient visits. Deaths are common in developing countries, with annual worldwide mortality estimated at 527,000 (rotavirus causes 29% of all diarrheal deaths among children <5 years of age).[7] Reinfection is common but results in mild or no disease, and repeated reinfections reduce the likelihood of subsequent infections. Outbreaks and nosocomial spread occur frequently in day care centers, pediatric hospital wards, and nurseries.

In the tropics, rotavirus may occur at any time of the year. In the prevaccine era in the United States, annual epidemics began in the late fall in the Southwest and spread to the North and East by the end of winter or early spring. From 1996 to 2005, G1P[8] strains accounted for 78.5% of infections, G2P[4] for 9.2%, G9P[8] for 3.6%, G3P[8] for 1.7%, and G4P[8] for 0.8%.[8] This is similar to the distribution of serotypes globally, although G9P[8] is more common in some regions outside the United States and other strains are seen in the Eastern Mediterranean and Africa.[9] The predominant types vary from year to year and within geographic regions.

Immunization Program

The first vaccine against rotavirus, rhesus rotavirus vaccine, tetravalent (RRV-TV), was licensed in 1998 under the trade name RotaShield (Wyeth, acquired by Pfizer in 2009). The vaccine included a G3-like rhesus rotavirus strain that was naturally attenuated for humans, as well as three rhesus-human reassortants representing serotypes G1, G2, and G4 (each strain also expressed the rhesus P[3]). The vaccine was administered orally at 2, 4, and 6 months of age, was 70% to 95% effective at preventing severe rotavirus gastroenteritis, and was recommended for all infants in the United States.[10] Within a year of licensure, RRV-TV was found to be associated with intussusception and the vaccine was pulled from the market (see *Chapter 7: Addressing Concerns About Vaccination—Do Rotavirus Vaccines Cause Intussusception?*).

The disease burden, however, continued to justify a vaccination program, as did the cost of rotavirus disease—>$1 billion each year in the United States alone in direct medical and societal costs. It was estimated that a universal vaccination program instituted in a single US birth cohort—assuming only 70% coverage and looking at outcomes over 5 years—would reduce the number of domiciliary episodes of rotavirus gastroenteritis by 48%, office visits by 60%, emergency department visits by 64%, hospitalizations by 66%, and deaths by 44%. The cost per case averted would be $138, cost per serious case averted would be $3024, and cost per year of life saved would be $197,190 (2004 dollars).[11]

RV5 was licensed in 2006 and was recommended for all infants in the United States.[5] Changes in the epidemiology of rotavirus gastroenteritis were seen almost immediately—rotavirus seasons started later, became shorter, and were less intense than they had been.[12] Laboratory surveillance data for 2009-2010 demonstrated that the North, Midwest, and West never even *had* a rotavirus season, at least not one defined as 2 consecutive weeks with at least 10% of laboratory tests positive for rotavirus.[13] Claims-based data showed 60% to 75% reductions in rotavirus hospitalizations among children <5 years of age; between 2007 and 2009, an estimated 64,855 hospitalizations were prevented, at a savings of $278 million in treatment costs.[14] Hospital-based surveillance in 18 states demonstrated similarly dramatic reductions in acute gastroenteritis discharges.[15] Active surveillance in three US counties in 2008 demonstrated an 87% reduction in rotavirus hospitalizations among infants 6 to 11 months of age, in whom vaccine coverage rates were 77%; there was also a 92% reduction among children 24 to 35 months of age, likely the result of herd immunity.[16] Further evidence of indirect effects came from a nationally-representative database of gastroenteritis admissions at US hospitals, which showed significant reductions in hospitalization of older children and even adults (this study also highlighted a previously unrecognized burden of disease).[17] Studies also showed sharp declines in rotavirus-associated outpatient visits,[18,19] and the spatiotemporal patterns of rotavirus activity changed such that the historical spread of disease from Southwest to Northeast was no longer evident.[20]

These changes in epidemiology occurred when RV5 was essentially the only vaccine being used, since RV1 was not licensed until April 2008. Updated recommendations for prevention of rotavirus disease were published in 2009,[21] and contraindications were updated in 2010[22] and 2011.[23]

Vaccines

Characteristics of the rotavirus vaccines licensed in the United States are given in **Table 22.1**. Both are live-attenuated vaccines that are given orally. RV5 is a mixture of five different reassortant viruses, each of which is a (naturally attenuated) bovine rotavirus strain that has been engineered to express a different immunogenic protein (G1, G2, G3, G4, or P[8]) from human rotavirus. RV1 is a single human rotavirus strain (G1P[8]) that was attenuated by serial passage in tissue culture, much the same way as the Sabin polio vaccine.

Efficacy and/or Immunogenicity

Prelicensure studies of RV5 involved >70,000 infants; half of the subjects were enrolled in the United States, a third in Finland, and the rest in Latin America, Europe, and Taiwan. Detailed information about efficacy came from about 7000 of these infants. The pivotal trial was a placebo-controlled study called the Rotavirus Efficacy and Safety Trial (REST).[24] Efficacy against rotavirus gastroenteritis of any severity due to serotypes G1 through G4 during the first season after vaccination was 74%, and efficacy against severe disease was 98%. Efficacy against disease of any severity was 71% through two seasons; in the second season alone, efficacy was 63% against disease of any severity and 88% against severe disease. Emergency department visits due to rotavirus serotypes G1 through G4 were reduced by 94% during the 2 years following Dose 3, and hospitalizations were reduced by 96%; in a separate post hoc analysis, efficacy against hospitalizations and emergency department visits due to G9P[8] strains was 100%. In an extension of REST conducted in Finland, efficacy against rotavirus-associated hospitalizations and emergency department visits, regardless of serotype, was 94% for >3 years following vaccination.[25]

A postlicensure study utilizing a national health insurance claims database compared 33,140 infants who received 3 doses of RV5 to 26,167 unimmunized controls. Effectiveness was estimated at 100% against rotavirus hospitalizations and emergency department visits and 96% against outpatient visits.[26] Case-control studies at children's hospitals yielded similarly high estimates of effectiveness.[27,28]

Prelicensure studies of RV1 also involved >70,000 infants. Two pivotal trials were done—one in Europe[29] and one in Latin America and Finland.[30,31] Efficacy in the European study against rotavirus gastroenteritis of any severity through one season was 87% and through two seasons was 79%; the respective efficacies against severe disease were 96% and 90%. Hospitalizations were reduced by 100% through one season and 96% through two seasons. In the Latin America/Finland study, efficacy against severe rotavirus gastroenteritis through one season was 85% and through two seasons was 81%; hospitalizations were reduced by 85% and 83%, respectively. The vaccine was highly effective against G1P[8] strains. For non-G1 strains, efficacy through one season against any severity of disease ranged from 76% for G9P[8] to 90% for G3P[8], but was not significant for G2P[4] (very few cases occurred). Efficacy through two seasons against any severity of disease ranged from 58% for G2P[4] to 85% for G3P[8]. Efficacy through one season against severe disease ranged from 95% for G9P[8] to 100% for G3P[8] and G4P[8], but was not significant for G2P[4] (again, very few cases occurred). Efficacy through two seasons against severe disease ranged from 85% for G9P[8] to 95% for G4P[8].

In an integrated analysis of all randomized, double-blind, placebo-controlled, phase 2 and 3 studies of RV1, efficacy against severe disease caused by G1P[8] strains (which share both G and P types with the vaccine) was estimated at 87.4%.[32] Efficacy against severe disease caused by G2P[4] strains was estimated at 71.4%; since these strains share neither G nor P types with the vaccine, these data indicate cross-protection. There are no data regarding postlicensure effectiveness of RV1 in the United States.

Efficacy of both RV1[33] and RV5[34,35] is lower in developing countries. Potential explanations include interference by maternal antibodies, breast-feeding, and coadministration of oral polio vaccine.

Safety

Prelicensure trials of RV5 showed a slight excess of vomiting (6.7% vs 5.4%) and diarrhea (10.4% vs 9.1%) after Dose 1 and a slight excess of diarrhea (8.6% vs 6.4%) after Dose 2.[24] In prelicensure trials of RV1, solicited adverse events occurred at similar rates among RV1 recipients and placebo recipients, although there were slightly increased unsolicited reports of irritability (11.4% vs 8.7%) and flatulence (2.2% vs 1.3%) compared with placebo.[30] An integrated safety summary of eight randomized, double-blind trials of RV1 involving a total of 71,209 infants demonstrated no differences in solicited adverse events or serious adverse events.[36]

RV1 is shed in about 50% of vaccinees, more commonly after Dose 1; RV5 is shed in about 10% of vaccinees after Dose 1 but very rarely after subsequent doses. Horizontal transmission has been documented for both vaccines. For a discussion of rotavirus vaccines and intussusception, see *Chapter 7: Addressing Concerns About Vaccines—Do Rotavirus Vaccines Cause Intussusception?*

TABLE 22.1 — Rotavirus Vaccines

Trade name	Rotarix	RotaTeq
Abbreviation	RV1 (rotavirus vaccine, monovalent)	RV5 (rotavirus vaccine, 5-valent)
Manufacturer/distributor	GlaxoSmithKline	Merck
Type of vaccine	Live-attenuated, classical	Live-attenuated, engineered
Composition:		
Virus strain	Human rotavirus strain 89-12, serotype G1P1[8]	5 naturally attenuated bovine rotavirus reassortants expressing the following serotypes: Human G1, bovine P7[5] Human G2, bovine P7[5] Human G3, bovine P7[5] Human G4, bovine P7[5] Bovine G6, human P1[8]
Propagation	Vero (African green monkey kidney) cells	Vero (African green monkey kidney) cells
Amount	10^6 median cell culture infective dose	2.0 to 2.8×10^6 infectious units of each virus
Adjuvant	None	None
Preservative	None	None
Excipients and contaminants	Lyophilized vaccine: Amino acids Dextran Dulbecco's Modified Eagle Medium Sorbitol Sucrose	Sucrose Sodium citrate Sodium phosphate monobasic monohydrate Sodium hydroxide Polysorbate 80 Cell culture media

	Diluent: Calcium carbonate Xanthan	Fetal bovine serum (trace)
Latex	Tip cap (and plunger for one presentation) contains latex	None
Labeled indications	Prevention of rotavirus gastroenteritis caused by serotype G1 and non-G1 serotypes G3, G4, and G9	Prevention of rotavirus gastroenteritis caused by serotypes G1, G2, G3, and G4
Labeled ages	6 to 24 weeks	6 to 32 weeks
Dose	1 mL	2 mL
Route of administration	PO[a]	PO[a]
Labeled schedule:		
Dose 1	6 to 20 weeks of age	6 to 12 weeks of age
Dose 2	≥4 weeks after Dose 1 but <24 weeks of age	≥4 weeks after Dose 1 but not <33 weeks of age
Dose 3	—	≥4 weeks after Dose 2 but not <33 weeks of age
Recommended schedule[b]:	2, 4 months of age	2, 4, 6 months of age
Dose 1	6 weeks to 14 weeks 6 days of age	6 weeks to 14 weeks 6 days of age
Dose 2	≥4 weeks after Dose 1 but <8 months 0 days of age	≥4 weeks after Dose 1 but <8 months 0 days of age
Dose 3	—	≥4 weeks after Dose 2 but <8 months 0 days of age
How supplied (number in package)	1-dose vial (10), lyophilized, with diluent in prefilled oral applicator	1-dose squeezable, plastic tube (10, 25)

Continued

TABLE 22.1 — *Continued*

Trade name	Rotarix	RotaTeq
Abbreviation	RV1 (rotavirus vaccine, monovalent)	RV5 (rotavirus vaccine, 5-valent)
Cost per dose ($US, 2011):		
Public	89.25	59.76
Private	102.50	72.34
Reference package insert	February 2011	July 2011

[a] The dose should not be repeated if it is spit out or regurgitated.

[b] The series should be completed with the same product, but vaccination should not be deferred if the same product is unknown or not available. If any dose in the series is RV5 or unknown, a total of 3 doses should be given.

- *Contraindications*
  - Severe allergic reaction (eg, anaphylaxis) to previous dose of vaccine or any vaccine component (risk of recurrent allergic reaction). Because RV1 may cause latex sensitization, some experts recommend RV5 for infants with spina bifida or bladder extrophy; however, if only RV1 is available, it should be given.
  - Severe combined immunodeficiency disease (risk of disease caused by live virus)
  - History of intussusception (risk of recurrent intussusception)
- *Precautions*
  - Moderate or severe acute illness (difficulty distinguishing illness from vaccine reaction)
  - Moderate or severe acute gastroenteritis (risk of impaired immune response)
  - Immunodeficiency or immunosuppression (risk of disease caused by live virus). Adverse events are unlikely in HIV-infected infants because the vaccine strains are attenuated and the vast majority of HIV-exposed infants in the United States will not have HIV infection.

Recommendations

All infants should be vaccinated against rotavirus. There is no preference for one vaccine over the other. The following circumstances *do not* preclude vaccination:

- Infants who have already had an episode of rotavirus gastroenteritis
- Breast-feeding
- Premature infants who are clinically stable and are being or have been discharged from the nursery (those who are remaining in the nursery or neonatal intensive care unit should not be vaccinated)
- Infants living in the home of immunocompromised or pregnant individuals (standard precautions should be followed to minimize the potential for transmission)
- Infants who have received antibody-containing blood products (there is the theoretical risk that passively acquired antibodies could inactivate a dose of the vaccine, but this should not be an issue since it is a multiple-dose series)
- Infants with pre-existing gastrointestinal conditions such as malabsorption syndromes, Hirschsprung's disease, or short-gut syndrome. The RV1 package insert lists as a contraindication uncorrected congenital malformation of the gastrointestinal tract that would predispose to intussusception.

The series should be completed with the same product, but vaccination should not be deferred if the same product is not available (if a mixed schedule is used, or if a previous product is unknown, a total of 3 doses should be given). It is not necessary to repeat a dose if the infant spits up. Standard precautions should be used for infants who are hospitalized after vaccination.

REFERENCES

1. Marshall GS. *Pediatr Infect Dis J.* 2009;28:355-362.
2. Coffin SE, et al. *Pediatr Infect Dis J.* 2006;25:584-589.
3. Dennehy PH, et al. *Pediatr Infect Dis J.* 2006;25:1123-1131.
4. Saulsbury FT, et al. *J Pediatr*. 1980;97:61-65.
5. Parashar UD, et al. *MMWR*. 2006;55(RR-12):1-13.
6. Payne DC, et al. *Pediatrics*. 2008;122:1235-1243.
7. Parashar UD, et al. *J Infect Dis*. 2009;200(suppl 1):S9-S15.
8. Gentsch JR, et al. *Clin Infect Dis*. 2009;200:S99-S105.
9. CDC. *MMWR.* 2008;57:1255-1257.
10. CDC. *MMWR*. 1999;48(RR-2):1-23.
11. Widdowson MA, et al. *Pediatrics*. 2007;119:684-697.
12. Panozzo CA, et al. *MMWR.* 2009;58:1146-1149.
13. Tate JE, et al. *Pediatr Infect Dis J.* 2011;30:S30-S34.
14. Cortes JE, et al. *N Engl J Med.* 2011;365:1108-1117.
15. Curns AT, et al. *J Infect Dis*. 2010;201:1617-1624.
16. Payne DC, et al. *Clin Infect Dis*. 2011;53:245-253.
17. Lopman BA, et al. *J Infect Dis*. 2011;204:980-986.
18. Cortese MM, et al. *Pediatr Infect Dis J.* 2010;29:489-494.
19. Begue RE, et al. *Pediatrics*. 2010;126:e40-e45.
20. Curns AT, et al. *Pediatr Infect Dis J.* 2011;30:S54-S55.
21. Cortese MM, et al. *MMWR*. 2009;58(RR-2):1-25.
22. CDC. *MMWR*. 2010;59:687-688.
23. CDC. *MMWR*. 2011;60:1427.
24. Vesikari T, et al. *N Engl J Med.* 2006;354:23-33.
25. Vesikari T, et al. *Pediatr Infect Dis J.* 2010;29:957-963.
26. Wang FT, et al. *Pediatrics*. 2010;125:e208-e213.
27. Boom JA, et al. *Pediatr Infect Dis J.* 2010;29:1133-1135.
28. Desai SN, et al. *Vaccine*. 2010;28:7501-7506.
29. Vesikari T, et al. *Lancet*. 2007;370:1757-1763.
30. Ruiz-Palacios GM, et al. *N Engl J Med.* 2006;354:11-22.
31. Linhares AC, et al. *Lancet*. 2008;371:1181-1189.
32. De Vos B, et al. *Pediatr Infect Dis J.* 2009;28:261-266.
33. Madhi SA, et al. *N Engl J Med.* 2010;362:289-298.
34. Armah GE, et al. *Lancet*. 2010;376:606-614.
35. Zaman K, et al. *Lancet*. 2010;376:615-623.
36. Cheuvart B, et al. *Pediatr Infect Dis J.* 2009;28:225-232.

23 Smallpox

The Pathogen

Variola virus is a very large, brick-shaped, enveloped DNA virus in the Poxviridae family (genus *Orthopoxvirus*) that replicates in the cytoplasm and is closely related to vaccinia, cowpox, and monkeypox. Direct organ damage by viral infection is unusual, as is secondary bacterial infection. Instead, morbidity results from toxemia associated with circulating immune complexes and viral antigens. Encephalitis can occur and is similar to the acute perivascular demyelination syndromes that may complicate measles and varicella infection or smallpox vaccination.

Clinical Features

Initial infection takes place at mucosal surfaces of the oropharynx or respiratory tract.[1] Three to 4 days later, viremia leads to visceral dissemination, but the patient remains asymptomatic. Secondary viremia leads to a marked *prodromal illness*, which begins 12 to 14 days after infection and is characterized by high fever, malaise, headache, backache, prostration, chills, vomiting, delirium, and/or abdominal pain. *Rash* begins 1 to 4 days into the prodrome and is coincident with a decrease in fever; maculopapular lesions initially appear in the mouth and on the face and forearms, spreading to the trunk and legs. The lesions evolve slowly into *vesicles* and *pustules*, which are characteristically deep-seated, round, firm, and discrete, although some may coalesce. Eventually, the lesions develop an umbilicated appearance with a central dimple. Fever usually continues until scabs form, about 2 weeks into the illness. Scars are evident after the scabs separate.

Variola major refers to the typical smallpox syndrome, which is easily recognized and accounts for the vast majority of cases; mortality rates approximate 30%. *Hemorrhagic smallpox* follows a shorter incubation period and is characterized by an extreme prodrome, the development of dusky erythema, and the eruption of petechiae and hemorrhage into skin and mucous membranes. Pregnant women are disproportionately affected and the syndrome is uniformly fatal. In *malignant (flat) smallpox*, the onset is equally abrupt, but the initial confluent lesions never evolve into pustules, instead remaining flat, soft, and velvety. Mortality approaches 100% as well. *Modified smallpox* occurs in previously vaccinated persons, and although the prodrome may be severe, the lesions are fewer in number, more superficial, and evolve more rapidly; death is rare. *Variola minor (alastrim)*, caused by a less-pathogenic strain of the virus, is differentiated by fewer constitutional symptoms, sparse rash, and excellent prognosis. *Variola sine eruptione* is asymptomatic or self-limited with fever and flu-like symptoms; it occurs in previously vaccinated persons or infants with maternal antibodies.

Failure to diagnose the first wave of cases during a smallpox attack would have grave consequences. For this reason, and given the fact that most practicing physicians today have never seen a case, attention has focused on recognizing the clinical signs and symptoms and differentiating smallpox from other conditions that bear similarities, most notably chickenpox. **Table 23.1** provides clues to accurate and timely diagnosis. Suspected cases should immediately be reported to state or local health departments. The CDC also maintains a 24/7 Emergency Operations Center that is available to health care providers at 770-488-7100.

Epidemiology and Transmission

Natural smallpox has been *eradicated* from the face of the earth, but the variola virus itself is not extinct, existing as it is in US and Russian government laboratory freezers (see *Chapter 1: Introduction to Vaccinology—Goals of Immunization Programs*). The possibility exists that the virus could get into the wrong hands and be used as a weapon of bioterrorism.[2]

Certain features of smallpox make it attractive as a weapon, including the small infectious dose, high mortality rate, absence of natural and vaccine-induced immunity at the population level, lack of established therapy, historical fear and panic related to the disease, and person-to-person spread, which would amplify the effect of a primary release by generating secondary and tertiary cases. Epidemic disease in developed countries today would have the potential for great devastation because of the high point prevalence of atopic skin disease, use of immunosuppressive therapies, chronic conditions, HIV infection, as well as aging of the population.

Fortunately, variola virus is labile, and <90% remains viable for 24 hours after aerosol release in the presence of ultraviolet light. Transmission occurs through direct contact with body fluids and inhalation of aerosols and droplet nuclei expelled from the oropharynx of infected persons. Close contact is usually required, and secondary attack rates vary from about 40% to 90% under these circumstances. Distant airborne transmission is rare, but fomites such as bedding or clothing can transmit the virus. Transmission does not occur through insects or animals. Patients are most infectious 7 to 10 days after the rash develops; since this occurs after a debilitating prodromal illness, patients are likely to be easily recognized and bedridden at the time they are most contagious. Transmission from subclinical cases is of little epidemiologic importance.

Immunization Program

Until 1972, smallpox vaccine was given in the United States at 1 year of age. This program was abandoned because of global eradication. The remaining interest in smallpox vaccination resides in protecting laboratory workers and preparing for the possibility of bioterrorism.

Universal pre-event vaccination would constitute an absolute deterrent to a smallpox attack and could be conducted under controlled conditions.[3,4] However, the overall risk of an attack is low, the population at risk cannot be determined, and the risks of vaccination are substantial. *Surveillance and containment*, or *ring vaccination*, involves the isolation of suspected and confirmed cases and the identification, vaccination, and monitoring of their contacts. Vaccination can be extended to household contacts of contacts as well, or other people with indirect exposure, and the strategy can be supplemented by local quarantine and travel restrictions. This strategy, which was highly successful during the global eradication campaign, is workable because vaccination is effective if given soon after exposure. Ring vaccination, however, might not work as well in a largely nonimmune, highly mobile population experiencing a multisite intentional aerosol release. In addition, the logistical complexity of this approach is daunting, especially in the face of the potential for public panic. *Universal postevent vaccination* would be logistically difficult and would provide little additional benefit to ring vaccination, although the CDC National Pharmaceutical Stockpile has protocols for simultaneous delivery of vaccine to every state and territory within 24 hours of an event. The current US vaccination plan combines limited pre-event vaccination with ring vaccination.[5]

As of June 2001, pre-event vaccination was recommended only for laboratory and HCP involved in orthopox research.[6] In the wake of the anthrax attacks of October 2001, recommendations were made to vaccinate smallpox response teams in each state and smallpox health care teams at predesignated isolation and care facilities, and, eventually, at each acute care hospital.[7]

The federal plan announced in December 2002 called for voluntary vaccination of up to 500,000 health and safety workers constituting local Smallpox Response Teams.[8] By mid-2003 it was clear that the federal plan to vaccinate civilians was proceeding much slower than anticipated; in all, only 40,000 civilians had been vaccinated, and the CDC had effectively ceased efforts to vaccinate additional people. The concomitant Department of

TABLE 23.1 — Diagnosis of Smallpox

Clinical Finding	Smallpox[a]	Chickenpox[b]
Major Criteria		
Prodrome	Fever ≥101°F (38.3°C) beginning 1 to 4 days before rash and at least one of the following: prostration, headache, backache, chills, vomiting, severe abdominal pain	None or mild
Lesion morphology	Deep-seated, firm, round, well-circumscribed vesicles or pustules, may be umbilicated or confluent	Superficial vesicles (resembling dewdrops on a rose petal)
Lesion development	Same stage of development on any one part of the body	Crops at different stages of development on any one part of the body
Minor Criteria		
Distribution	Centrifugal (concentrated on face and distal extremities)	Centripetal (concentrated on trunk)
Initial lesions	Oral mucosa, palate, face, forearms	Face or trunk
General appearance	Toxic or moribund	Well
Evolution	Slow (from macules to papules to pustules over days)	Rapid (from macules to papules to vesicles to pustules to crusts in <24 hours)
Palms and soles	Involved	Spared

[a] If the patient has all three major criteria, the risk of smallpox is high and authorities should be notified immediately. If the patient has a febrile prodrome and one other major criterion or ≥ 4 minor criteria, the risk is moderate and urgent evaluation is indicated. Other conditions to be considered in the differential diagnosis include disseminated herpes zoster or herpes simplex, impetigo, drug eruptions, erythema multiforme, Stevens-Johnson syndrome, enterovirus infection, scabies, secondary syphilis, bullous pemphigoid, and molluscum contagiosum. Cowpox and monkeypox resemble smallpox but can only be acquired directly from the respective animals. The differential diagnosis of hemorrhagic smallpox includes meningococcemia, hemorrhagic varicella, Rocky Mountain spotted fever, ehrlichiosis, and gram-negative sepsis.

[b] Other clues to the diagnosis of chickenpox include absence of a personal history of varicella or varicella vaccination and exposure to chickenpox or shingles. Most cases will occur in children because most adults are immune. The lesions are usually intensely pruritic and scarring is unusual.

Adapted from Centers for Disease Control and Prevention Web site. Evaluating patients for smallpox. http://www.bt.cdc.gov/agent/smallpox/diagnosis/pdf/spox-poster-full.pdf. Accessed January 9, 2012.

Defense plan called for stepwise, compulsory vaccination, first involving up to 5000 members of smallpox epidemic response teams, then 10,000 to 25,000 medical team members, then up to 500,000 mission-critical forces. As of January 2005, >700,000 service members had been vaccinated.

Vaccines

The origin of vaccinia virus is not clear, but it appears to be a hybrid between cowpox and smallpox that is not found in nature. In October 2002, the FDA relicensed Dryvax (Smallpox Vaccine, Dried, Calf Lymph Type), a product manufactured by Wyeth (acquired by Pfizer in 2009) until 1982 but held in storage at the CDC since then. Relicensure was intended to facilitate administration of the vaccine outside of investigational protocols. Dryvax was a lyophilized preparation of the New York City Board of Health strain of vaccinia harvested from lymph contained in skin lesions that develop after scarification of calves. A cell culture derived smallpox vaccine called ACAM2000 was licensed in August 2007 and has replaced Dryvax in the Strategic National Stockpile.[9,10] Characteristics of this vaccine are given in **Table 23.2**. ACAM2000 consists of live vaccinia virus that was plaque purified from Dryvax.

Handling and administration of smallpox vaccine is different from all other vaccines, as summarized below.

- *Reconstitution*
  - Wear gloves, use aseptic technique, and avoid contact of the vaccine with skin, eyes, and mucous membranes.
  - Bring the vaccine up to room temperature.
  - Lift up the cap seals on the vaccine and diluent vials.
  - Wipe off the rubber stopper with alcohol and allow it to dry.
  - Draw up 0.3 mL of diluent in the 1-mL tuberculin syringe fitted with a 25-gauge 5/8-inch needle that is provided with the vaccine.
  - Transfer the contents of the syringe to the vaccine vial.
  - Gently swirl without letting the liquid get on the rubber stopper. The reconstituted vaccine is clear to slightly hazy, colorless to straw-colored, and free from particulates.
- *Administration*
  - Providers must be properly educated on administration technique and must provide vaccinees with an FDA-approved Medication Guide.[11]
  - Wear gloves, use aseptic technique, and avoid contact of the vaccine with skin, eyes, and mucous membranes.
  - Preparation of the skin with alcohol is not required (this may inactivate the virus). Use soap and water if the site is grossly contaminated. If alcohol is used, the skin must be allowed to dry thoroughly before inoculation.

TABLE 23.2 — Smallpox Vaccine

Trade name	ACAM2000[a]
Abbreviation	—
Manufacturer/distributor	Sanofi Pasteur (formerly Acambis)
Type of vaccine	Live-attenuated, classical
Composition	Vaccinia, New York Board of Health strain Propagated in Vero (African green monkey kidney) cells 2.5 to 12.5 × 10^5 PFU/dose
Adjuvant	None
Preservative	None
Excipients and contaminants	HEPES (pH 6.5 to 7.5) (6 to 8 mM) Human serum albumin (2%) Sodium chloride (0.5% to 0.7%) Mannitol (5%) Neomycin (trace) Polymyxin B (trace) Glycerin (50% v/v) Phenol (0.25% v/v)
Latex	None
Labeled indications	Prevention of smallpox
Labeled ages	All ages
Dose	15 punctures *(see text)*
Route of administration	Percutaneous (scarification)
Labeled schedule	1 dose Booster doses every 3 years (for persons at continued high risk of exposure)
Recommended schedule	See text
How supplied (number in package)	100-dose vial, lyophilized, with diluent, bifurcated needles, and tuberculin syringe for reconstitution
Reference package insert	September 2009

[a] ACAM2000 is not commercially available but rather is purchased by the federal government for inclusion in the Strategic National Stockpile. Dryvax (Smallpox Vaccine, Dried, Calf Lymph Type; Pfizer [formerly-Wyeth]) is no longer available in the United States.

– Remove the vaccine vial cap (maintain sterile conditions for later recapping).
– Remove the bifurcated needle from its individual wrapping. Dip the bifurcated needle into the reconstituted vaccine and withdraw. A sufficient amount of liquid (approximately 0.0025 mL) is retained between the prongs by capillary action.
– Hold the needle between the thumb and first finger, perpendicular to the vaccinee's skin. Lay your wrist on the vaccinee's arm below the deltoid region. Use your other hand to pull the skin taut from underneath.
– Deposit the drop of vaccine on the skin. Using firm strokes from the wrist, make 15 rhythmic perpendicular insertions through the drop into the skin within a 5-mm area. A trace of blood should be visible after each puncture. *Do not* reinsert the needle into the vial between punctures or after the whole procedure.
– Discard the bifurcated needle immediately in a leak-proof, puncture-proof biohazard waste container. When ready for disposal, the vaccine vial, stopper, diluent syringe, and vented needle should be placed in a similar container. The container can be disposed of in the usual way.
– Absorb excess vaccine and blood with sterile gauze and discard in a biohazard container.
– Close the vaccine vial by reinserting the cap and return it to the refrigerator.
– Cover the site with gauze and adhesive tape. If the vaccinee will have direct patient contact, cover the gauze with a semipermeable dressing such as OpSite (Smith & Nephew) or Tegaderm (3M) (some of these products are supplied with attached gauze pads). Semipermeable dressings should not be used alone because they macerate the skin.

• *Postvaccination Care*
– Vaccinees should make sure a layer of clothing covers the dressing and should exercise meticulous hand hygiene after touching the site or dressings.
– Change the dressing every 3 to 5 days or more often if exudates accumulate (dressings can be discarded in the household trash if sealed in a plastic bag).
– Avoid rubbing and scratching.
– Do not put salves or ointments on the site.
– Keep the site dry. Showering or bathing can continue. If the site is uncovered, it should not be touched. The site should be blotted dry with gauze, which should then be discarded in a sealed plastic bag in the household trash. If a towel is used for drying the site, it should not be used on the rest of the body.

– Separately wash clothing or other material that comes into contact with the site, using hot water with detergent and/or bleach.

- *Assessing Response*
  – The subject should return for examination in 7 days.
  – A red, pruritic papule should form 2 to 5 days after vaccination. This becomes vesicular then pustular and reaches a maximum size by 8 to 10 days. The pustule dries and forms a scab, which separates by 14 to 21 days, leaving a pitted scar.
  – Failure to develop a skin lesion as described indicates failure of vaccination, and revaccination should be considered, unless the vaccinee had been previously vaccinated (pre-existing immunity can modify the cutaneous reaction). Images of appropriate primary and revaccination responses are shown in the package insert, and images of normal and adverse reactions can be viewed on the CDC Web site.[12]

Efficacy and/or Immunogenicity

Studies with Dryvax suggest that protection persists for at least 5 years after primary vaccination. Antibody levels steadily decline 5 to 10 years following vaccination, and although detectable cellular responses may persist, it must be assumed that immunity to smallpox wanes. Revaccination even one time results in boosted antibody levels that may persist for 30 years.

Two randomized, multicenter studies were conducted comparing ACAM2000 with Dryvax. One study looked at 1647 persons who had been vaccinated over 10 years earlier; 1242 received ACAM2000 and 405 received Dryvax. Successful revaccination was slightly less common in the ACAM2000 group, but antibody titers were not inferior. The second study looked at 1037 vaccinia-naïve subjects; 780 received ACAM2000 and 257 received Dryvax. In this case, vaccination success rates were not inferior, although antibody titers were lower. Overall, ACAM2000 was noninferior to Dryvax where it counts most—major cutaneous reaction in vaccinia-naïve subjects and strength of antibody response in vaccinia-experienced subjects (whose pre-existing immunity might have modified the cutaneous reaction).

Safety

Smallpox vaccine is the most reactogenic and dangerous of all licensed vaccines. By definition, successfully vaccinated persons develop a pustule at the inoculation site that lasts several weeks. Many experience additional local reactions and associated systemic complaints. In about one third of patients, these symptoms may lead to missed work, school, or recreational activities, or to trouble sleeping. Common side effects for ACAM2000 include itching, soreness, fever, headache, rash, and fatigue. As with Dryvax, transmission to individuals who are pregnant, immunocompromised, or have chronic skin problems can lead to serious complications. In order to prevent serious adverse events, a Risk Minimization Action Plan was implemented for ACAM2000.[13]

Potential complications of vaccination include inadvertent inoculation, generalized vaccinia, erythema multiforme, eczema vaccinatum, post-vaccinal encephalitis or encephalomyelitis, progressive vaccinia, contact vaccinia, and fetal infection. The safety of the post-9/11 civilian and military smallpox vaccination program (in which Dryvax was used) has been reviewed.[8] Nearly 800,000 vaccinees were included. No cases of eczema vaccinatum, progressive vaccinia, fetal vaccinia, or workplace contact transmission were reported, suggesting that education and screening procedures were successful. Anticipated reactions included 43 cases of generalized vaccinia, later determined to be hypersensitivity reactions, and 2 cases of encephalitis. Inadvertent infection of the skin occurred in 62 vaccinees and 50 contacts of vaccinees. Cardiac ischemic events (including 3 fatal myocardial infarctions) occurred in 33 persons, which was below the expected background rate. A total of 107 cases of myopericarditis were reported. Among military personnel alone, the observed incidence within 30 days of vaccination (16.11 per 100,000) was 7.5-fold higher than the background rate (for unknown reasons, the increased risk was seen among primary vaccinees in the military program but among revaccinees in the civilian program). A causal relationship was further suggested by temporal clustering as well as wide geographic and cross-seasonal distribution. The risk of myocarditis and/or pericarditis after vaccination with ACAM2000 is estimated to be 1 in 175 previously unvaccinated adults.

- *Contraindications (postexposure)*
  - In the event of exposure to smallpox, there are no contraindications to vaccination.
- *Contraindications (pre-event, applies to potential vaccinees and their household or sexual contacts)*—most of these involve risk of disease caused by live virus
  - *Eczema, atopic dermatitis, other acute, chronic, or exfoliative skin conditions*: burns, impetigo, chickenpox, contact dermatitis, shingles, herpes, severe acne, psoriasis, Darier's disease (keratosis follicularis), even if currently inactive. Two screening questions have been suggested (a *yes* to either question means *no* vaccine): Have you or a member of your household ever been diagnosed with eczema or atopic dermatitis? Have you or a family member ever had an itchy, red, scaly rash that lasts for >2 weeks and often comes and goes?

- *Immunodeficiency or immunosuppression*: solid organ or bone marrow transplantation, generalized malignancy, leukemia, lymphoma, agammaglobulinemia, autoimmune disease, treatment with radiation, antimetabolites, alkylating agents, corticosteroids (in similar doses to those outlined in *Chapter 6: Vaccination in Special Circumstances—Medication-Induced Immunosuppression*), chemotherapy agents or organ transplant medications, and HIV infection (routine testing is not recommended, but should be done in persons with risk factors, those who are unsure of their status and those who are concerned that they could have HIV infection)
- *Pregnancy*: Vaccinated women should not be pregnant and should not become pregnant for 4 weeks (Pregnancy Category D—vaccine can cause fetal harm, so use only if the potential benefits outweigh the potential risks). For reassurance, women can perform a urine pregnancy test on the first morning void on the day of vaccination. Routine pregnancy testing is not recommended. Inadvertent vaccination during pregnancy is not ordinarily a reason to terminate the pregnancy, although the mother should be aware of the extremely rare occurrence of fetal vaccinia.

• *Contraindications (pre-event, applies to potential vaccinees only)*
- Severe allergic reaction (eg, anaphylaxis) to previous dose of vaccine or any vaccine component (risk of recurrent allergic reaction)
- Infants <12 months of age (risk of disease caused by live virus; ACIP advises against pre-event vaccination of persons <18 years of age)
- Breast-feeding (risk of disease caused by live virus)
- Cardiac risk, including underlying heart disease with or without symptoms, persons with three or more risk factors such as hypertension, diabetes, hypercholesterolemia, first-degree relative under age 50 years with heart disease, and smoking (risk of myocarditis). Verbal screening for risk factors is recommended. Special follow-up for persons with risk factors who have already been vaccinated is not recommended.

• *Precautions (postexposure)*
- In the event of exposure to smallpox, there are no precautions to vaccination.

• *Precautions (pre-event)*
- Moderate or severe acute illness (difficulty distinguishing illness from vaccine reaction)
- Inflammatory eye disease requiring steroid therapy (risk of disease from live virus)

Vaccinia immune globulin intravenous, a polyclonal immune globulin product made from blood of recently vaccinated blood donors, is available from the CDC under an Investigational New Drug (IND) protocol to treat complications of vaccination.[14] Cidofovir may help limit viral replication and is also available from the CDC under an IND.[15] Civilian providers seeking access to these drugs should first contact their state health department.

The Public Readiness and Emergency Preparedness Act, enacted in December 2005, provides compensation to persons for serious physical injuries or deaths resulting from pandemic, epidemic, or security countermeasures in the event of designated public health emergencies. Smallpox vaccine injuries are covered under this program.[16]

Recommendations

For those who receive pre-event vaccination today, a single dose is recommended, with booster doses every 10 years. Revaccination every 3 years should be considered for workers with occupational exposure to orthopox viruses. The vaccine will completely prevent or significantly modify smallpox if given 3 to 4 days after exposure; vaccination 4 to 7 days postexposure probably modifies the severity of the disease.

The US Civilian Smallpox Preparedness and Response Program was implemented in 2003.[17] This called for acute care hospitals to establish Smallpox Health Care Teams that would provide hospital-based, in-room evaluation and management for the first 7 to 10 days. Team members were to include emergency department and intensive care unit staff; general medical and primary care staff; residents; medical subspecialists; infection control professionals; respiratory therapists; radiology technicians; security personnel; and housekeeping staff. Clinical laboratory workers were not included because clinical specimens are expected to contain low levels of virus and standard precautions are considered to be protective. Emergency medical technicians (EMTs) were not routinely included, but hospital-based EMTs could be vaccinated if included on the response teams. Designated vaccinated staff were to examine all vaccinated HCP each day after vaccination, assess vaccine take, and change the dressings if indicated. Persons handling the vaccine were also to be vaccinated.

Routine leave for vaccinated HCP was not recommended. However, leave was indicated for systemic illness, extensive lesions that could not be covered, or inability to adhere to infection control precautions. A phased-in, staggered approach to vaccination was recommended, beginning with groups of previously vaccinated persons. Rigorous screening for contraindications was recommended, but routine pregnancy and HIV testing was not.

Revaccination of persons who were initially vaccinated under the civilian program is recommended only on an "out-the-door" basis, ie, only after there is determination of a credible threat to public health and prior to engaging in activities involving a risk for exposure to smallpox.[18] Revaccination is recommended every 10 years, however, for persons who routinely administer vaccine to others.

Smallpox vaccination is recommended for laboratory workers who directly handle cultures or animals infected with non-highly attenuated vaccinia viruses or vaccinia recombinants, as well as other orthopoxviruses that infect humans (eg, monkeypox and cowpox). Vaccination should also be considered for HCP who may contact materials contaminated with such viruses.

Smallpox vaccine may be administered simultaneously with all inactivated vaccines and live vaccines except for VAR, in which case ≥4 weeks should separate the 2 inoculations. Tuberculin skin tests should be deferred at least 1 month following smallpox vaccination to minimize the risk of false-negatives. Blood donation by vaccinees (as well as persons with contact vaccinia) should be deferred until the scab spontaneously separates or 21 days postvaccination, whichever is later.

Under all circumstances, *pre-event* vaccination of civilians is voluntary. A complete information packet for potential vaccinees is available at the CDC Web site.[5]

REFERENCES

1. Moore ZS, et al. *Lancet*. 2006;367:425-435.
2. Henderson DA, et al. *JAMA*. 1999;281:2127-2137.
3. Halloran ME, et al. *Science*. 2002;298:1428-1432.
4. Bozzette SA, et al. *N Engl J Med*. 2003;348:416-425.
5. Emergency preparedness and response: smallpox. Centers for Disease Control and Prevention Web site. http://www.bt.cdc.gov/agent/smallpox. Accessed January 9, 2012.
6. Rotz LD, et al. *MMWR*. 2001;50(RR-10):1-25.
7. Wharton M, et al. *MMWR*. 2003;52(RR-7):1-16.
8. Poland GA, et al. *Vaccine*. 2005;23:2078-2081.
9. CDC. *MMWR*. 2008;57:207-208.
10. Nalca A, et al. *Drug Design Dev Ther*. 2010;4:71-79.
11. Medication Guide ACAM2000™. Centers for Disease Control and Prevention Web site. http://www.bt.cdc.gov/agent/smallpox/vaccination/pdf/ACAM2000MedicationGuide-31Aug2007.pdf. Accessed January 10, 2012.
12. Smallpox vaccination and adverse events training module. Centers for Disease Control and Prevention Web site. http://www.bt.cdc.gov/training/smallpoxvaccine/reactions. Accessed January 9, 2012.
13. ACAM2000 (smallpox vaccine) questions and answers. US Food and Drug Administration Web site. http://www.fda.gov/BiologicsBloodVaccines/Vaccines/QuestionsaboutVaccines/ucm078041.htm. Accessed January 9, 2012.
14. Smallpox vaccination and adverse events training module. Centers for Disease Control and Prevention Web site. http://www.bt.cdc.gov/training/smallpoxvaccine/reactions/vig_current.html. Accessed January 9, 2012.
15. Investigational Vistide (cidofovir) information. Centers for Disease Control and Prevention Web site. http://emergency.cdc.gov/agent/smallpox/vaccination/cidofovir.asp. Accessed January 9, 2012.
16. Countermeasures Injury Compensation Program. Health Resources and Services Administration Web site. http://www.hrsa.gov/gethealthcare/conditions/countermeasurescomp/. Accessed January 9, 2012.
17. Strikas RA, et al. *Clin Infect Dis*. 2008;46:S157-S167.
18. CDC interim guidance for revaccination of eligible persons who participated in the US Civilian Smallpox Preparedness and Response Program. Centers for Disease Control and Prevention Web site. http://www.bt.cdc.gov/agent/smallpox/revaxmemo.asp. Accessed January 9, 2012.

24 *Streptococcus pneumoniae*

The Pathogen

S pneumoniae is a facultatively anaerobic, catalase-negative gram-positive bacterium that looks like lancet-shaped diplococci on Gram stain.[1] The organism produces a polysaccharide capsule that is the basis for serotyping (there are >90 known serotypes, although most invasive disease is caused by <20 of these). The capsule contributes to virulence by inhibiting complement-mediated lysis and phagocytosis by neutrophils (antibodies to the capsular polysaccharide are protective). Other virulence factors include pneumolysin and pneumococcal surface protein A. *S pneumoniae* often colonizes the nasopharynx—disease results from contiguous spread to respiratory tract structures such as the middle ear space or lungs, hematogenous seeding of distant sites such as the meninges, or from bacteremia without focal infection. Resistance to penicillin and other antibiotics has increased dramatically since the early 1990s.

Clinical Features

Before the conjugate-vaccine era, *bacteremia* without focal infection accounted for 70% of invasive disease in those <2 years of age; *bacteremic pneumonia* accounted for another 12% to 16%.[2] With the disappearance of invasive *H influenzae* type b disease from the United States in the 1990s, *S pneumoniae* became the leading cause of bacterial meningitis among young children (collectively, bacteremia, meningitis, and infection of other normally sterile body sites is referred to as *invasive pneumococcal disease* or IPD). *S pneumoniae* was also a common cause of noninvasive respiratory syndromes including *acute otitis media* (AOM), where it accounted for 28% to 55% of cases. By 12 months of age, 62% of children had at least one episode of AOM, making this one of the more common reasons for sick visits to pediatric offices. Complications of otitis media include mastoiditis and suppurative intracranial infection.

Pneumonia is the most common presentation of pneumococcal disease in adults. Classically, there is abrupt onset of fever and an episode of rigors. Other symptoms include pleuritic chest pain, productive cough yielding mucopurulent, rusty sputum, dyspnea, tachypnea, hypoxia, tachycardia, malaise, and weakness. Nausea, vomiting, and headaches occur less frequently. Complications include empyema, pericarditis, and abscess. Pneumococcal meningitis also occurs in adults. Symptoms include headache, lethargy, vomiting, irritability, fever, nuchal rigidity, cranial nerve signs, seizures, and coma. The spinal fluid profile and neurologic complications are similar to those seen in other forms of bacterial meningitis. One quarter of patients with pneumococcal meningitis also have pneumonia.

Mortality is highest in patients with bacteremia or meningitis, in patients with underlying medical conditions, and in the very young and the very old. In some high-risk groups, mortality from bacteremia is as high as 40% despite antibiotic therapy.

Epidemiology and Transmission

Humans are the only natural hosts and transmission occurs by direct person-to-person contact or via respiratory droplets. Spread within the household is facilitated by crowding and occurs more often in the late winter and early spring, when respiratory viral disease is more prevalent. In general, higher rates of nasopharyngeal carriage lead to higher rates of disease.

It is estimated that 1 million children worldwide die from IPD each year. In 1999, the year before the introduction of PCV7 in the United States, the overall incidence of IPD was 24 per 100,000 population.[3] The rate was as high as 205 per 100,000 in children 1 year of age and as low as 4 per 100,000 in children between 5 and 17; adults ≥65 years of age had a rate of 62 per 100,000. At the time, it was estimated that there were a total of 64,400 cases of IPD and 7300 deaths. The most common serious clinical syndrome was bacteremic pneumonia (54%), followed by bacteremia without a focus (38%) and meningitis (5%), and pneumococcus was estimated to cause over one third of community-acquired and half of hospital-acquired pneumonia cases in adults. In addition, an estimated 5 million cases of AOM due to pneumococcus occurred each year in children <5 years of age. Children with functional or anatomic asplenia and children with HIV infection were at particularly high risk for IPD, with rates in some studies >50 times those in age-equivalent children without these conditions. Alaska Native, American Indian, and African American children were also at increased risk. The reason for this is not known, but a similar racial and ethnic predilection was seen for invasive *H influenzae* type b. Day care attendance was associated with a 2- to 3-fold increased risk of IPD and AOM among children <5 years of age.

Immunization Program

A 14-valent pneumococcal polysaccharide vaccine was licensed in the United States in 1977. In 1983, this was replaced by 23-valent vaccines, which were recommended for all persons ≥65 years of age as well as high-risk persons from 2 to 64 years of age.[4] PCV7 was introduced in 2000 and was recommended for all infants, with a booster dose in the second year of life.[2] At that time, PCV7 covered 80% of the serotypes causing IPD in young children in the United States. By 2005, universal infant immunization had resulted in a 77% reduction in IPD among children <5 years of age.[5] The largest percentage decline was in children 1 year of age. During 2001-2005, 62,000 children <5 years of age were spared IPD—59% through direct effects of the vaccine and the remainder through herd immunity, the result of decreased nasopharyngeal carriage. Rates of hospitalization for pneumococcal meningitis in children <2 years of age declined from 7.7 per 100,000 in the prevaccine era to 2.6 per 100,000 in 2001-2004 (there was also a 33% decrease among adults ≥65 years of age).[6]

By 2004, all-cause pneumonia admission rates had declined by 39% in children <2 years of age; admissions for pneumococcal pneumonia declined 65%[7] and outpatient visits for otitis media declined by 20%.[8] Rates of infection due to drug-resistant strains also declined[9]; possible mechanisms for this include direct effects on vaccine serotypes, which are disproportionately resistant, as well as global decreases in antibiotic use.[10] Considering only direct effects of PCV7 on IPD, pneumonia, and otitis media in children <5 years of age, PCV7 is estimated to have cost $201,000 per life-year saved, with a net cost of $145 per child vaccinated (2006 dollars).[11] However, with the inclusion of indirect effects in all age groups, PCV7 was estimated to be cost saving, to the tune of $503 per child vaccinated. Studies demonstrated significant decreases in nasopharyngeal carriage of vaccine serotypes among vaccinated children and their adult contacts, but there was an increase in colonization with nonvaccine serotypes.[12,13] This was accompanied by relative increases in IPD due to those serotypes (so called *replacement disease*), particularly serotype 19A.[14]

Declines in IPD due to vaccine serotypes also were seen among older persons as a result of herd immunity (**Figure 1.9**). In fact, by 2003 the incidence of IPD caused by PCV7 serotypes declined 50% among persons ≥50 years of age, with no change in disease caused by the 14 serotypes contained in PPSV23 that are not in PCV7.[15] In 2008, ACIP extended the recommendations for PPSV23 to include adults 19 to 64 years of age who smoke or have asthma and revoked a previous recommendation for routine immunization of American Indians and Alaska Natives.[16] Most studies show that routine vaccination of adults ≥65 years of age is cost-effective, at <$50,000 per life-year or QALY gained.[17]

PCV7 was routinely used from 2000 through 2009. Despite the successes outlined above, it was estimated that in 2004 pneumococcus was still responsible for 4 million episodes of illness, 22,000 deaths, nearly a half-million hospitalizations, three-quarters of a million emergency department visits, and 5 million outpatient visits.[18] In 2008, a dose of PCV7 was recommended for all incompletely immunized children 24 to 59 months of age.[19] PCV13, which covers 6 additional pneumococcal serotypes, was licensed in 2010. Shortly thereafter, PCV13 replaced PCV7 in the routine schedule,[20] and additional recommendations were made for supplemental dosing in children who had already completed the PCV7 series, as well as for immunizing high-risk children.[21] As of 2007, 64% of IPD occurring in children <5 years of age was caused by serotypes contained in PCV13 but not in PCV7 (mostly, serotypes 3, 7F, and 19A); of the estimated 4600 cases that occurred that year, 2900 were potentially preventable by PCV13.[22] The switch to routine use of PCV13 was estimated to prevent 106,000 incremental IPD cases, 2.9 million cases of pneumonia, and save $11.6 billion over a 10-year period (2008 dollars).[23] A catch-up program was estimated to prevent an additional 12,600 IPD cases, 404,000 cases of pneumonia, and save an additional $737 million.

In December 2011, the label for PCV13 was extended to include adults ≥50 years of age, but recommendations for use had not been published as of February 2012.

Vaccines

Characteristics of pneumococcal vaccines licensed in the United States are given in **Table 24.1**. PPSV23 is a 23-valent pure polysaccharide vaccine. PCV13 is a protein-polysaccharide conjugate vaccine, made much the same way as Hib and MCV4. Biologic differences between conjugate and polysaccharide vaccines are discussed in *Chapter 1: Introduction to Vaccinology—The Germinal Center Reaction* and are summarized in **Table 1.3**.

Efficacy and/or Immunogenicity

In a controlled clinical trial involving nearly 40,000 children, PCV7 reduced IPD caused by vaccine serotypes by 97%.[24] The vaccine also reduced X-ray–confirmed pneumonia by 73%, and children who received PCV7 had 7% fewer episodes of AOM and underwent 20% fewer tympanostomy tube placements than unvaccinated children. In a Finnish study, efficacy against AOM caused by vaccine-related serotypes was 57%, but there was an increase of 33% in otitis episodes caused by nonvaccine serotypes[25]; despite this, there was a net reduction of 34% in AOM caused by *S pneumoniae*. In a 2009 meta-analysis of clinical trials in children <24 months of age, efficacy against IPD due to vaccine serotypes was approximately 90% and efficacy against otitis media due to vaccine serotypes was just over 50%.[26] Efficacy against radiographically confirmed pneumonia (serotypes largely unknown) was about 30%. A case-control study done after licensure demonstrated that ≥1 dose of PCV7 was 96% effective in preventing IPD in healthy children 3 to 59 months of age and 81% effective in those with coexisting disorders.[27]

PCV13 was compared with PCV7 in a clinical trial involving over 600 infants.[28] The proportion of subjects achieving ≥0.35 mcg/mL of anticapsular antibody to the shared serotypes after 3 doses was similar, except for 6B and 9V, where the PCV13 responses did not meet this prespecified noninferiority criterion. However, geometric mean concentrations (GMCs) of antibody were similar, as were functional (opsonophagocytic) antibody levels. Robust responses to the 6 nonshared serotypes, as well as to all 13 serotypes after the toddler dose, were demonstrated. On the basis of these data, PCV13 was given indications for the prevention of IPD and otitis media caused by the 7 serotypes shared with PCV7, as well as an indication for prevention of IPD caused by the additional 6 serotypes. A 2011 meta-analysis suggested that most infants are protected against IPD after 2 doses of the primary series.[29]

In studies involving approximately 400 adults 60 to 64 years of age, PCV13 elicited opsonophagocytic antibody titers that were noninferior to PPSV23 for the 12 shared serotypes; for 6A, which is unique to PCV13, 89% of subjects demonstrated at least a 4-fold increase in antibody titer. Among approximately 400 adults 50 to 59 years of age, responses to PCV13 were noninferior to those in the older adults. On the basis of these data, PCV13 was given an indication for prevention of pneumonia and IPD due to all 13 serotypes in adults ≥50 years of age.

Protective efficacy of pneumococcal polysaccharide vaccines was initially demonstrated in healthy gold miners in South Africa. Postlicensure case-control studies estimate the efficacy of PPSV23 in preventing serious pneumococcal disease in immunocompetent persons to be 56% to 81%, and a meta-analysis suggested efficacy against bacteremic pneumococcal pneumonia in low-risk, but not high-risk, adults.[30] A surveillance study demonstrated 57% overall effectiveness against IPD caused by vaccine serotypes; effectiveness was 65% to 84% in persons with underlying high-risk conditions and 75% in immunocompetent adults ≥65 years of age.[31] A recent Cochrane Review placed the efficacy of PPSV23 at 80% based on randomized controlled trials and 52% based on observational studies.[32] Antibody levels decline 5 to 10 years after vaccination and may decline faster in the elderly. At least one study suggested that protection may last as long as 9 years. PPSV23 does not reduce nasopharyngeal carriage and does not protect children from otitis media.

TABLE 24.1 — *S pneumoniae* Vaccines[a]

Trade name	Pneumovax 23	Prevnar 13
Abbreviation	PPSV23	PCV13 (PCV13-CRM)
Manufacturer/distributor	Merck	Pfizer (formerly Wyeth)
Type of vaccine	Inactivated, purified subunits	Inactivated, engineered subunits
Composition[b]	Capsular polysaccharides (25 mcg each) from *S pneumoniae* serotypes 1, 2, 3, 4, 5, 6B, 7F, 8, 9N, 9V, 10A, 11A, 12F, 14, 15B, 17F, 18C, 19A, 19F, 20, 22F, 23F, 33F	Capsular polysaccharides from *S pneumoniae* serotypes 1, 3, 4, 5, 6A, 7F, 9V, 14, 18C, 19A, 19F, 23F (2.2 mcg each) and 6B (4.4 mcg), conjugated to CRM_{197}, a nontoxic mutant diphtheria toxin (34 mcg)
Adjuvant	None	Aluminum phosphate (0.125 mg aluminum)
Preservative	Phenol (0.25%)	None
Excipients and contaminants	None reported	Polysorbate 80 (100 mcg) Succinate buffer (295 mcg)
Latex	None	None
Labeled indications	Prevention of pneumococcal disease caused by vaccine serotypes	Children: prevention of IPD caused by all 13 vaccine serotypes and prevention of otitis media caused by the PCV7[a] serotypes Adults: prevention of pneumonia and IPD caused by all 13 serotypes
Labeled ages	≥2 years	Children: 6 weeks to 5 years Adults: ≥50 years

Dose	0.5 mL	0.5 mL
Route of administration	Intramuscular or subcutaneous	Intramuscular
Labeled schedule	1 dose	Children: 2, 4, 6, 12 to 15 months of age, and 1 dose for children 15 months to 5 years of age who have received 4 doses of PCV7 Adults: 1 dose
Recommended schedule	65 years of age High-risk Revaccination in 5 years	Children: 2, 4, 6, 12 to 15 months of age, and 1 dose for children 15 months to 4 years of age who have received 4 doses of PCV7 or have incomplete schedules Adults: pending as of February 2012
How supplied (number in package)	1-dose vial (10) 5-dose vial (1)	Prefilled syringe (10)
Cost per dose ($US, 2011):		
Public	20.57	97.21
Private	48.97	114.15
Reference package insert	October 2011	January 2012

[a] Pnu-Imune 23 (PPSV23; Wyeth) and Prevnar (PCV7-CRM, containing serotypes 4, 6B, 9V, 14, 18C, 19F, and 23F; Wyeth), are no longer available.
[b] The Danish nomenclature for serotypes is given. The corresponding American nomenclature is as follows: 1=1; 2=2; 3=3; 4=4; 5=5; 6B=26; 7F=51; 8=8; 9N=9; 9V=68; 10A=34; 11A=43; 12F=12; 14=14; 15B=54; 17F=17; 18C=56; 19A=57; 19F=19; 20=20; 22F=22; 23F=23; 33F=70.

Safety

The safety of PCV13 was evaluated in over 4700 vaccinees across 13 clinical trials. Serious adverse events, most commonly bronchiolitis, gastroenteritis, and pneumonia, were rare and occurred with similar frequency to rates seen after PCV7. The frequency of solicited local reactions, reported in approximately 1500 infants, included redness in 24% to 42% (reactions increased with incremental doses), swelling in 20% to 32%, and tenderness in around 60%; very few reactions were considered severe. Fever occurred in 24% to 32%, but was generally ≤102.2°F (≤39°C); fever is less common among older children receiving a catch-up dose. Serious adverse events were also rarely reported among over 6000 adults who received PCV13 in clinical trials. Solicited local reactogenicity, assessed among several hundred adults, included redness (16% to 20%), swelling (about 20%), and pain (about 80%); very few reactions were considered severe. Fever ≥100.4°F (≥38°C) occurred in <5% of subjects.

For persons ≥65 years of age receiving PPSV23, overall injection-site adverse experiences occur in about 50% after primary vaccination and in 80% after revaccination; moderate-severe pain and/or significant induration occur in about 10% of primary vaccinees and in 30% of revaccinees. Systemic adverse experiences such as fatigue, myalgia, and headache, are reported after primary vaccination in approximately 22% and after revaccination in 33%.

- *Contraindications*
  - Severe allergic reaction (eg, anaphylaxis) to previous dose of vaccine or any vaccine component (risk of recurrent allergic reaction; for PCV7 and PCV13, this includes reactions to any diphtheria toxoid-containing vaccine, since these vaccines contain CRM_{197}, a mutant diphtheria toxin)
- *Precautions*
  - Moderate or severe acute illness (difficulty distinguishing illness from vaccine reaction)

Recommendations

All children should be vaccinated against *S pneumoniae*. The primary series of PCV13 consists of doses at 2, 4, and 6 months of age, with a booster dose given at 12 to 15 months of age. For previously unimmunized infants and children, the number of doses depends on the age at which the series is initiated (**Figure 8.4**). A single (supplemental) dose of PCV13 is recommended for healthy children 14 months to 4 years of age who have completed a PCV7 schedule, as well as those 24 months to 4 years of age with any incomplete PCV7 or PCV13 schedule, including those who have never been immunized (in high-risk children, the supplemental dose is recommended to 5 years of age).

All adults ≥65 years of age should be vaccinated against *S pneumoniae*. One dose of PPSV23 is usually given at 65 years of age, and routine revaccination is not recommended (those who received a dose before 65 years of age should receive a second dose if ≥5 years have elapsed since the first dose).

Immunization of high-risk persons is discussed in *Chapter 6: Vaccination in Special Circumstances* and is outlined in **Table 6.2**. It should be noted that PPSV23 is often used to assess the adequacy of polysaccharide antibody responses in persons ≥2 years of age who are suspected of having immune deficiency.[33]

REFERENCES

1. Catterall JR. *Thorax*. 1999;54:929-937.
2. CDC. *MMWR*. 2000;49(RR-9):1-35.
3. ABCs report: *Streptococcus pneumoniae*, 1999. Centers for Disease Control and Prevention Web site. http://www.cdc.gov/abcs/reports-findings/survreports/spneu99.html. Accessed February 27, 2012.
4. CDC. *MMWR*. 1997;46(RR-8):1-24.
5. CDC. *MMWR*. 2008;57:144-148.
6. Tsai CJ, et al. *Clin Infect Dis*. 2008;46:1664-1672.
7. Grijalva CG, et al. *Lancet*. 2007;369:1179-1186.
8. Grijalva CG, et al. *Pediatrics*. 2006;118:865-873.
9. Kyaw MH, et al. *N Engl J Med*. 2006;354:1455-1463.
10. Dagan R, et al. *Lancet Infect Dis*. 2008;8:785-795.
11. Ray GT, et al. *Vaccine*. 2009;27:6483-6494.
12. O'Brien KL, et al. *J Infect Dis*. 2007;196:1211-1220.
13. Millar EV, et al. *Clin Infect Dis*. 2008;47:989-996.
14. Kaplan SL, et al. *Pediatrics*. 2010;125:429-436.
15. Lexau CA, et al. *JAMA*. 2005;294:2043-2051.
16. Nuorti JP, et al. *MMWR*. 2010;59:1102-1106.
17. Ogilvie I, et al. *Vaccine*. 2009;27:4891-4904.
18. Huang SS, et al. *Vaccine*. 2011;29:3398-3412.
19. CDC. *MMWR*. 2008;57:343-344.
20. CDC. *MMWR*. 2010;59:258-261.
21. Nuorti JP, et al. *MMWR*. 2010;59(RR-11):1-19.
22. Farley MM, et al. *MMWR*. 2010;59:253-257.
23. Rubin JL, et al. *Vaccine*. 2010;28:7634-7643.
24. Black S, et al. *Pediatr Infect Dis J*. 2000;19:187-195.
25. Eskola J, et al. *N Engl J Med*. 2001;344:403-409.
26. Pavia M, et al. *Pediatrics*. 2009;123:e1103-e1110.
27. Whitney CG, et al. *Lancet*. 2006;368:1495-1502.
28. Yeh SH, et al. *Pediatrics*. 2010;126:e493-e505.
29. Rückinger S, et al. *Vaccine*. 2011;29:9600-9606.
30. Fine MJ, et al. *Arch Intern Med*. 1994;154:2666-2677.
31. Butler JC, et al. *JAMA*. 1993;270:1826-1831.
32. Moberley SA, et al. *Cochrane Database Syst Rev*. 2008;(1):CD000422.
33. Paris K, et al. *Ann Allergy Asthma Immunol*. 2007;99:462-464.

25 Typhoid Fever

The Pathogen

Salmonella typhi (also known as *Salmonella enterica* subspecies *enterica* serotype Typhi) is a motile, nonlactose-fermenting, gram-negative bacillus. Infection begins in the gut, where the organism invades Peyer's patches, multiplies in macrophages, and disseminates to the mesenteric lymph nodes, reticuloendothelial organs, and ultimately the bloodstream. The Vi capsular antigen interferes with complement binding and enhances virulence. *S typhi* produces a cholera-like toxin that causes efflux of electrolytes and water into the intestinal lumen.

Clinical Features

Typhoid fever refers to enteric fever caused by *S typhi*, although other salmonella species can cause a less-severe form of enteric fever.[1] The incubation period is 5 to 21 days depending on inoculum size and health of the host. The onset is insidious, with fever and abdominal pain accompanied by malaise and anorexia. Fever climbs each day, reaching 104°F (40°C) by the end of the first week; adults display relative bradycardia for the level of fever. Early on, up to 50% of patients have constipation and 30% have diarrhea. Diarrhea is more common in infants and is typically of small volume and pea soup-like, containing red blood cells and leukocytes but not gross blood. During the first week of illness, children complain of headache and often are irritable, drowsy, or delirious. Adults may display psychosis or delirium, and arthralgia and back pain are common. Patients may appear toxic, have meningismus, a coated tongue with musty odor, and a tender doughy abdomen with guarding. During the second week of illness, a rash may appear on the abdomen or chest consisting of crops of salmon-colored, blanching, slightly raised lesions measuring 2 to 4 mm, referred to as *rose spots*. The spleen may be palpable and tender and respiratory symptoms may develop. Untreated, the illness lasts 4 to 6 weeks.

Complications generally occur during the third or fourth week and may include intestinal hemorrhage or perforation. The patient's mental status may progress to coma. Additional complications include hepatitis, cholecystitis, arthritis, osteomyelitis, parotitis, endocarditis, myocarditis, pericarditis, pneumonia, meningitis, pyelonephritis, pancreatitis, and orchitis. Laboratory abnormalities include anemia, leukopenia or leukocytosis, thrombocytopenia, and elevated hepatic and muscle enzymes. Relapses occur in 5% to 20% of cases even after appropriate therapy, although they are usually milder than the initial illness. Infants are more likely than adults to develop massive hepatosplenomegaly and thrombocytopenia, and they have a higher mortality rate. However, young children may have *S typhi* bacteremia with mild disease manifestations. Typhoid fever during pregnancy increases the risk of premature labor and spontaneous abortion. Up to 4% of patients who recover from typhoid fever become chronic carriers of *S typhi* and are potential sources of infection for others.

S typhi can also cause nontyphoidal gastroenteritis, bacteremia, and extraintestinal focal infection.

Epidemiology and Transmission

There are an estimated 12 to 33 million cases of typhoid fever each year in the world, with the highest incidence in Asia (especially the Indian subcontinent), Central and South America, and Africa. In endemic areas, the annual incidence is as high as 500 to 900 cases per 100,000 people, and the peak is in school-aged children. In developed countries, the incidence is only 0.2 to 3.7 cases per 100,000. Four hundred cases are reported in the United States each year, with the highest risk among international travelers.[2]

Humans are the only reservoir of *S typhi* and transmission is by the fecal-oral route; the infectious dose is about 10^7 organisms. Patients with cholecystitis or gallstones are especially vulnerable to chronic carriage and may excrete up to 10^9 organisms per gram of stool. Direct person-to-person transmission is unusual; rather, disease spreads through feces-contaminated food or water. For this reason, countries with inadequate sanitation systems, overcrowded living conditions, and limited potable water have the highest rates of disease. Laboratory workers have acquired infection through accidents and HCP have acquired infection from patients because of poor handwashing. Occasionally, transplacental transmission occurs from a bacteremic mother to the fetus, and infants may be infected at the time of birth through exposure to bacteria shed in the mother's stool.

Immunization Program

Worldwide, approximately 500,000 people die each year of typhoid fever. In endemic areas, aside from the human costs, the direct medical and indirect societal costs are high. Interest in vaccination is highest in areas where antibiotic treatment is not readily available and where antibiotic-resistant strains have increased in prevalence. Outbreaks of multidrug-resistant *S typhi* infection have occurred in the Indian subcontinent, Southeast Asia, and Africa and have been associated with high rates of complications and death. Vaccination might be beneficial for persons at high risk for disease, including children, international travelers, and military personnel. Persons who travel from low-risk to high-risk areas are particularly susceptible because they have not developed immunity through repeated exposure to low doses of *S typhi* over time.

Recommendations for use of typhoid vaccine were published in 1978, 1990, and most recently in 1994.[3]

Vaccines

Characteristics of the typhoid fever vaccines licensed in the United States are given in **Table 25.1**. One of these is a parenterally administered pure polysaccharide vaccine, analogous to MPSV4 and PPSV23. The other is an orally administered live-attenuated bacterium.

Efficacy and/or Immunogenicity

In a clinical trial of TViPSV conducted in Nepal, 3454 subjects received a liquid formulation of the vaccine and 3454 controls received a pneumococcal polysaccharide vaccine; most subjects were adults.[4] Efficacy against blood culture-confirmed typhoid fever was 74% during the 20-month follow-up period. In a second trial conducted in South Africa, a lyophilized formulation was evaluated in school children who received the vaccine (N=5692) or a meningococcal (serogroups A and C) polysaccharide vaccine as placebo (N=5692).[5] Efficacy was 55% against blood culture-confirmed typhoid fever during a 3-year follow-up period. Four-fold or greater increases in antibody to the Vi polysaccharide were seen in 88% to 96% of US adults who received one dose of the vaccine.

A large-scale effectiveness trial was conducted in Kolkata, India from 2004 to 2006 using TViPSV manufactured by GlaxoSmithKline (Typherix).[6] Slum-dwelling residents ≥2 years of age were randomized by geographic cluster to receive TViPSV (N=18,869) or HepA as control (N=18,804). Vaccine effectiveness was 61% in general but as high as 80% among children 2 to 5 years of age. Effectiveness was 44% among unvaccinated persons living in TViPSV clusters, an indication of herd immunity that was achieved with only 60% vaccine coverage.

25

The efficacy of Ty21a was first evaluated in Egypt, where 16,486 children aged 6 to 7 years were given 3 doses of a liquid formulation on alternate days; 15,902 children were given placebo. Efficacy was 95% during a 3-year surveillance period.[7] A series of field trials were then performed in Santiago, Chile. The first one, which compared 1 or 2 doses given 1 week apart,

TABLE 25.1 — Typhoid Vaccines[a]

Trade name	Typhim Vi	Vivotif
Abbreviation	TViPSV	Ty21a
Manufacturer/distributor	Sanofi Pasteur	Crucell (formerly Berna Biotech)
Type of vaccine	Inactivated, purified subunit	Live-attenuated, engineered
Composition	Capsular polysaccharide Vi extracted from strain *Salmonella enterica serovar typhi*, *S typhi* Ty2 Vi polysaccharide (25 mcg)	Strain *Salmonella typhi* Ty21a mutagenized and selected for attenuation 2 to 6.8 × 10^9 colony-forming units
Adjuvant	None	None
Preservative	Phenol (0.25%)	None
Excipients and contaminants	Polydimethylsiloxane (residual) Fatty-acid ester-based antifoam (residual) Sodium chloride (4.15 mg) Disodium phosphate (0.065 mg) Monosodium phosphate (0.023 mg)	Sucrose (26 to 130 mg) Ascorbic acid (1 to 5 mg) Amino acid mixture (1.4 to 7 mg) Lactose (100 to 180 mg) Magnesium stearate (3.6 to 4.4 mg)
Latex	None	None
Labeled indications	Prevention of typhoid fever	Prevention of typhoid fever
Labeled ages	≥2 years	≥7 years[b]
Dose	0.5 mL	1 capsule
Route of administration	Intramuscular	PO (swallow 1 hour before meal with a cold or lukewarm drink)

Labeled schedule	1 dose Booster doses every 2 years (for persons with continued exposure)	0, 2, 4, 6 days[c] Booster series of 4 doses every 5 years (for persons with continued exposure)
Recommended schedule	Same	Same
How supplied (number in package)	20-dose vial (1)	4 capsules in a single foil blister package
Cost per dose ($US, 2011):		
Public	—	—
Private	48.12	55.04
Reference package insert	December 2005	August 2006

[a] Typhoid Vaccine USP (Pfizer [formerly Wyeth]), a phenol-inactivated, whole-cell vaccine for parenteral administration, is no longer produced.
[b] The ACIP recommends use at ≥6 years of age.
[c] Some experts recommend repeating the series if all 4 doses are not given within 3 weeks.

25

involved 82,543 school-aged children. Efficacy at 24 months was 29% and 59%, respectively.[8] Another trial, which compared three doses on alternate days to three doses given 21 days apart, involved 109,594 school-aged children.[9] Efficacy was best in the group that received the shorter schedule, reaching 69% over 4 years and with persistent efficacy demonstrated at 5 years. Subsequent studies established that efficacy was best using a 4-dose, alternate-day regimen.

Safety

TViPSV causes local tenderness in 97% to 98% of vaccinees, pain in 27% to 41%, induration in 5% to 15%, and erythema in 4% to 5%. Systemic signs and symptoms include malaise (4% to 24%), headache (16% to 20%), myalgia (3% to 7%), and nausea (2% to 8%). Fever ≥100°F occurs in <2% of vaccinees. Reactogenicity is similar after repeat immunization but is less pronounced in children. Postmarketing surveillance in countries where >14 million doses were distributed demonstrated some systemic reactions but very few serious adverse events. From 1995 to 2002, the reporting rate to VAERS for adverse events was 4.5 per 100,000 doses distributed, and for serious adverse events, it was 0.34 per 100,000 doses distributed.

Ty21a is less reactogenic than TViPSV. Symptoms reported during clinical studies included abdominal pain (6%), nausea (6%), headache (5%), fever (3%), diarrhea (3%), vomiting (2%), and rash (1%), but only nausea occurred more frequently than in placebo groups. In field trials involving >500,000 school children, this vaccine did not cause serious adverse reactions. Postmarketing surveillance in the early 1990s, during which time 60 million doses were distributed, revealed only a handful of adverse events and only one serious allergic reaction.[10] From 1991 to 2002, the reporting rate to VAERS for adverse events was 9.7 per 100,000 doses distributed, and for serious adverse events, was 0.59 per 100,000 doses distributed.

- *Contraindications*
  - Both vaccines: severe allergic reaction (eg, anaphylaxis) to previous dose of vaccine or any vaccine component (risk of recurrent allergic reaction)
  - Ty21a: immune impairment (risk of disease caused by live bacterium)
- *Precautions*
  - Both vaccines: moderate or severe acute illness (difficulty distinguishing illness from vaccine reaction)
  - Ty21a: concomitant antibiotics or proguanil therapy (inactivation of live bacterial vaccine). Mefloquine and chloroquine may be given.

Recommendations

Routine immunization is *not* recommended in the United States, not even for sewage sanitation workers, persons attending rural summer camps, or people living in areas in which natural disasters such as floods have occurred. There is also no evidence that typhoid vaccine is useful in controlling common-source outbreaks.

Vaccination *is*, however, recommended for the following groups:

- Travelers to endemic areas (especially developing countries in Latin America, Asia, and Africa) who will have prolonged exposure to potentially contaminated food and water. People should be cautioned that vaccination is not a substitute for careful avoidance of contaminated food and drink. Typhoid vaccine is not *required* for international travel, but is *recommended*. See **Table 6.6** for region-specific recommendations.
- Persons with intimate exposure (eg, household contact) to a documented carrier of *S typhi* (the vaccine cannot be used to *treat* chronic carriers)
- Microbiology laboratory workers who are in frequent contact with *S typhi*
- Persons living in endemic areas outside the United States

There are no data on interchangeability of typhoid vaccines. However, if a booster series is necessary in a person who previously received the inactivated whole-cell vaccine, it is reasonable to give 4 doses of Ty21a or 1 dose of TViPSV. There is no evidence that concomitant administration of either vaccine with other live oral or live or inactivated parenteral vaccines impairs immune responses.

REFERENCES

1. Parry CM, et al. *N Engl J Med*. 2002;347:1770-1782.
2. Taylor DN, et al. *J Infect Dis*. 1983;148:599-602.
3. Cieslak PR, et al. *MMWR*. 1994;43(RR-14):1-7.
4. Acharya IL, et al. *N Engl J Med*. 1987;317:1101-1104.
5. Klugman KP, et al. *Vaccine*. 1996;14:435-438.
6. Sur D, et al. *N Engl J Med*. 2009;361:335-344.
7. Wahdan MH, et al. *J Infect Dis*. 1982;145:292-296.
8. Black RE, et al. *Vaccine*. 1990;8:81-84.
9. Levine MM, et al. *Lancet*. 1987;1:1049-1052.
10. Begier EM, et al. *Clin Infect Dis*. 2004;38:771-779.

26 Varicella

The Pathogen

Varicella-zoster virus (VZV) is a large, enveloped virus in the Herpesviridae family, a hallmark feature of which is the ability to establish *latency* and to undergo *reactivation*.[1] After inoculation at mucosal surfaces, replication occurs in the regional lymph nodes, resulting in a primary viremia that seeds the liver and other reticuloendothelial organs. A secondary mononuclear cell-associated viremia then ensues, which distributes virus to the skin, resulting in the vesicular lesions of *chickenpox*, as well as to the respiratory mucosa, facilitating contagion through respiratory droplets. Latent infection is invariably established in the dorsal root ganglia, where the linear, double-stranded DNA genome takes on a closed circular configuration. With reactivation, the genome linearizes, viral proteins are made, and virions are assembled; these are transported along sensory nerves to the skin, where replication causes *herpes zoster*, also known as *shingles*.

Cellular immunity is critical to limiting primary infection and preventing reactivation. Periodic re-exposure to exogenous natural varicella and/or subclinical reactivation of endogenous VZV may lead to boosts in immunity.

Clinical Features

The incubation period ranges from 10 to 21 days.[1] In children, *rash* is often the first sign of disease, but adults may have a 1- to 2-day prodrome of fever and malaise. The rash is pruritic, usually beginning on the scalp or hairline, moving to the trunk and the extremities. Lesions are 1 to 4 mm in diameter and appear in successive crops over several days; at any given time these crops are in different stages of development. Lesions characteristically evolve from macules to papules and then to superficial, delicate vesicles containing clear fluid on an erythematous base, so-called "dew drops on rose petals." They rapidly become pustules that crust and fall off, leaving shallow ulcers. Lesions can occur on mucous membranes and the cornea. The average patient with primary varicella has malaise and fever for 2 to 3 days and develops 200 to 500 lesions, some of which may form a scar.[2]

Varicella in vaccinated persons, termed *breakthrough* or *vaccine-modified varicella*, is generally characterized by a shorter duration of illness and the absence of systemic symptoms and complications.[3] There are usually <50 lesions; these are often maculopapular rather than vesicular and are difficult to recognize as chickenpox. However, up to 30% of children with breakthrough disease may have an illness that is similar to mild primary varicella.

In the prevaccine era, 5% to 10% of otherwise healthy children experienced complications. Half of these were secondary bacterial infections, usually caused by *Staphylococcus aureus* or group A beta-hemolytic streptococcus (GABHS). Varicella increased the risk of severe GABHS infection among previously healthy children by 40- to 60-fold, and it was estimated that preventing varicella could prevent at least 15% of cases of severe pediatric GABHS infection. Otitis media occurs in up to 5% of cases. Serious secondary infections, such as pneumonia, bacteremia, osteomyelitis, septic arthritis, endocarditis, necrotizing fasciitis, and toxic shock syndrome occur much less frequently. Other complications include cerebellar ataxia, encephalitis, and Reye syndrome, which is associated with aspirin use during the illness. Although the case-fatality rate in children is very low, the absolute number of childhood deaths in the prevaccine era was high (about 50 per year in the early 1990s) because there were so many cases.[4] Ninety percent of children who died had no identifiable risk factors for severe varicella.

Adults have more severe disease and higher complication rates. Slightly over 1% of all adults with varicella are admitted to the hospital, and the case-fatality rate is 25 times higher than in children.[4] In the prevaccine era, only 5% of cases, but 35% of annual deaths, occurred in adults; the majority of these had no identifiable risk factor for severe disease.

Immunocompromised persons may develop *progressive varicella*, characterized by high fever, extensive vesicular eruption, and a high complication rate. Mild hepatitis occurs in 20% to 50% of cases, but is usually asymptomatic. Similarly, 5% to 16% of patients develop thrombocytopenia, but bleeding is rare. *Hemorrhagic varicella* is characterized by thrombocytopenia and extensive purpuric lesions. Although rare, *congenital varicella syndrome*, characterized by birth defects and neurologic devastation, occurs in 1% of pregnancies complicated by varicella in the first or second trimester. Maternal varicella in the peripartum period can lead to severe *neonatal varicella* because of the high inoculum and absence of transplacental maternal antibodies; the fatality rate is as high as 30%.

When immunity wanes, as it does with aging, reactivation of latent VZV can result in herpes zoster (see *Chapter 28: Zoster*).

Epidemiology and Transmission

Humans are the only natural hosts. Transmission occurs via respiratory droplets or by direct contact with or aerosolization of virus from vesicular skin lesions. Natural chickenpox is highly contagious, with attack rates among susceptible household contacts approaching 90%; contagiousness begins 1 to 2 days before onset of rash and lasts until the last lesion has crusted. Shingles is less contagious because there is less virus in the lesions and the respiratory tract is not involved. Vaccine-modified varicella also is less contagious than primary chickenpox, unless the number of lesions is >50, in which case contagiousness approaches that of primary disease.[5]

Varicella is less common in tropical than in temperate areas. In the United States, the incidence is highest between March and May and lowest between September and November. Before universal immunization, essentially every child got chickenpox, most often by 4 years of age. Every year there were 4 million cases, 11,000 hospitalizations, and 100 deaths.[6]

Immunization Program

VAR was licensed in the United States in 1995. Initial recommendations called for universal immunization of children 12 to 18 months of age and catch-up for children 19 months to 12 years of age who had not had chickenpox.[7] Vaccination of susceptible persons ≥13 years of age (with 2 doses) was recommended if they were anticipated to have close contact with persons at high risk for serious complications; catch-up for other adolescents was considered desirable, but was not strongly recommended. It was suggested that vaccination also be considered for certain susceptible persons at high risk for exposure, and consideration was given to vaccination of susceptible nonpregnant women of childbearing age, who would be at risk for complications if they became pregnant and developed varicella. In 1999, stronger recommendations for these persons were issued, essentially changing the language from "should be considered" to "recommended."[8] Vaccination of all susceptible adolescents and adults living in households with children was recommended; so was postexposure vaccination, use of VAR for outbreak control, and vaccination of asymptomatic or mildly symptomatic HIV-infected children without evidence of immunosuppression. Recommendations for HCP, including the definition of evidence of immunity, were updated in 2011.[9]

Between 1997 and 2005, vaccine uptake among 2-year-olds increased to nearly 90%. Surveillance indicated approximately 90% declines in disease incidence, and the most affected age shifted from 3 to 6 years to 9 to 11 years. Between 1995 to 1998 and 2002 to 2005, overall varicella-related hospitalizations declined from 2.54 per 100,000 to 0.62 per 100,000; this included a 77% decrease among persons <20 years of age and 60% decrease among those ≥20.[10] From 2000 to 2006, an estimated 50,000 varicella-related hospitalizations were prevented.[11] The rate of varicella-related ambulatory visits decreased 66% in the 8 years after licensure.[12] Within 5 years, the annual number of varicella-related deaths in the United States declined from 145 to 66[13]; by 2007, deaths from chickenpox had been nearly eliminated.[14]

Despite these successes, and in the face of high immunization rates, outbreaks of varicella continued to occur, especially among elementary school students. Possible explanations for this include the fact that some children fail to seroconvert after 1 dose, and that immunity may wane with time.[15] Thus, it became clear that a 1-dose strategy would not eliminate indigenous transmission, something that is especially critical to protecting those who, because of medical contraindications, cannot be vaccinated. Therefore, in 2007, a routine 2-dose strategy was adopted.[16] A case-control study in Connecticut a few years later showed that vaccine effectiveness was 86% for 1 dose and 98% for 2 doses[17]; during the same time period, the incidence of varicella in that state decreased by approximately 50%.[18]

In 1995, it was estimated that every dollar spent on varicella vaccination would result in a savings of $5.40, when both direct medical and indirect societal costs were considered. For the 2006 birth cohort (4.1 million children) followed over 40 years, it was estimated that without a vaccination program there would be $333 million in direct costs from varicella and $1.5 billion in societal costs (2006 dollars).[19] A 1-dose program would prevent 3.6 million cases and result in a net savings of $1.1 billion. A 2-dose program would prevent 375,000 additional cases at an incremental cost of $104 million; the cost per quality-adjusted life year saved would be $109,000.

Vaccines

Characteristics of the VAR licensed in the United States are given in **Table 26.1**. This is a single human varicella strain (originally isolated in Japan from a child named Oka) that was attenuated by serial passage in tissue culture, much the same way as the Sabin polio vaccine. VAR is the only herpesvirus vaccine to be licensed and is the first live vaccine that can establish latency.

Efficacy and/or Immunogenicity

Prelicensure studies showed seroconversion rates after 1 dose of 97% among children 1 to 12 years of age and 79% among adolescents. Adolescents and adults who received 2 doses separated by 4 to 8 weeks had seroconversion rates of 99%. In a study of children 12 months to 12 years of age, 86% of those who received 1 dose developed antibody levels of ≥5 glycoprotein ELISA units/mL, the presumed correlate of protection; nearly 100% achieved

TABLE 26.1 — Varicella Vaccine[a]

Trade name	Varivax
Abbreviation	VAR
Manufacturer/distributor	Merck
Type of vaccine	Live-attenuated, classical
Composition	Oka/Merck strain Propagated in human diploid (MRC-5) cells At least 1350 plaque-forming units
Adjuvant	None
Preservative	None
Excipients and contaminants	Sucrose (25 mg) Hydrolyzed gelatin (12.5 mg) Sodium chloride (3.2 mg) Monosodium L-glutamate (0.5 mg) Sodium phosphate dibasic (0.45 mg) Potassium phosphate monobasic (0.08 mg) Potassium chloride (0.08 mg) Residual components of MRC-5 cells, including DNA and protein Sodium phosphate monobasic (trace) EDTA (trace) Neomycin (trace) Fetal bovine serum (trace)
Latex	None
Labeled indications	Prevention of varicella
Labeled ages	≥12 months
Dose	0.5 mL
Route of administration	Subcutaneous
Labeled schedule	12 months to 12 years: 1 dose, with revaccination ≥3 months later ≥13 years: 1 dose, with revaccination 4 to 8 weeks later
Recommended schedule	12 to 15 months, 4 to 6 years Catch-up
How supplied (number in package)	1-dose vial (1, 10), lyophilized, with diluent
Cost per dose ($US, 2011):	
Public	69.73
Private	87.10
Reference package insert	August 2011

[a] VAR is also available in combination with MMR (ProQuad; Merck).

26

this level after a second dose, whether that was given 3 months or several years after the first dose. Long-lived humoral and cellular immune responses have been seen in vaccinees, although persistence of immunity in the absence of boosting from exposure to natural virus cannot be studied until indigenous transmission is eliminated.

In prelicensure trials, efficacy of 1 dose was 70% to 90% against any disease and 95% against severe disease. A case-control study set in pediatric offices from 1997 to 2003 demonstrated 1-dose effectiveness of 85%,[20] and a study of household exposures demonstrated 79% effectiveness at preventing secondary disease.[5] Severe varicella, characterized by >500 lesions, hospitalization, and complications, is extremely rare in vaccinees. A randomized trial in children showed 94% efficacy of 1 dose over 10 years, compared with 98% efficacy of 2 doses given 3 months apart; in this study, the breakthrough rate was reduced 3.3-fold.[21]

In three controlled trials involving a total of 110 healthy susceptible children with household varicella exposure, the attack rate among children receiving postexposure vaccination was 18% compared with 78% among controls.[22] Most children were vaccinated within 3 days of exposure, and most breakthrough disease was mild. In a study involving 77 household contacts vaccinated within 5 days of exposure, effectiveness of VAR in preventing any disease was estimated at 62% and in preventing moderate to severe disease at 79%.[23] None of the breakthrough cases were severe.

Safety

Injection-site reactions are reported in about 20% of vaccinees, and 15% may have low-grade fever. About 3% of children and 1% of adults get a few vesicles at the injection site, and up to 5% may experience a generalized varicella-like rash, with a median of 5 lesions, mostly maculopapular. The vaccine virus establishes latency, and herpes zoster caused by the vaccine virus can occur. However, the risk of herpes zoster is 4 to 12 times lower in vaccinated young children than in those with a history of natural disease.[24] Transmission of the vaccine virus from healthy vaccinees to susceptible persons is extremely rare and is only known to occur when the vaccinee develops a rash after vaccination. When transmission does occur, disease is mild and there is no evidence of reversion to virulence.

Ten years after licensure and the distribution of 55.7 million doses worldwide, 16,683 reports of adverse events (5054 of which were breakthrough disease) had been received, for a reporting rate of 3.4 per 10,000 doses distributed.[25] Vesicular rashes occurring in the first 2 weeks after vaccination were mostly due to wild-type VZV, indicating that vaccinees had been exposed to or were incubating the natural infection when they were vaccinated. Among 95 reports of herpes zoster for which specimens were available, 57 were due to the vaccine strain and 38 were wild-type VZV. There were no primary neurologic events associated with vaccination. Household transmission was reported in 3 instances, and in each case the vaccinee had developed a vesicular rash. Disseminated infection was seen in 7 patients, all but 6 of whom were immunocompromised.

- *Contraindications*
  - Severe allergic reaction (eg, anaphylaxis) to previous dose of vaccine or any vaccine component (risk of recurrent allergic reaction; this includes reactions to gelatin and neomycin)
  - Severe immunodeficiency or immunosuppression (risk of disease caused by live virus)
  - Pregnancy (theoretical risk to the fetus of live-virus vaccine or attribution of birth defects to vaccination). ACIP recommends that vaccinated women avoid pregnancy for 1 month; the package insert says 3 months (ACIP recommendations are usually followed in practice).
- *Precautions*
  - Moderate or severe acute illness (difficulty distinguishing illness from vaccine reaction)
  - Recent receipt of antibody-containing blood product (risk of impaired response to vaccine)
  - Salicylate therapy in children and adolescents (theoretical risk of Reye syndrome; the manufacturer recommends withholding salicylates at least 6 weeks after administration of vaccine, but other nonsteroidal anti-inflammatory agents can be used)
  - Active, untreated tuberculosis (risk of exacerbation of tuberculosis; note that the package insert lists this as a contraindication)
  - MMRV: personal, sibling or parent history of seizures (risk of febrile seizure)

Recommendations

All people without evidence of immunity to varicella should be vaccinated. The criteria for evidence of immunity are listed in **Table 26.2**; importantly, for children born after 1994, a reported history of chickenpox is no longer a reliable indicator of immunity.[26]

For children, Dose 1 is usually given at 12 to 15 months of age and Dose 2 at 4 to 6 years of age. Dose 2 may be given any time ≥3 months following Dose 1. For persons ≥13 years of age, 2 doses are given 4 to 8 weeks apart. Anyone who received 1 dose in the past should receive a second dose. Evidence of immunity

TABLE 26.2 — Evidence of Immunity to Varicella

Any one of the following criteria constitute evidence of immunity:

1. Written documentation of age-appropriate vaccination[a]:
   - Preschool-aged children: 1 dose
   - School-aged children, adolescents, and adults: 2 doses
2. Laboratory evidence of immunity[b]
3. Laboratory confirmation of disease
4. Birth in the United States before 1980 (exception: HCP, pregnant women, and immunocompromised individuals)
5. History of typical varicella: diagnosis or verification of history by any health care professional (eg, school or occupational clinic nurse, nurse practitioner, physician assistant, physician)[c]
6. History of atypical or mild varicella: diagnosis or verification of history by a physician or physician's designee, utilizing the following information:
   - Epidemiologic link to a typical or laboratory-confirmed case
   - Laboratory confirmation performed at the time of acute disease
7. Herpes zoster: diagnosis or verification of history by any health care professional

[a] Appropriately vaccinated persons who become immunosuppressed later in life are considered immune, except for hematopoietic stem-cell transplant recipients.

[b] Serologic testing of adults before vaccination may be cost-effective since approximately 80% will be found to be seropositive. Receipt of blood products can cause false-positive serologic test results because of passive transfer of antibodies.

[c] In general, immunocompromised individuals with a verified history of varicella are considered immune. The exception is hematopoietic stem-cell transplant recipients, who are considered susceptible, regardless of their own personal history of varicella or a history of varicella in the donor. Transplant recipients who develop herpes zoster are subsequently considered immune.

Adapted from Marin M, et al. *MMWR*. 2007;56 (RR-4):1-40, and Shefer A, et al. *MMWR*. 2011;60(RR-7):1-45.

should be assessed in all individuals, and those without evidence of immunity should be vaccinated. Special attention should be paid to assessment of school-aged children, students in college and other postsecondary educational institutions, HCP, household contacts of immunosuppressed persons, teachers, day care employees, residents and staff in institutional settings, inmates and staff of correctional facilities, military personnel, nonpregnant women of childbearing age, persons living in homes with children, and international travelers.

While there are no official recommendations, infants who had chickenpox before 6 months of age, and possibly before 9 months, should probably be vaccinated once they reach 12 months (there is no harm in giving the vaccine to someone who has already had chickenpox). This is because the immunity imparted by natural disease in infants who have maternal antibodies may be suboptimal. Pregnant women without evidence of immunity should be vaccinated beginning in the postpartum period. HIV-infected persons without evidence of *severe* immunosuppression should be vaccinated (see *Chapter 6: Vaccination in Special Circumstances—HIV Infection*). Susceptible household and other close contacts of immunocompromised persons also should be vaccinated; if the vaccinee develops a rash, contact with the immunocompromised person should be avoided until the rash resolves.

Vaccination of persons without evidence of immunity is recommended for outbreak control. Vaccination can also be used as postexposure prophylaxis for healthy, susceptible persons if given within 3 to 5 days of exposure (off-label recommendation).

Exposed persons who lack evidence of immunity (**Table 26.2**), have contraindications to vaccination, and are at high risk for complications of varicella should receive passive immunoprophylaxis with varicella zoster immune globulin (VariZIG). Exposure is constituted by living in the same household as an infectious person with either chickenpox or herpes zoster; direct, indoor, face-to-face contact with an infectious person for >5 minutes (some experts say 1 hour); or sharing the same hospital room. A special case of exposure that carries high risk is the neonate whose mother develops chickenpox in the peripartum period. The following persons should receive passive immunoprophylaxis if susceptible and exposed:

26

- Immunocompromised patients, including those with primary and acquired immunodeficiencies, those receiving immunosuppressive medications, and those with cancer. Patients who receive regular immune globulin infusions do not need prophylaxis unless the last dose was ≤3 weeks before exposure.
- Neonates whose mothers have signs and symptoms of varicella from 5 days before to 2 days after delivery
- Preterm neonates who are exposed postnatally:

– ≥28 weeks gestation whose mothers lack evidence of immunity
– <28 weeks gestation or birth weight ≤1000 g, regardless of maternal immunity

- Pregnant women (VariZIG is given to protect the mother from complications of varicella; whether it will protect the fetus is not known).

The only high-titer immune globulin product available in the United States is VariZIG, but this must be obtained under an investigational new-drug protocol (FFF Enterprises, phone number 800-843-7477; http://www.fffenterprises.com/Products/VariZIG.aspx. Accessed February 4, 2012).[27] VariZIG is supplied in 125-unit vials, and the dose is 125 units/10 kg intramuscularly; the minimum dose is 125 units and the maximum dose is 625 units. Intravenous immune globulin can be used if VariZIG is not available.

After intramuscular administration of VariZIG, varicella antibodies persist for about 6 weeks. Onset of action is prompt, but the duration of protection is unknown. When given within 96 hours of exposure, VariZIG significantly reduces the morbidity and mortality from varicella among immunocompromised individuals. Attack rates are about one fifth as high as those in untreated, exposed persons, and the severity of disease is reduced. Receipt of VariZIG may extend the incubation period of varicella to 28 days. If the patient develops varicella, antiviral therapy should be instituted.

The most frequent local adverse reactions to VariZIG are pain, redness, or swelling at the injection site, occurring in about 1% of patients. Systemic reactions are less frequent and include gastrointestinal symptoms, malaise, headache, rash, and respiratory symptoms. Certain safety issues are common to all immune globulin products, including the possibility of transmission of blood-borne pathogens that are not killed in the manufacturing process. In addition, patients with selective IgA deficiency may be at increased risk for anaphylactic reactions to VariZIG because it may contain minute amounts of IgA.

REFERENCES

1. Arvin AM. *Clin Microbiol Rev*. 1996;9:361-381.
2. Balfour HH, et al. *J Pediatr*. 1990;116:633-639.
3. Watson BM, et al. *Pediatrics*. 1993;91:17-22.
4. Meyer PA, et al. *J Infect Dis*. 2000;182:383-390.
5. Seward JF, et al. *JAMA*. 2004;292:704-708.
6. Seward JF, et al. *JAMA*. 2002;287:606-611.
7. CDC. *MMWR*. 1996;45(RR-11):1-36.
8. CDC. *MMWR*. 1999;48(RR-6):1-5.
9. Shefer A, et al. *MMWR*. 2011;60(RR-7):1-45.
10. Reynolds MA, et al. *J Infect Dis*. 2008;197(suppl 2):S120-S126.
11. Lopez AS, et al. *Pediatrics*. 2011;127:238-245.
12. Shah SS, et al. *Pediatr Infect Dis J*. 2010;29:199-204.
13. Nguyen HQ, et al. *N Engl J Med*. 2005;352:450-458.
14. Marin M. et al. *Pediatrics*. 2011;128:214-220.
15. Chaves SS, et al. *N Engl J Med*. 2007;356:1121-1129.
16. Marin M, et al. *MMWR*. 2007;56(RR-4):1-40.
17. Shapiro ED, et al. *J Infect Dis*. 2011;203:312-315.
18. Kattan JA, et al. *J Infect Dis*. 2011;203:509-512.
19. Zhou F, et al. *J Infect Dis*. 2008;197(suppl 2):S156-S164.
20. Vázquez M, et al. *JAMA*. 2004;291:851-855.
21. Kuter B, et al. *Pediatr Infect Dis J*. 2004;23:132-137.
22. Macartney K, et al. *Cochrane Database Syst Rev*. 2008;(3): CD001833.
23. Brotons M, et al. *Pediatr Infect Dis J*. 2010;29:10-13.
24. Civen R, et al. *Pediatr Infect Dis J*. 2009;28:954-959.
25. Galea SA, et al. *J Infect Dis*. 2008;197(suppl 2):S165-S169.
26. Perella D, et al. *Pediatrics*. 2009;123:e820-e828.
27. CDC. *MMWR*. 2006;55:209-210.

27 Yellow Fever

The Pathogen

Yellow fever (YF) virus, a member of the Flaviviridae family, consists of a single-stranded RNA genome surrounded by a protein nucleocapsid and a lipid envelope.[1] After inoculation by the bite of an infected mosquito, the virus spreads through lymphatics to the viscera, and viremia ensues. The liver is particularly affected, with the appearance of necrotic masses (Councilman's bodies) in hepatocytes; the resulting bleeding diathesis that can occur is the basis for classifying YF as a *hemorrhagic fever*. Cytokine storm contributes to the pathogenesis of life-threatening disease.

Clinical Features

Infection may be asymptomatic or present as a viral syndrome of varying severity.[2] The classic triad of *jaundice*, *hemorrhage*, and *albuminuria* occurs in 10% to 20% of patients, and the associated case fatality rate is 20% to 50%. The onset of symptoms is abrupt, with fever, headache, backache, malaise, myalgia, nausea, vomiting, prostration, photophobia, restlessness, irritability, and dizziness; epistaxis and bleeding from the gums may also occur. Children may experience febrile seizures. Examination reveals congestion of the skin, conjunctivae, and mucous membranes. Leukopenia, albuminuria, and elevated serum transaminase levels may be present. After about 3 days of illness, most patients experience a remission of symptoms, but this may be brief and relapse can occur, with prostration, marked venous congestion, extreme bradycardia, severe nausea, vomiting, epigastric pain, jaundice, marked albuminuria, anuria, hematemesis (referred to as *vomito negro*), and melena. The hemorrhagic manifestations may be so severe as to cause hypotension, shock, acidosis, myocardial dysfunction, arrhythmias, and death, usually after 7 to 10 days. Central nervous system signs include delirium, agitation, seizures, stupor, and coma, and complications include pneumonia, parotitis, skin infections, and renal abscesses.

Epidemiology and Transmission

Transmission of *jungle* YF involves tree hole-breeding mosquitoes and nonhuman primates in the rain forests of Africa and South America. Humans exposed to the mosquitoes in this environment, such as forestry workers, soldiers, and settlers, may acquire the infection and travel to urban areas where *Aedes aegypti* mosquitoes become infected after feeding on them. These mosquitoes may in turn infect other persons, leading to epidemics of *urban* YF ("jungle" and "urban" describe the epidemiology—the clinical manifestations are identical). *A aegypti* breeds in and around houses and thereby sustains interhuman transmission. YF virus is also transmitted vertically from infected female mosquitoes to their offspring. This mode of transmission is important to survival of the virus during prolonged dry periods.

YF occurs throughout sub-Saharan Africa, where epidemics are common, as well as in tropical South America. Nearly 20,000 cases were reported between 1987 and 1991, with 4500 deaths.[3] After accounting for underreporting, the true number of cases is thought to be about 200,000 per year. The case-fatality rate in Africa is as high as 75% and in South America as high as 40%. Epidemics of YF have reappeared in the urban centers of West Africa and there is concern that it may reappear in tropical urban centers in the Americas. In South America, approximately 100 cases are reported each year in forested areas. Mass vaccination campaigns and mosquito-control programs have been instituted in South America in an attempt to prevent urban outbreaks. Interestingly, YF has never been reported in Asia.

Immunization Program

As with Japanese encephalitis, control of mosquito populations can reduce the risk of transmission. Mosquito bites can be minimized through the use of insect repellent, permethrin-impregnated clothing, and staying in screened-in or air-conditioned rooms. Immunization is recommended, however, because these measures provide no guarantee against exposure. One of the most important rationales for vaccination is the risk of reemergence of YF carried by *A aegypti* mosquitoes in urban areas of the Americas. This is a possibility because *A aegypti* infests many areas that are currently free of YF, including coastal regions of South America, the Caribbean, North America, the Middle East, coastal eastern Africa, the Indian subcontinent, Asia, and Australia.

YF vaccination recommendations were published in 2002[4] and updated in 2010.[5]

Vaccines

Characteristics of the YFV licensed in the United States are given in **Table 27.1**. This is a live vaccine that was attenuated by serial passage in vitro, much the same way as the Sabin polio vaccine. Because continued serial passage can result in strains with higher rates of adverse events, vaccine lots are prepared from a large pool of secondary seed lots.

TABLE 27.1 — Yellow Fever Vaccine

Trade name	YF-Vax
Abbreviation	YFV
Manufacturer/distributor	Sanofi Pasteur
Type of vaccine	Live-attenuated, classical
Composition	YF virus strain 17D-204 Propagated in chick embryos ≥4.74 $\log_{10}$ plaque-forming units
Adjuvant	None
Preservative	None
Excipients and contaminants	Sorbitol Gelatin Sodium chloride
Latex	Vial stopper contains latex
Labeled indications	Prevention of YF
Labeled ages	≥9 months
Dose	0.5 mL
Route of administration	Subcutaneous
Labeled schedule	1 dose Booster dose every 10 years (for persons with continued exposure)
Recommended schedule	Same See text regarding vaccination of infants 6 to 8 months of age
How supplied (number in package)	1-dose vial (5), lyophilized, with diluent 5-dose vial (1), lyophilized, with diluent
Cost per dose ($US, 2011):	
Public	—
Private	68.08
Reference package insert	January 2010

Efficacy and/or Immunogenicity

While the efficacy of YFV has never been tested in a controlled clinical trial, numerous observations suggest efficacy. For example, neutralizing antibodies can be demonstrated in 90% of vaccinees after 10 days and in 99% by 30 days.[6] Infection of laboratory workers disappeared after vaccination became routine, and in Brazil and other South American countries, YF only occurs in people who have not been immunized. Immunization during outbreaks results in rapid disappearance of new cases, and high rates of coverage in endemic areas are followed by marked reductions in disease incidence. During an epidemic in Nigeria in 1986, vaccine efficacy was estimated at 85%. Immunity following vaccination persists for at least 30 to 35 years and probably for life.[7]

Safety

Reactions to YFV are typically mild. Studies between 1953 and 1994 showed that <5% of vaccinees experience erythema and pain at the infection site, headaches, and fever, typically 5 to 7 days after immunization. A study in 2001 among 715 adults demonstrated mild systemic reactions such as headache, myalgia, malaise, and asthenia in 10% to 30% of subjects.[6] The rate of systemic adverse events appears to be higher in older vaccinees.

Two important serious adverse events have been described[9]:

- *Vaccine-associated viscerotropic disease*: Formerly known as *febrile multiple organ-system failure*, this begins within 10 days of vaccination and is characterized by fever, nausea, vomiting, malaise, diarrhea, myalgia, or dyspnea along with evidence of end-organ damage, including jaundice, hepatic dysfunction, renal impairment, myocarditis, rhabdomyolysis, and thrombocytopenia. Progression to cardiorespiratory failure and death may occur. The liver pathology resembles that seen with wild-type YF, but the disease appears to be related to host factors rather than reversion to virulence of the vaccine virus. The overall incidence of this adverse event in the United States is estimated at 1 in 250,000 doses administered, but the rate is higher in persons ≥60 years of age.[10]
- *Vaccine-associated neurotropic disease*: Formerly known as *postvaccination encephalitis*, symptoms begin within 30 days of vaccination and include fever, headache, and focal or global neurological dysfunction. Signs of inflammation or encephalopathy are seen on CSF examination, EEG, or imaging studies. The overall incidence of this adverse event in the United States is estimated at 1 in 125,000 doses administered, but the rate is higher in persons ≥60 years of age.[10]
- *Contraindications*
  - Severe allergic reaction (eg, anaphylaxis) to previous dose of vaccine or any vaccine component, including eggs (risk of recurrent allergic reaction). Being able to eat lightly cooked (eg, scrambled) eggs without a reaction is reasonable evidence of a very low risk of anaphylaxis. Being able to eat eggs in baked products is not a reliable predictor because heat can denature egg proteins. Mild or local manifestations of allergy to eggs or feathers are not a contraindication. Skin testing can be done and desensitization may be possible (the procedure is described in the package insert).

– Age <6 months (risk of disease caused by live virus)
– Immune impairment (risk of disease caused by live virus). This includes symptomatic HIV infection or CD4 count <15% (<6 years if age) or <200 cells/mcL (≥6 years of age); thymic disorder including thymoma; primary immunodeficiencies; malignant neoplasms; transplantation; and immunosuppressive or immunomodulatory therapies, including radiation. Corticosteroid use is not a contraindication in the following situations: administration of <20 mg prednisone or equivalent (<2 mg/kg for persons ≤10 kg) per day; short-term (<2 weeks) therapy; long-term, alternate-day administration of short-acting preparations; physiologic replacement; topical or inhaled preparations; intra-articular, bursal, or tendon injection.

- *Precautions*
  – Moderate or severe acute illness (difficulty distinguishing illness from vaccine reaction)
  – Age 6 to 8 months or ≥60 years (risk of disease caused by live virus)
  – Asymptomatic HIV infection and CD4 count 15% to 24% (<6 years of age) or 200 to 499 cells/mcL (≥6 years of age) (risk of disease caused by live virus)
  – Pregnancy (theoretical risk to the fetus of live-virus vaccine or attribution of birth defects to vaccination).
  – Breast-feeding (risk of disease caused by live virus[11])

Recommendations

Vaccination is recommended for persons ≥9 months of age who are traveling to or living in areas of South America and Africa where YF transmission is possible (see *Chapter 6: Vaccination in Special Circumstances—Travel*). Vaccination should be limited to situations where exposure to YF is likely or where vaccination is required for entry into the country. If international travel requirements are the *only* reason for vaccination of an individual at high risk for vaccine complications, consideration should be given to writing a waiver letter. Laboratory personnel who might be exposed to virulent YF virus or to concentrated preparations of vaccine strains should be vaccinated.

YFV can only be administered at a site approved by the WHO (the CDC's Division of Global Migration and Quarantine and state and territorial health departments can designate nonfederal vaccination centers). Vaccinees must receive an *International Certificate of Vaccination or Prophylaxis* that has been completed, signed, and validated with the center's stamp; the certificate is valid from 10 days to 10 years after vaccination. New certificates have been produced since December 15, 2007, in response to a revision of the International Health Regulations; persons vaccinated before that date may use the old certificate until it expires.[12] Certain countries in Africa require evidence of vaccination from all entering travelers. Some countries waive the requirements for travelers who will be staying <2 weeks and come from areas with little risk of YF transmission. Other countries require persons, even if only in transit, to have a valid certificate if they have been in countries either known or thought to have YF, or even where YF does not exist but where *A aegypti* mosquitoes are found. The CDC[13] and WHO[14] web sites contain information on YF endemic areas and countries that require certificates.

Because of the risk of vaccine-associated encephalitis, infants <6 months of age should not be vaccinated under any circumstances. Travel of infants 6 to 8 months of age to endemic areas should be deferred; if travel is unavoidable, vaccination is acceptable (off-label recommendation), but the risk of adverse events may be higher than in infants ≥9 months of age. Pregnant women may be vaccinated if travel cannot be postponed and if exposure is very likely; while there is no definitive evidence of fetal harm from maternal vaccination, there is the possibility of decreased immune response, and testing for seroconversion should be considered.

REFERENCES

1. Monath TP, et al. *Adv Virus Res*. 2003;60:343-395.
2. Barnett ED. *Clin Infect Dis*. 2007;44:850-856.
3. Robertson SE, et al. *JAMA*. 1996;276:1157-1162.
4. Cetron MS, et al. *MMWR*. 2002;51(RR-17):1-11.
5. CDC. *MMWR*. 2010;59(RR-7):1-27.
6. Monath TP, et al. *Am J Trop Med Hyg*. 2002;66:533-541.
7. Poland JD, et al. *Bull World Health Organ*. 1981;59:895-900.
8. CDC. *MMWR*. 2001;50:643-645.
9. Kitchener S. *Vaccine*. 2004;22:2103-2105.
10. Gershman M, Staples JE. Yellow fever, in *Traveler's Health- Yellow Book*. Centers for Disease Control and Prevention Web site. http://wwwnc.cdc.gov/travel/yellowbook/2012/chapter-3-infectious-diseases-related-to-travel/yellow-fever.htm. Accessed February 5, 2012.
11. Couto AM, et al. *MMWR*. 2010;59:130-132.
12. CDC. *MMWR*. 2008;56:1345-1346.
13. Yellow fever. Centers for Disease Control and Prevention Web site. http://www.cdc.gov/yellowfever. Accessed February 5, 2012.
14. Yellow fever. World Health Organization Web site. http://www.who.int/topics/yellow_fever/en/index.html. Accessed February 5, 2012.

28 Zoster

The Pathogen

The biology of varicella-zoster virus (VZV) is described in *Chapter 26: Varicella. Herpes zoster*, or *shingles*, results from reactivation of latent VZV from sensory dorsal root or cranial nerve ganglia.[1] The virus initially reaches these ganglia by retrograde axonal transport from the skin during an episode of chickenpox. In latency, which may last for many decades, there is restricted gene transcription and limited protein expression, and intact virions are not produced. What triggers release from latency into active, lytic infection is not clear, but it is known that reduced VZV-specific (T-cell) responder cell frequency characterizes all conditions associated with reactivation.

Normally there is enough constitutive immune surveillance for antigens associated with lytic infection that when active replication begins, infected cells are destroyed or replication is otherwise shut down. When immune surveillance wanes, lytic infection in neuronal cell bodies can progress, and virions are transported back along sensory nerves to the skin, where lesions much like those of chickenpox are produced. Unlike with chickenpox, however, the lesions are restricted to a single dermatome (more than one dermatome may be involved in immunocompromised individuals). Moreover, they are associated with significant pain, the result of cell destruction and inflammation in the sensory ganglion. Pain often persists after regression of the lesions, a condition termed *postherpetic neuralgia* (PHN). This is associated with degeneration of primary afferent neuronal cell bodies and axons, scarring in the dorsal root ganglion, and *central sensitization*, which refers to changes in the dorsal horn of the spinal cord that generalize and perpetuate pain impulses.

Zoster is a re-immunizing event—immunity to VZV is boosted, and for this reason most people only have one lifetime episode.

Clinical Features

A prodrome of headache, photophobia, and malaise without fever may occur.[2] Pain (often described as burning, shooting, stabbing, or throbbing), itching, or tingling precede skin lesions by 1 to 5 days. Lesions form over 3 to 5 days, beginning as clusters of erythematous macules in one dermatome that rapidly become papules with superimposed clear vesicles, and—much like chickenpox—evolve to pustules and shallow ulcers with crusts that fall off within 2 to 4 weeks, often leaving scars and permanent changes in pigmentation. Thoracic, cervical, and ophthalmic dermatomes are most often involved, and the lesions do not cross the midline. Systemic symptoms occur in <20% of patients, and occasionally there are a few lesions outside the dermatome. Motor nerve involvement with associated paresis may be seen in 5% to 15% of patients (the mechanism for this is not clear). Involvement of the geniculate ganglion can lead to facial nerve paralysis (sensory and motor nerves are joined in nerve VII); the combination of lesions on the ear, hard palate, or tongue and facial paralysis is termed *Ramsay Hunt syndrome* and is associated with vertigo, hearing loss, tinnitus, and loss of taste. Occasionally, pain occurs without skin lesions—this is called *zoster sine herpete*.

Zoster tends to be more severe with advancing age. Subclinical involvement of the central nervous system is common in immunocompetent individuals; there may be cerebrospinal fluid (CSF) pleocytosis in up to half of patients and VZV can be detected in CSF in a third. Immunocompromised patients may experience severe localized zoster or *disseminated zoster* due to hematogenous spread of the infection outside of the original dermatome. The spectrum of illness ranges from generalized rash to life-threatening pneumonia, hepatitis, encephalitis, and disseminated intravascular coagulopathy.

PHN lasting ≥1 month occurs in 20% to 30% of patients with zoster, and about 10% have pain lasting ≥3 months. Pain may last for months or years and may be constant, intermittent, or triggered by trivial stimuli; half of patients describe it as excruciating. Quality of life may be dramatically affected, leading to social withdrawal, depression, and even suicide. Advanced age correlates with the severity of PHN, and PHN is rare in children.

Other complications of zoster include secondary bacterial infection, eye involvement with keratitis or retinitis, myelitis, and granulomatous angiitis.

Epidemiology and Transmission

Zoster only occurs in people who have had been infected with VZV; this includes >99.5% of the US population ≥40 years of age. It is contagious in the sense that VZV from the lesions can cause chickenpox in a susceptible individual; however, zoster cannot directly cause zoster in another person, nor can chickenpox, because latency must first be established. Of note, the risk of contagion from zoster is less than that from chickenpox because there is less virus that can aerosolize from the lesions and there is no transmission from respiratory sections before the lesions erupt.

Estimates of age-adjusted incidence rates in the United States vary from 3.2 to 4.2 per 1000 population, or about 1 million cases annually.[3] The rate is much higher—about 10 per 1000—in persons ≥60 years of age. About one third of people in the United

States will experience an episode of zoster in their lifetime. The most important risk factors are increasing age and conditions or medications that impair cell-mediated immunity; other risk factors include psychological stress, female gender, white race, mechanical trauma, and genetic susceptibility.[1] Exposure to varicella (eg, living or working in environments with young children) may protect against zoster by providing a boost to immunity *(see discussion below)*. Varicella vaccination is also protective—while the vaccine virus establishes latency and can reactivate, the rate of zoster is lower in vaccinated persons than in naturally infected persons.[4] Zoster in children may be up to 10 times less common than in adults; when it does occur, a history of maternal varicella during pregnancy or chickenpox in the first year of life is often elicited (these are situations that can lead to immune tolerance, ie, blunting of immune memory to VZV).

Questions have been raised about how the universal varicella vaccination program will affect the incidence of zoster. Several competing factors are involved. First, as more and more people are vaccinated, fewer and fewer will become latently infected with wild-type VZV, which is prone to reactivate more readily than the vaccine strain; this might result in fewer people developing zoster as they age. However, less circulating virus in the community may mean fewer opportunities for boosted immunity in those who are already infected with wild-type VZV. Therefore, episodes of zoster could increase in one generation (those who are already infected with wild-type VZV and will not have the "benefit" of exposure to natural virus) while they decrease in another (those who received VAR and never become latently infected with wild-type VZV). Some studies suggest decreased rates of zoster among people exposed to young children (a proxy for exposure to varicella),[5,6] although a study from France showed that monks without exposure to varicella had no greater risk of zoster than the general population,[7] challenging the notion that circulating wild-type virus is important in preventing zoster. Studies have shown conflicting results regarding changes in the incidence of zoster in the VAR era.[8] For example, one study showed a striking increase in incidence of zoster among US veterans >40 years of age, from 3.10 episodes per 1000 in 2000 to 5.22 per 1000 in 2007.[9] On the other hand, a population-based study from Canada that included 212,521,806 person-years of observation showed decreases in zoster among children, as one might expect, but no increases among older persons.[10]

Immunization Program

It is estimated that each case of zoster results in up to three outpatient visits and from one to five medication prescriptions. Up to 4% of episodes result in hospitalization, with a mean duration of 5 days and average cost of $3221 to $7206 (2006 dollars).[3] Annualized health care costs for PHN are as high as $5000 per episode. Assuming a vaccine cost of $150, a 1-dose vaccination program for healthy persons ≥60 years of age would cost from $27,000 to $112,000 per QALY gained. This places ZOS in the intermediate-to-high end of cost-benefit compared with other vaccination programs.

The rationale for a zoster vaccine program is simple: vaccination boosts cellular immune responses, thereby preventing reactivation.[11,12] ZOS was licensed in 2006, and recommendations for routine use in persons ≥60 years of age were published in 2008.[3] In 2011, the labeled age indication was extended to include adults 50 through 59 years of age, although the recommended age for routine vaccination was not changed.[13]

Vaccines

Characteristics of the herpes zoster vaccine licensed in the United States are given in **Table 28.1**. ZOS consists of the same live-attenuated strain of VZV that is used in VAR, only in sufficiently high amount (14 times that in VAR) to overcome existing antibody and replicate in previously infected persons.

Efficacy and/or Immunogenicity

ZOS was evaluated in a double-blind, randomized, placebo-controlled trial (the Shingles Prevention Study) involving 38,546 healthy adults ≥60 years of age who either had a personal history of varicella or who had resided in the United States for ≥30 years (and were therefore very likely to have been infected with VZV).[14] The majority of suspected cases were confirmed by PCR. The mean duration of follow-up was 3.1 years, and patients with confirmed zoster were followed for at least 6 months.

Overall, there was a 51% reduction in cases of zoster among vaccinees and a 67% reduction in cases of PHN, defined as ≥30 days of pain. Among subjects who developed zoster, the risk of PHN was reduced by 39%. Other complications, such as allodynia (a painful response to a normally nonpainful stimulus), bacterial superinfection, disseminated zoster, impaired vision, peripheral motor-nerve palsies, ptosis, scarring, and sensory loss were less common among vaccinees than placebees, but occurred with similar frequency among vaccine and placebo cases of zoster—these results indicate that the main benefit of ZOS is in preventing zoster rather than in modifying the severity and/or complication rate, should zoster occur. Efficacy for prevention of zoster was highest among those 60 to 69 years of age, but the greatest effect in reducing the severity of illness was among persons 70 to 79

TABLE 28.1 — Zoster Vaccine

Trade name	Zostavax
Abbreviation	ZOS
Manufacturer/distributor	Merck
Type of vaccine	Live-attenuated, classical
Composition	Oka/Merck strain Propagated in human diploid (MRC-5) cells 19,400 plaque-forming units
Adjuvant	None
Preservative	None
Excipients and contaminants	Sucrose (31.16 mg) Hydrolyzed porcine gelatin (15.58 mg) Sodium chloride (3.99 mg) Monosodium L-glutamate (0.62 mg) Sodium phosphate dibasic (0.57 mg) Potassium phosphate monobasic (0.10 mg) Potassium chloride (0.10 mg) Residual components of MRC-5 cells, including DNA and protein Neomycin (trace) Bovine calf serum (trace)
Latex	None
Labeled indications	Prevention of herpes zoster (shingles)
Labeled ages	≥50 years
Dose	0.65 mL
Route of administration	Subcutaneous
Labeled schedule	1 dose
Recommended schedule	60 years of age
How supplied (number in package)	1-dose vial (1, 10), lyophylized, with diluent
Cost per dose ($US, 2011):	
Public	118.73
Private	161.50
Reference package insert	June 2011

years of age. Efficacy declined during the first year following vaccination but stabilized thereafter at around 50%.

Anamnestic antibody and T-cell responses were seen in vaccinated subjects and persisted for 3 to 6 years. Immune responses were inversely related to the risk of zoster. Subsequent studies have shown ZOS to be safe and immunogenic among persons with a history of zoster.[15]

Safety

Erythema and pain at the injection site occur in about 35% of vaccinees; swelling occurs in 26%, and pruritus in 7%. Most of these reactions are mild and resolve within 4 days. A varicella-like rash occurs at the injection site within 3 to 4 days in 0.1% of vaccinees, and fever occurs in <1%. In the Shingles Prevention Study, serious adverse events such as death (which might have been expected given the advanced age of the subjects) occurred with equal frequency among vaccinees and placebees. Horizontal transmission of vaccine virus is a theoretical concern; standard precautions should be adequate to protect susceptible persons who are in contact with vaccinees who develop lesions.

- *Contraindications*
  - Severe allergic reaction (eg, anaphylaxis) to previous dose of vaccine or any vaccine component (risk of recurrent allergic reaction)
  - Immunodeficiency or immunosuppression (risk of disease caused by live virus). The following may receive ZOS: patients with leukemia in remission who have not had chemotherapy or radiation for ≥3 months; patients receiving systemic steroids for <14 days or <20 mg/day; patients receiving low doses of methotrexate (≤0.4 mg/kg/week), azathioprine (≤3 mg/kg/day), or 6-mercaptopurine (≤1.5 mg/kg/day); HIV-infected persons with CD4 count ≥200/mcL and CD4 percentage ≥15% of total lymphocytes; and persons with humoral immune deficiencies. Providers may consider immunizing hematopoietic stem-cell transplant recipients who are immunocompetent and who are ≥24 months post-transplant.
  - Pregnancy (theoretical risk of live virus vaccine to the fetus or attribution of birth defects to vaccination). ACIP recommends that vaccinated women avoid pregnancy for 1 month, although pregnancy is unlikely in the age group targeted for routine immunization; the package insert says 3 months (ACIP recommendations are usually followed in practice).
- *Precautions*
  - Moderate or severe acute illness (difficulty distinguishing illness from vaccine reaction)
  - Active, untreated tuberculosis (risk of exacerbation of tuberculosis)

Recommendations

All persons ≥60 years of age should be vaccinated against zoster. The usual schedule is 1 dose of ZOS at 60 years of age, but catch-up vaccination is recommended (there is no upper age limit). Vaccination is recommended regardless of the personal history with respect to varicella. Patients who have had zoster should be vaccinated; while there is no minimum interval between an episode of zoster and vaccination, it would seem prudent to wait at least a year to vaccinate since immunity presumably will have been boosted by the episode. Patients with chronic medical conditions may be vaccinated, as long as those conditions are not associated with immunosuppression. ZOS is not indicated to treat acute zoster, prevent PHN in patients who already have zoster, or to treat PHN. ZOS is not recommended for persons who have received VAR, but few persons today who are ≥60 years of age will fit into that category.

If immunosuppression is anticipated, vaccination should occur at least 14 days earlier. Persons taking antiviral medications such as acyclovir, famciclovir, and valacyclovir should discontinue those medications at least 24 hours before vaccination and remain off medication for at least 14 days. Receipt of antibody-containing blood products is not a contraindication to vaccination.

ZOS is labeled for use at 50 to 59 years of age but is not routinely recommended. Providers may consider vaccinating persons in this age group who might not be expected to tolerate an episode of zoster or PHN very well, such as persons with chronic pain syndromes, severe depression, other comorbid conditions, inability to take treatment medications, and those in certain occupations.

The package insert says to consider separating ZOS and PPSV23 by ≥4 weeks because the antibody response to VZV might be impaired with simultaneous administration. Simultaneous administration is acceptable, however, because lower antibody levels are unlikely to translate into reduced protection.[16]

REFERENCES

1. Gershon AA, et al. *J Clin Virol.* 2010;48:S2-S7.
2. Gnann JW Jr, et al. *N Engl J Med.* 2002;347:340-346.
3. Harpaz R, et al. *MMWR.* 2008;57(RR-5):1-30.
4. Civen R, et al. *Pediatr Infect Dis J.* 2009;28:954-959.
5. Thomas SL, et al. *Lancet.* 2002;360:678-682.
6. Salleras M, et al. *Vaccine.* 2011;29:7602-7605.
7. Gaillat J, et al. *Clin Infect Dis.* 2011;53:405-410.
8. Reynolds MA, et al. *J Infect Dis.* 2008;197(suppl 2):S224-S227.
9. Rimland D, et al. *Clin Infect Dis.* 2010;50:1000-1005.
10. Tanuseputro P, et al. *Vaccine.* 2011;29:8580-8584.
11. Kimberlin DW, et al. *N Engl J Med.* 2007;356:1338-1343.
12. Oxman MN. *Clin Infect Dis.* 2010;51:197-213.
13. Harpaz R, et al. *MMWR.* 2011;60:1529.
14. Oxman MN, et al. *N Engl J Med.* 2005;352:2271-2284.
15. Mills R, et al. *Vaccine.* 2010;28:4204-4209.
16. Oxman MN, et al. *Vaccine.* 2011;29:3625-3627.

29 Combination Vaccines

Background

Some of the first vaccines licensed in the United States were combinations of antigens. For example, the influenza vaccine (first licensed in 1945) contains antigens from three different strains of influenza virus. Likewise, the hexavalent pneumococcal polysaccharide vaccine (1947), DTwP vaccine (1948), trivalent IPV (1955), and trivalent OPV (1963) were also combinations. Today, the term *combination vaccine* refers to a vaccine whose components could be given as separately available products (referred to herein as *component vaccines*). The modern era of combination vaccines began in the 1990s, when combinations of routinely administered childhood vaccines such as DTwP, DTaP, Hib, and HepB were developed.

Most immunizations are concentrated in the first 2 years of life. Depending on how vaccine visits are scheduled, as many as 9 shots may be due on 1 day (eg, a 15-month-old may be due for HepB, DTaP, Hib, PCV13, IPV, IIV, MMR, VAR, and HepA). Scheduling many shots for 1 day causes distress for parents,[1] let alone health care professionals—enough so that compliance with universal vaccine programs may be threatened. Combination vaccines reduce the number of shots necessary without reducing the delivery of antigens, and thus are a logical solution to this problem.

Development, Evaluation, and Licensure

Producing safe and effective combination vaccines is far more complex than simply mixing antigens together in a single vial.[2] Adjuvants, buffers, stabilizers, and excipients can have *physical* or *chemical interactions* with antigens that reduce immunogenicity, and many of these interactions cannot be predicted a priori. *Antigenic competition* can occur as vaccine components vie for position in binding to major histocompatibility molecules on antigen-presenting cells at the site of injection. This may explain in part the decreased anti-PRP responses that were seen with initial attempts to combine Hib with DTaP (importantly, even though the antibody titers were lower, the quality of the response in terms of avidity, opsonic activity, and memory may have been similar to the component Hib[3]). *Carrier-induced epitopic suppression* may cause decreased antibody responses to protein-polysaccharide conjugates (such as Hib) when there has been prior or simultaneous immunization with free (homologous) carrier protein.[4] Interference can be seen when different conjugates containing the same carrier protein are given at the same time, although the effects are unpredictable—for example, coadministration of Hib- and meningococcal serogroup C-tetanus toxoid conjugate vaccines results in enhanced Hib responses.[5] When live viral vaccines are given together, *viral interference* may limit responses as the replication of one virus is inhibited by the replication of the other; this is why MMRV contains higher amounts of mumps virus and VZV than what is present in MMR and VAR—so that the mumps virus and VZV can replicate in the setting of measles virus replication. While these interactions are important considerations, they must be differentiated from "immune overload," a popular concept that has no scientific basis (see *Chapter 7: Addressing Concerns About Vaccines—Can Multiple Vaccines Overload the Immune System?*).

Once compatibility issues are worked out in laboratory and animal models, extensive clinical trials are required to prove that a new combination vaccine is safe and effective. FDA guidelines require that such trials compare the combination to separately but simultaneously administered component vaccines. Reactogenicity is compared with the most reactogenic of the individual components. For antigens that have an established serologic correlate of protection, it may be enough to demonstrate that the combination induces protective antibody responses. However, the FDA generally requires that *noninferiority* with component vaccines be demonstrated, generally meaning no more than a 10% reduction in seroprotection (seroprotection may be measured by a variety of ways, such as the proportion of vaccinees achieving a specific antibody titer, the proportion of vaccinees with a ≥4-fold rise in titer, the proportion of seroconverters, the geometric mean concentration of antibody, or some combination of these; the criteria are usually agreed upon before the clinical trials are performed). Efficacy against disease is inferred for most new combination vaccines rather than directly demonstrated.

Effect on Quality

The more shots that are due on a given day, the more likely it is that one or more vaccinations will be deferred to another day.[6] In recent years, it has become clear that such deferrals may lead to reduced coverage rates and poor immunization timeliness. Several studies now suggest that use of combination vaccines, by reducing the number of shots due, can lead to improvements in coverage and timeliness. A study of administrative claims from the Georgia Medicaid program demonstrated higher coverage rates among children who had received a combination vaccine (either HepB-Hib-OMP or DTaP-HepB-IPV) compared with children who had received the component vaccines, an effect that was independent of other determinants of coverage.[7] In another analysis of the same database, 2-year-olds who had received 3 doses of DTaP-HepB-IPV had markedly fewer cumulative days undervaccinated (125 days) than did control children (334 days) for the series of 4 DTaP, 3 IPV, 1 MMR, 3 Hib, 3 HepB, and 1 VAR.[8] Similar findings have been seen in managed-care populations.[9]

Barriers to the adoption of combination vaccines include cost, loss of administration fees, perceptions about adverse events, and the complexity of having so many multivalent choices.[10-12] Antigen-based reimbursement, as opposed to reimbursement based on injections per se, is designed to remove financial disincentives to adoption of combination vaccines (see *Chapter 4: Vaccine Practice—Coding, Billing and Costs*).

Vaccines

Modern combination vaccines available in the United States that are based on DTaP are listed in **Table 29.1**; others are listed in **Table 29.2**. The following generalizations are offered:

- *Efficacy and/or immunogenicity*—Licensure by the FDA ensures that the immunogenicity (and presumably the protective efficacy) of a given combination vaccine is noninferior to that of the component vaccines given separately.
- *Safety*—Licensure by the FDA ensures that, in all clinically meaningful respects, a given combination vaccine is as safe as the separately administered components. However, a few issues are noteworthy. For example, DTaP-HepB-IPV causes higher rates of fever (when coadministered with Hib and PCV) than do the component vaccines. However, most of these fevers are low-grade (only 0.4% in one study were >103.1°F) and most (98.8% in the same study) do not result in medical attention. In a postlicensure study involving approximately 61,000 infants who received a total of 120,000 doses of DTaP-HepB-IPV, postvaccination fevers prompting medical visits occurred in <0.3% of both vaccinees and historical controls.[13] DTaP-IPV/Hib is not associated with increased rates of fever.[14] Prelicensure clinical trials demonstrated higher rates of fever following the first dose of MMRV compared to MMR plus VAR, and postlicensure studies show that this can lead to febrile seizures in in about 1 out of every 2300 to 2600 vaccinees (see *Chapter 7: Addressing Concerns About Vaccines—Can Vaccines Cause Febrile Seizures?*).
- *Contraindications and precautions*—Contraindications and precautions for combination vaccines are the same as for the individual components. One exception is MMRV, where a

TABLE 29.1 — DTaP-Based Combination Vaccines[a]

Trade name	Kinrix	Pediarix	Pentacel
Abbreviation	DTaP-IPV	DTaP-HepB-IPV	DTaP-IPV/Hib-T
Manufacturer/distributor	GlaxoSmithKline	GlaxoSmithKline	Sanofi Pasteur
Diseases prevented:			
Diphtheria	√	√	√
Tetanus	√	√	√
Pertussis	√	√	√
Hepatitis B	—	√	—
H influenzae type b	—	—	√
Polio	√	√	√
Type of vaccine	Inactivated, purified subunits, toxoids, and whole agent	Inactivated, purified subunits, toxoids, engineered subunit, and whole agent	Inactivated, purified subunits, toxoids, engineered subunit, and whole agent
Component vaccines[b]:			
DTaP	Infanrix	Infanrix	Similar to Daptacel
HepB	—	Engerix-B	—
Hib	—	—	ActHIB[c]
IPV	IPV[d]	IPV[d]	Poliovax[e]
Composition:			
Diphtheria toxoid	25 Lf units	25 Lf units	15 Lf units
Tetanus toxoid	10 Lf units	10 Lf units	5 Lf units
Inactivated pertussis toxin	25 mcg	25 mcg	20 mcg

Filamentous hemagglutinin	25 mcg	25 mcg	20 mcg
Pertactin	8 mcg	8 mcg	3 mcg
Fimbriae types 2 and 3	—	—	5 mcg
HBsAg	—	Expressed in yeast (*S cerevisiae*) (10 mcg)	—
Polyribosylribitol phosphate	—	—	10 mcg conjugated to tetanus toxoid (24 mcg)
Poliovirus type 1 (Mahoney)	40 D antigen units	40 D antigen units	40 D antigen units
Poliovirus type 2 (MEF-1)	8 D antigen units	8 D antigen units	8 D antigen units
Poliovirus type 3 (Saukett)	32 D antigen units	32 D antigen units	32 D antigen units
Poliovirus propagation	Vero (African green monkey kidney) cells	Vero (African green monkey kidney) cells	Human diploid (MRC-5) cells
Poliovirus inactivation	Formaldehyde	Formaldehyde	Formaldehyde
Adjuvant	Aluminum hydroxide (≤0.6 mg aluminum)	Aluminum hydroxide Aluminum phosphate (≤0.85 mg aluminum)	Aluminum phosphate (0.33 mg aluminum)
Preservative	None	None	None
Excipients and contaminants	Sodium chloride (4.5 mg) Formaldehyde (≤100 mcg) Polysorbate 80 (≤100 mcg) Neomycin sulfate (≤0.05 ng) Polymyxin B (≤0.01 ng)	Sodium chloride (4.5 mg) Formaldehyde (≤100 mcg) Polysorbate 80 (≤100 mcg) Neomycin sulfate (≤0.05 ng) Polymyxin B (≤0.01 ng)	Polysorbate 80 (10 ppm) Formaldehyde (≤5 mcg) Glutaraldehyde (<50 ng) Bovine serum albumin (≤50 ng) 2-phenoxyethanol (3.3 mg)[f]

Continued

TABLE 29.1 — *Continued*

Trade name	Kinrix	Pediarix	Pentacel
Abbreviation	DTaP-IPV	DTaP-HepB-IPV	DTaP-IPV/Hib-T
Excipients and contaminants *(continued)*		Yeast protein (≤5%)	Neomycin (<4 pg) Polymyxin B sulfate (<4 pg)
Latex	Tip cap (and plunger for one presentation) of prefilled syringe contains latex	Tip cap (and plunger for one presentation) of prefilled syringe contains latex	None
Labeled ages	4 to 6 years	6 weeks to 6 years[g]	6 weeks to 4 years
Dose	0.5 mL	0.5 mL	0.5 mL
Route of administration	Intramuscular	Intramuscular	Intramuscular
Labeled schedule	Dose 5 of DTaP and Dose 4 of IPV in previous recipients of Pediarix and Infanrix	2, 4, 6 months of age[h]	2, 4, 6, 15 to 18 months of age[i]
Recommended schedule[j]	Same	Same	Same
Total reduction in shots[k]	1	5	6 or 7[l]
How supplied (number in package)	1-dose vial (10) Prefilled syringe (5, 10)	1-dose vial (10) Prefilled syringe (5, 10)	1-dose vial (5) of ActHIB, lyophilized, with 1-dose vial (5) of DTaP-IPV as diluent

Cost per dose ($US, 2011):			
Public	34.25	51.15	52.55
Private	48.00	70.72	77.48
Reference package insert	November 2011	November 2011	July 2011

[a] TriHIBit (DTaP/Hib-T; Sanofi Pasteur) is no longer available as of early 2012.

[b] The combination vaccines may not be strict mixtures of the component vaccines. In some cases, the amount of antigen or the method of production may be different than the separate components.

[c] The liquid DTaP-IPV combination is used to reconstitute the lyophilized ActHIB.

[d] Not licensed separately in the United States.

[e] Not distributed separately in the United States.

[f] Not present as a preservative.

[g] Only labeled for the primary series (not booster doses). Not labeled for use in infants of HBsAg-positive or -unknown mothers, but use in these infants is considered acceptable.

[h] With the birth dose of HepB, use of this combination vaccine will result in four total doses of HepB. This does not increase reactogenicity or compromise immunogenicity. Patients who receive Pediarix according to this schedule will need DTaP boosters at 15 to 18 months and 4 to 6 years of age, as well as an IPV booster at 4 to 6 years of age.

[i] Patients who receive Pentacel according to this schedule do not need further doses of Hib but they *do* need DTaP and IPV boosters at 4 to 6 years of age. Dose 4 may be given as early as 12 months of age if the opportunity to vaccinate later may be missed and if ≥6 months have elapsed since Dose 3.

[j] ACIP expresses a preference for the same DTaP product for the entire series, but vaccination should not be deferred if the same product is not immediately available or if the previous products are not known.

[k] Reduction in shots across the complete routine immunization schedule if the practice uses component vaccines and switches to the combination.

[l] The lower number applies if the provider uses PedvaxHIB (Hib-OMP), because a dose of that vaccine is not given at 6 months (there is one less shot saved).

TABLE 29.2 — Other Combination Vaccines

Trade name	Comvax	ProQuad	Twinrix
Abbreviation	HepB-Hib-OMP	MMRV	HepA-HepB
Manufacturer/distributor	Merck	Merck	GlaxoSmithKline
Diseases prevented	Hepatitis B Invasive *H influenzae* type b	Measles Mumps Rubella Varicella	Hepatitis A Hepatitis B
Type of vaccine	Inactivated, engineered subunits	Live-attenuated, classical	Inactivated, whole agent, and engineered subunit
Component vaccines[a]	Recombivax HB (HepB) PedvaxHIB (Hib-OMP)	M-M-R_{II} (MMR)[b] Varivax (VAR)[c]	Havrix (HepA) Engerix-B (HepB)
Composition	HBsAg expressed in yeast (*S cerevisiae*) (5 mcg) Polyribosylribitol phosphate (7.5 mcg) conjugated to *N meningitidis* serogroup B (strain B11) outer membrane protein (125 mcg)	Measles virus, Moraten strain (derived from the Edmonston B strain), propagated in chick embryo cells, at least 1000 $TCID_{50}$ Mumps virus, Jeryl Lynn strain (actually consists of two distinct strains), propagated in chick embryo cells, at least 19,950 $TCID_{50}$	HAV, HM175 strain, propagated in human diploid (MRC-5) cells and inactivated with formalin (720 ELISA units) HBsAg expressed in yeast (*S cerevisiae*) (20 mcg)

		Rubella virus, RA 27/3 strain, propagated in human diploid lung fibroblast (WI-38) cells, at least 1000 $TCID_{50}$ Varicella virus, Oka/Merck strain, propagated in human diploid (MRC-5) cells, at least 9770 plaque-forming units	
Adjuvant	Aluminum hydroxyphosphate sulfate (0.225 mg aluminum)	None	Aluminum phosphate, aluminum hydroxide (0.45 mg aluminum)
Preservative	None	None	None
Excipients and contaminants	Yeast protein (≤5%) Sodium borate decahydrate (35 mcg) Sodium chloride (0.9%) Formaldehyde (≤0.0004%)	Sucrose (21 mg) Hydrolyzed gelatin (11 mg) Sodium chloride (2.4 mg) Sorbitol (1.8 mg) Monosodium L-glutamate (0.40 mg) Sodium phosphate dibasic (0.34 mg) Human albumin (0.31 mg) Sodium bicarbonate (0.17 mg) Potassium phosphate monobasic (72 mcg)	Amino acids Sodium chloride Phosphate buffer Polysorbate 20 Formalin (≤0.1 mg) Residual MRC-5 proteins (≤2.5 mcg) Neomycin sulfate (≤20 ng) Yeast protein (≤5%)

Continued

TABLE 29.2 — *Continued*

Trade name	Comvax	ProQuad	Twinrix
Abbreviation	HepB-Hib-OMP	MMRV	HepA-HepB
Excipients and contaminants *(continued)*		Potassium chloride (60 mcg) Potassium phosphate dibasic (36 mcg) Residual components of MRC-5 cells, including DNA and protein Neomycin (<16 mcg) Bovine calf serum (0.5 mcg) Other buffer and media ingredients	
Latex	Vial stopper contains latex	None	Tip cap (and plunger for one presentation) of prefilled syringe contains latex
Labeled ages	6 weeks to 15 months[d]	12 months to 12 years	≥18 years
Dose	0.5 mL	0.5 mL	1 mL
Route of administration	Intramuscular	Subcutaneous	Intramuscular
Labeled schedule	2, 4, 12 to 15 months of age[e]	12 to 15 months of age Revaccination at 4 to 6 years of age	0, 1, 6 months Alternative schedule: 0, 7, 21 to 30 days; booster at 12 months

Recommended schedule	Same	Same	Same
Total reduction in shots[f]	2 or 3[g]	1 or 2[h]	2 (alternative schedule: 1)
How supplied (number in package)	1-dose vial (10)	1-dose vial (10), lyophilized, with diluent	1-dose vial (10) Prefilled syringe (1, 5, 10)
Cost per dose ($US, 2011):			
Public	29.50	—	47.50
Private	43.56	139.12	89.85
Reference package insert	December 2010	August 2011	November 2011

[a] The combination vaccines may not be strict mixtures of the component vaccines. In some cases, the amount of antigen or the method of production may be different than the separate components.
[b] The amount of mumps virus in MMRV is 1.6-times higher than in MMR (M-M-R_{II}; Merck).
[c] The amount of varicella virus in MMRV is 7-times higher than in VAR (Varivax; Merck).
[d] Not labeled for use in infants of HBsAg-positive or -unknown mothers, but use in these infants is considered acceptable.
[e] With the birth dose of HepB, use of this combination vaccine will result in four total doses of HepB. This does not increase reactogenicity or compromise immunogenicity. Patients who receive Comvax according to this schedule do not need further doses of HepB or Hib.
[f] Reduction in shots across the complete routine immunization schedule if the provider uses component vaccines and switches to the combination.
[g] The higher number applies if ActHIB is currently in use, because switching to Comvax reduces the total number of Hib doses needed to complete the primary series from 3 to 2.
[h] The number of shots is reduced by 2 if ProQuad is used at both 12 to 15 months of age and 4 to 6 years of age.

personal or family (ie, sibling or parent) history of seizures is listed an incremental precaution.[15]

Recommendations

In 1999, the ACIP, AAP, and AAFP issued a statement expressing a clear preference for combination vaccines over separate injections of the component vaccines.[16] In 2009, the preference for combination vaccines was reworded to state that combination vaccines are "generally" preferred, and that the following factors should be considered in deciding whether or not to use them: patient preference, potential for adverse events, number of injections, vaccine availability, likelihood of improved coverage, likelihood of patient return, storage, and costs.[17] ACIP has also offered guidance for integrating particular combination vaccines into the schedule (**Figure 8.2**).[18,19]

One exception to the preference for combination vaccines is MMRV. The ACIP recommends that either MMR plus VAR or MMRV can be used for the first dose when given at 12 to 47 months of age; however, the former is preferred unless the parents expressed a preference for the combination.[15] The AAP maintains that either option is acceptable, as long as the caregivers are fully informed about the risks and benefits of either approach.[20] MMRV is generally preferred for the first dose in children 4 through 12 years of age as well as for second doses.

Use of combination vaccines may result in *overimmunization* because unnecessary doses of an antigen may be given. For example, an infant who receives the birth dose of HepB and then receives DTaP-HepB-IPV at 2, 4, and 6 months of age will receive 4 total doses of HepB, when only 3 doses are required. As another example, a child who receives DTaP-IPV/Hib at 2, 4, 6, and 15 months of age will need DTaP and IPV at 4 to 6 years of age—a total of 5 doses of IPV will be given, when only 4 are required. These extra doses are not harmful and are an accepted consequence of using combination vaccines.

Providers are warned not to combine vaccines in the same syringe unless the products are specifically labeled for this purpose.

REFERENCES

1. Kennedy A, et al. *Pediatrics*. 2011;127:S92-S99.
2. International Symposium on Combination Vaccines. *Clin Infect Dis*. 2001;33(suppl 4):S261-S375.
3. Poolman J, et al. *Vaccine*. 2001;19:2280-2285.
4. Dagan R, et al. *Infect Immun*. 1998;66:2093-2098.
5. Pöllabauer EM, et al. *Vaccine*. 2009;27:1674-1679.
6. Meyerhoff AS, et al. *Prevent Med*. 2005;41:540-544.
7. Marshall GS, et al. *Pediatr Infect Dis J*. 2007;26:496-500.
8. Happe LE, et al. *Pediatr Infect Dis J*. 2009;28:98-101.
9. Happe LE, et al. *Am J Manag Care*. 2007;13:506-512.
10. Gidengil CA, et al. *Clin Pediatr*. 2009;48:539-547.
11. Gidengil CA, et al. *Arch Pediatr Adolesc Med*. 2010;164:1138-1144.
12. Shen AK, et al. *Pediatrics*. 2011;128:1087-1093.
13. Zangwill KM, et al. *Pediatrics*. 2008;122:e1179-e1185.
14. Black S, et al. *Expert Rev Vaccines*. 2005;4:793-805.
15. CDC. *MMWR*. 2010;59(RR-3):1-12.
16. Advisory Committee on Immunization Practices (ACIP), et al. *Pediatrics*. 1999;103:1064-1077.
17. Kroger AT, et al. *MMWR*. 2011;60(RR-2):1-61.
18. CDC. *MMWR*. 2008;57:1078-1079.
19. CDC. *MMWR*. 2008;57:1079-1080.
20. American Academy of Pediatrics Committee on Infectious Diseases. *Pediatrics*. 2011;128:630-632.

30

Appendix

(All web sites accessed February 28, 2012)

Governmental Agencies

Centers for Medicare & Medicaid Services (CMS)
http://www.cms.hhs.gov

Department of Defense (DOD)
http://www.defense.gov

National Institute of Allergy and Infectious Diseases (NIAID)
http://www.niaid.nih.gov

Food and Drug Administration (FDA)
http://www.fda.gov

Centers for Disease Control and Prevention (CDC)
http://www.cdc.gov/vaccines

Health Resources and Services Administration (HRSA)
http://www.hrsa.gov

National Vaccine Program Office (NVPO)
http://www.hhs.gov/nvpo

National Vaccine Advisory Committee (NVAC)
http://www.hhs.gov/nvpo/nvac

US Agency for International Development (USAID)
http://www.usaid.gov

International Agencies

Pan American Health Organization (PAHO)
http://new.paho.org

World Health Organization (WHO)
http://www.who.int/en

Professional Associations

American Academy of Family Physicians (AAFP)
http://www.aafp.org

American Academy of Pediatrics (AAP)
http://www.aap.org

American College Health Association (ACHA)
http://www.acha.org

American College of Physicians (ACP)
http://www.acponline.org

American Medical Association (AMA)
http://www.ama-assn.org

American Nurses Association (ANA)
http://nursingworld.org

American Pharmacists Association (APhA)
http://www.pharmacist.com

American Public Health Association (APHA)
http://www.apha.org

Association for Prevention Teaching and Research (APTR)
(formerly the Association of Teachers of Preventive Medicine)
http://www.atpm.org

Association of State and Territorial Health Officials (ASTHO)
http://www.astho.org

Infectious Diseases Society of America (IDSA)
http://www.idsociety.org

Pediatric Infectious Diseases Society (PIDS)
http://www.pids.org

Advocacy, Implementation, and Safety

Allied Vaccine Group
http://www.vaccine.org

American Immunization Registry Association
http://www.immregistries.org

Brighton Collaboration
http://www.brightoncollaboration.org

Children's Hospital of Philadelphia Vaccine Education Center
http://www.vaccine.chop.edu

Children's Vaccine Program at PATH
http://www.path.org

Clinical Immunization Safety Assessment (CISA) Network
http://www.cdc.gov/vaccinesafety/Activities/cisa.html

Every Child by Two (ECBT)
http://www.ecbt.org

Families Fighting Flu
http://www.familiesfightingflu.org

Global Alliance for Vaccines and Immunization (GAVI)
http://www.gavialliance.org

Immunization Action Coalition (IAC)
http://www.immunize.org

Institute for Vaccine Safety, Johns Hopkins Bloomberg School of Public Health
http://www.vaccinesafety.edu

Meningitis Angels
http://www.meningitis-angels.org

National Foundation for Infectious Diseases (NFID)
http://www.nfid.org

National Meningitis Association
http://www.nmaus.org

National Network for Immunization Information (NNii)
http://www.immunizationinfo.org

Parents of Kids With Infectious Diseases (PKIDs)
http://www.pkids.org

Sabin Vaccine Institute (SVI)
http://www.sabin.org

Society of Teachers of Family Medicine (STFM) Group on Immunization Education
http://www.immunizationed.org
See also Shots by STFM On-Line: http://www.immunizationed.org/ShotsOnline.aspx

Texas Children's Hospital Center for Vaccine Awareness and Research
http://www.texaschildrens.org/carecenters/vaccine/Default.aspx

Vaccinate Your Baby
http://www.vaccinateyourbaby.org

Vaccines.gov
http://www.vaccines.gov

Voices for Vaccines
http://www.voicesforvaccines.org

Coverage and Assessment

Behavioral Risk Factor Surveillance System (BRFSS)
http://www.cdc.gov/brfss

Comprehensive Clinic Assessment Software Application (CoCASA)
http://www.cdc.gov/vaccines/programs/cocasa/index.html

Healthcare Effectiveness Data and Information Set (HEDIS)
http://web.ncqa.org/tabid/59/Default.aspx

National Health Interview Survey (NHIS)
http://www.cdc.gov/nchs/nhis.htm

National Immunization Survey (NIS)
http://www.cdc.gov/nis

National Notifiable Diseases Surveillance System (NNDSS)
http://www.cdc.gov/osels/ph_surveillance/nndss/nndsshis.htm

Books

Allen A. *Vaccine: The Controversial Story of Medicine's Greatest Lifesaver*. New York, NY: WW Norton; 2008.

Atkinson W, Wolfe C, Hamborsky J. *Epidemiology and Prevention of Vaccine-Preventable Diseases (The Pink Book)*. 12th ed. Washington, DC: Public Health Foundation; 2011.

Brunette GW, Kozarsky PE, Magill AJ, Shlim DR. *CDC Health Information for International Travel 2012*. New York, NY: Oxford University Press; 2012.

Colgrove J. *State of Immunity: The Politics of Vaccination in Twentieth-Century America*. Berkeley, CA: University of California Press; 2006.

Cunningham RM, Boom JA, Baker CJ. *Vaccine-Preventable Disease: The Forgotten Story*. Houston, TX: Texas Children's Hospital; 2009.

Fields D, Brown A. *Baby 411: Clear Answers and Smart Advice for Your Baby's First Year*. 4th ed. Boulder, CO: Windsor Peak Press; 2009.

Mnookin S. *The Panic Virus: A True Story of Medicine, Science, and Fear*. New York, NY: Simon and Schuster; 2011.

Myers MG, Pineda D. *Do Vaccines Cause That?! A Guide for Evaluating Vaccine Safety Concerns*. Galveston, TX: Immunizations for Public Health; 2008.

Offit PA. *The Cutter Incident: How America's First Polio Vaccine Led to the Growing Vaccine Crisis*. New Haven, CT: Yale University Press; 2007.

Offit PA. *Vaccinated: One Man's Quest to Defeat the World's Deadliest Diseases*. New York, NY: Harper Collins Publishers; 2007.

Offit PA. *Autism's False Prophets: Bad Science, Risky Medicine, and the Search for a Cure*. New York, NY: Columbia University Press; 2008.

Offit PA. *Deadly Choices: How the Anti-Vaccine Movement Threatens Our Children*. New York, NY: Basic Books; 2011.

Offit PA, Moser CA. *Vaccines and your Child: Separating Fact from Fiction*. New York, NY: Columbia University Press; 2011.

Oshinsky DM. *Polio: An American Story*. New York, NY: Oxford University Press; 2006.

Pickering, LK, ed. *Red Book: 2009 Report of the Committee on Infectious Diseases*. 28th ed. Elk Grove Village, IL: American Academy of Pediatrics; 2009.

Plotkin SA, Orenstein WA, Offit PA. *Vaccines*. 5th ed. St Louis, MO: Elsevier; 2008.

Smith MJ, Bouck L. *The Complete Idiot's Guide to Vaccinations: A Balanced Look at the Pros and Cons*. Indianapolis, IN: Alpha Books; 2009.

Manufacturers and Distributors

GlaxoSmithKline
http://www.gsk.com

MedImmune (*acquired by AstraZeneca in 2007*)
http://www.medimmune.com

Merck
http://www.merck.com

Novartis
http://www.novartis.com

Pfizer *(acquired Wyeth in 2009)*
http://www.pfizer.com

Sanofi Pasteur *(acquired Acambis in 2008)*
http://www.sanofipasteur.com

State Health Department Immunization Programs

State health department web sites can be accessed through the following URL: http://www.cdc.gov/mmwr/international/relres.html.

Abbreviations

AAFP ....American Academy of Family Physicians
AAP ....American Academy of Pediatrics
ACCV..................Advisory Commission on Childhood Vaccines
ACHA ....American College Health Association
ACIP....................Advisory Committee on Immunization Practices
AIDS ....acquired immune deficiency syndrome
AOM ....acute otitis media
ANA....................American Nurses Association
APC ....antigen-presenting cell
APhA...................American Pharmaceutical Association
APHA..................American Public Health Association
ASD ....autistic-spectrum disorder
ATPM..................Association of Teachers of Preventive Medicine
AVG ....Allied Vaccine Group
BCG ....Bacille Calmette-Guérin (tuberculosis vaccine)
BLA ....Biologics License Application
BRFSS.................Behavioral Risk Factor Surveillance System
CBER ....Center for Biologics Evaluation and Research
CDC ....Centers for Disease Control and Prevention
CHD ....congenital heart disease
CI ....confidence interval
CISA....................Clinical Immunization Safety Assessment (Network)
CLD ....chronic lung disease (bronchopulmonary dysplasia)
CMS ....Centers for Medicare and Medicaid Services, formerly known as the Health Care Financing Administration (HCFA)
CMV....................cytomegalovirus
CMV-IGIV ....cytomegalovirus immune globulin, intravenous
CNS ....central nervous system
CoCASA ....Comprehensive Clinic Assessment Software Application
CPT ....Current Procedural Terminology
CRM_{197} ....cross-reactive material (a mutant diphtheria toxin)
CRS ....congenital rubella syndrome
CSF ....cerebrospinal fluid
CTL ....cytotoxic T lymphocyte
DHHS..................Department of Health and Human Services
DMARD..............disease-modifying antirheumatic drug
DMEM ....Dulbecco's Modified Eagle Medium
DMID..................Division of Microbiology and Infectious Diseases
DNA....................deoxyribonucleic acid
DOD....................Department of Defense
DT ....diphtheria, tetanus vaccine (infant/child formulation)
DTaP...................diphtheria, tetanus, acellular pertussis vaccine (infant/child formulation)
DTwP...................diphtheria, tetanus, whole-cell pertussis vaccine
EDTA ....ethylene diamine tetraacetic acid

EMLA ....eutectic mixture of local anesthetic
EMT ....emergency medical technician
EPA ....Environmental Protection Agency
FDA ....(US) Food and Drug Administration
FHA ....filamentous hemagglutinin
FIM ....fimbriae (also known as agglutinogens)
FQHC..................federally qualified health center
GABHS .... group A beta-hemolytic streptococcus
GCP ....Good Clinical Practices
GLP ....Good Laboratory Practices
GMP....................Good Manufacturing Practices
GVHD.................graft-versus-host disease
H ....hemagglutinin
HAV ....hepatitis A virus
HBIG...................hepatitis B immune globulin
HBsAb.................antibody to hepatitis B surface antigen
HBsAg.................hepatitis B surface antigen
HBV ....hepatitis B virus
HCFA ....Health Care Financing Administration, now known as the Centers for Medicare and Medicaid Services (CMS)
HCP ....health care personnel
HEDIS.................Healthcare Effectiveness Data and Information Set
HepA ....hepatitis A vaccine
HepB ....hepatitis B vaccine
HEPES ....N-2-hydroxyethylpiperazine-N'2-ethanesulfonic acid
HHS ....(Department of) Health and Human Services
Hib ....*Haemophilus influenzae* type b conjugate vaccine
Hib-CRM ....*Haemophilus influenzae* type b vaccine, CRM_{197} conjugate
Hib-D ....*Haemophilus influenzae* type b vaccine, diphtheria toxoid conjugate
Hib-OMP.............*Haemophilus influenzae* type b vaccine, (*N meningitidis*) outer membrane protein conjugate
Hib-T...................*Haemophilus influenzae* type b vaccine, tetanus toxoid conjugate
HICPAC ....Healthcare Infection Control Practices Advisory Committee
HIV ....human immunodeficiency virus
HPV ....human papillomavirus vaccine
HPV2...................human papillomavirus vaccine, 2-valent
HPV4...................human papillomavirus vaccine, 4-valent
HRIG...................human rabies immune globulin
hSBA...................serum bactericidal assay using human complement
HSCT ....hematopoietic stem-cell transplant
IAC ....Immunization Action Coalition
IBD ....inflammatory bowel disease
ICD-9-CM...........International Classification of Diseases, 9th Revision, Clinical Modification

30

IDSA ....Infectious Diseases Society of America
IG ....immune globulin
IgE ....immunoglobulin E
IgG ....immunoglobulin G
IGIM ....(polyclonal) immune globulin, intramuscular
IGIV ....(polyclonal) immune globulin, intravenous
IgM ....immunoglobulin M
IGRA....................interferon-gamma release assay (for tuberculosis)
IIV ....inactivated influenza vaccine
IIS ....Immunization Information Systems (also known as registries)
IM ....intramuscular
IN ....intranasal
IOM ....Institute of Medicine
IPD ....invasive pneumococcal disease
IPV ....inactivated poliovirus vaccine
IS ....intussusception
ISRC....................Immunization Safety Review Committee
ITP ....immune thrombocytopenic purpura
IU ....international unit
IV ....intravenous
JE ....Japanese encephalitis
JEV ....Japanese encephalitis vaccine
JE-MB ....Japanese encephalitis vaccine, mouse brain-derived
JE-VC..................Japanese encephalitis vaccine, Vero cell-derived
LAIV ....live-attenuated influenza vaccine
LEP ....low egg passage
LRI ....lower respiratory infection
MCD ....mad cow disease
MCV....................meningococcal conjugate vaccine
MCV4 ....meningococcal conjugate vaccine, 4-valent
MCV4-CRM ....meningococcal vaccine, 4-valent, CRM_{197} conjugate
MCV4-D ....meningococcal vaccine, 4-valent, diphtheria toxoid conjugate
MHC ....major histocompatibility complex
MMR...................measles, mumps, rubella vaccine
MMRV ....measles, mumps, rubella, varicella vaccine
MPSV..................meningococcal polysaccharide vaccine
MPSV4................meningococcal polysaccharide vaccine, 4-valent
MRI ....magnetic resonance imaging
MS ....multiple sclerosis
NCES ....National Childhood Encephalopathy Study
NCIRD ....National Center for Immunization and Respiratory Diseases
NCQA ....National Committee on Quality Assurance
NCVIA ....National Childhood Vaccine Injury Act
NDC ....National Drug Code
NHIS ....National Health Interview Survey

NIAID ....National Institute of Allergy and Infectious Diseases
NIH ....National Institutes of Health
NIP ....National Immunization Program
NIS ....National Immunization Survey
NNDSS ....National Notifiable Disease Surveillance System
NNii ....National Network for Immunization Information
NREVSS ....National Respiratory and Enteric Surveillance System
NRSSS ....National Rotavirus Strain Surveillance System
NVAC..................National Vaccine Advisory Committee
NVPO..................National Vaccine Program Office
NVSN..................New Vaccine Surveillance Network
OMP....................(*N meningitidis*) outer membrane protein
OPV ....oral polio vaccine
OSHA..................Occupational Safety and Health Administration
PAHO ....Pan American Health Organization
PCV ....pneumococcal conjugate vaccine
PCV1...................porcine circovirus 1
PCV2...................porcine circovirus 2
PCV7...................pneumococcal conjugate vaccine, 7-valent
PCV13.................pneumococcal conjugate vaccine, 13-valent
PCV7-CRM.........pneumococcal vaccine, 7-valent, CRM_{197} conjugate
PCV13-CRM.......pneumococcal vaccine, 13-valent, CRM_{197} conjugate
PDD ....pervasive developmental disorder
PDUFA................Prescription Drug User Fee Act
PFU ....plaque-forming units
PHN....................postherpetic neuralgia
PHS ....(US) Public Health Service
PI ....package insert (also known as product information)
PO ....per os (orally by mouth)
PPSV...................pneumococcal polysaccharide vaccine
PPSV23 ....pneumococcal polysaccharide vaccine, 23-valent
PRN ....pertactin
PRP ....polyribosylribitol phosphate
PS ....(capsular) polysaccharide
PT ....pertussis toxin
QALY..................quality-adjusted life year
RAB ....rabies vaccine
RAB-HDC...........rabies vaccine, human diploid cell
RAB-PCEC.........rabies vaccine, purified chick embryo cell
RET ....Reportable Events Table
RHC ....rural health clinic
RhoGAM.............Rho(D) immune globulin
RIG ....rabies immune globulin
RNA ....ribose nucleic acid
RR ....relative risk
RRV-TV ....rhesus-human reassortant rotavirus vaccine, tetravalent
rSBA....................serum bactericidal assay using rabbit complement
RSV ....respiratory syncytial virus

RSV-IGIV ....respiratory syncytial virus immune globulin, intravenous
RSVmAB ....respiratory syncytial virus monoclonal antibody
RV ....rotavirus vaccine
RV1 ....rotavirus vaccine, monovalent (live-attenuated human rotavirus vaccine)
RV5 ....rotavirus vaccine, 5-valent (pentavalent bovine rotavirus vaccine)
SC ....subcutaneous
SCHIP ....State Children's Health Insurance Program
SIDS....................sudden infant death syndrome
SIV ....simian immunodeficiency virus
SLV ....school-located vaccination
sp ....species
Tc ....cytotoxic T-cells
$TCID_{50}$ ....median tissue culture infective dose
TCR ....T-cell receptor
Td ....tetanus, diphtheria vaccine (adolescent/adult formulation)
Tdap ....tetanus, diphtheria, acellular pertussis vaccine (adolescent/adult formulation)
TIG ....tetanus immune globulin
tRNA ....transfer ribonucleic acid
TST ....tuberculin skin test, formerly referred to as PPD (purified protein derivative)
TT ....tetanus toxoid
TViPSV ....typhoid Vi polysaccharide vaccine
Ty21a...................(oral) typhoid vaccine
URI ....upper respiratory infection
US$ ....United States currency
USAID ....US Agency for International Development
USAMRIID.........US Army Medical Research Institute of Infectious Diseases
USP ....United States Pharmacopoeial Convention
v/v ....percent by volume in volume (mL per 100 mL of solution)
VAERS ....Vaccine Adverse Event Reporting System
VAR ....varicella vaccine
VariZIG ....varicella-zoster immune globulin
VFC ....Vaccines for Children (Program)
VICP....................(National) Vaccine Injury Compensation Program
VIG ....vaccinia immune globulin
VIS ....Vaccine Information Statement
VIT ....Vaccine Injury Table
VLP ....virus-like particle
VRBPAC ....Vaccines and Related Biological Products Advisory Committee
VRC ....(Dale and Betty Bumpers) Vaccine Research Center
VSD ....Vaccine Safety Datalink
VTEU ....Vaccine and Treatment Evaluation Unit
VZV ....varicella-zoster virus
WHO ....World Health Organization

WIC ....(US Department of Agriculture's Special Supplemental Nutrition Program for) Women, Infants and Children
XLA ....X-linked agammaglobulinemia
YF ....yellow fever
YFV ....yellow fever vaccine
ZOS ....zoster vaccine

Nomenclature

(See *Appendix Table*, next page)

APPENDIX TABLE — Vaccine and Infectious Agent Nomenclature

Disease	Infectious Agents Name	Abbreviation	Vaccine Designation(s)[a]
Anthrax	*Bacillus anthracis*	*B anthracis*	Anthrax vaccine
Diphtheria, tetanus (lockjaw), pertussis (whooping cough)	*Corynebacterium diphtheriae* *Clostridium tetani* *Bordetella pertussis*	*C diphtheriae* *C tetani* *B pertussis*	DTwP, DTaP, Tdap, DT, Td, TT
H influenzae type b (invasive)	*Haemophilus influenzae* type b	*H influenzae* type b	Hib (Hib-OMP, Hib-T)
Hepatitis A	Hepatitis A virus	HAV	HepA
Hepatitis B	Hepatitis B virus	HBV	HepB
Human papillomavirus-induced cervical cancer, anal cancer, genital warts	Human papillomavirus	—	HPV (HPV2, HPV4)
Influenza	Influenza virus	—	IIV, LAIV
Japanese encephalitis	Japanese encephalitis virus	JE virus	JEV (JEV-MB, JEV-VC)
Measles, mumps, rubella	Measles virus, mumps virus, rubella virus	—	MMR
N meningitidis (invasive)	*Neisseria meningitidis*	*N meningitidis*	MCV (MCV4-CRM, MCV4-D), MPSV4
Polio	Poliovirus	—	IPV
Rabies	Rabies virus	—	RAB (RAB-HDC, RAB-PCEC)
Rotavirus gastroenteritis	Rotavirus	—	RV (RV1, RV5)

S pneumoniae (invasive, otitis media, pneumonia)	*S pneumoniae*	*S pneumoniae*	PCV (PCV7-CRM, PCV13-CRM), PPSV23
Smallpox	Variola virus	—	Smallpox vaccine (vaccinia)
Typhoid fever	*Salmonella typhi*	*S typhi*	TViPSV, Ty21a
Varicella (chickenpox)	Varicella zoster virus	VZV	VAR
Yellow fever	Yellow fever virus	YF virus	YFV
Zoster (shingles)	Varicella zoster virus	VZV	ZOS
Modern combination vaccines			HepB-Hib-OMP
			DTaP-IPV
			DTaP-IPV/Hib-T
			DTaP-HepB-IPV
			MMRV
			HepA-HepB

[a] For conjugate vaccines, "-CRM," "-D," "-OMP," and "-T," indicate the protein carrier to which the polysaccharide is conjugated (respectively, CRM_{197} [a mutant diphtheria toxin]; diphtheria toxoid; *N meningitidis* outer membrane protein; and tetanus toxoid). Numbers following the abbreviations indicate the valency of the vaccine (eg, HPV2 contains two serotypes whereas HPV4 contains four serotypes). For combination vaccines, dashes indicate that the components are premixed (eg, DTaP-HepB-IPV); slash marks indicate that the components must be combined prior to administration (eg, DTaP-IPV/Hib-T, where liquid DTaP-IPV is used to reconstitute the lyophilized Hib-T).

Note: Page numbers in *italics* indicate figures.
Page numbers followed by a "t" indicate tables.

31

31